Regional Anaesthesia

Sioned Phillips · Amit Dixit
Chetan Mehra
Arunangshu Chakraborty
Nishkarsh Gupta · Anju Gupta
Editors

Regional Anaesthesia

A Guide to Clinical Exams

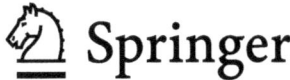 Springer

Editors
Sioned Phillips
Department of Anaesthesia
Frimley Park Hospital
Camberley, UK

Amit Dixit
Department of Anaesthesia
Ruby Hall Hospital
Pune, India

Chetan Mehra
Department of Anaesthesia
Indraprastha Apollo Hospital
New Delhi, Delhi, India

Arunangshu Chakraborty
Department of Anaesthesia
Sultan Qaboos Comprehensive Cancer
Care and Research Centre
Muscat, Oman

Nishkarsh Gupta
Onco-Anesthesia and Palliative
Medicine
All India Institute of Medical Sciences
New Delhi, India

Anju Gupta
Anesthesiology Pain and Critical Care
All India Institute of Medical Sciences
New Delhi, India

ISBN 978-3-032-05164-6   ISBN 978-3-032-05165-3   (eBook)
https://doi.org/10.1007/978-3-032-05165-3

This Springer imprint is published by the registered company Springer Nature Switzerland AG
The registered company address is: Gewerbestrasse 11, 6330 Cham, Switzerland

If disposing of this product, please recycle the paper.

Acknowledgement

We sincerely acknowledge the Anaesthesia Sonoanatomy (Anso) App for granting permission to use their images in various chapters of this book (Regional Anaesthesia, A Guide to clinical exams). Their innovative visual resources greatly enhanced the clarity and educational value of our work.

Contents

Part III   Individual Regional Anaesthesia Techniques

Part I

Regional Anesthesia Strategies for Various Surgical Procedures

Analgesia for Shoulder Surgery

Aditya Pal

Case Scenario

A 75-year-old female with a BMI of 38 kg m^{-2} is listed for arthroscopic rotator cuff repair. Her past medical history includes chronic obstructive pulmonary disease (COPD), hypertension, previous stroke, and ischaemic heart disease requiring coronary artery stenting. Her medication includes aspirin, ramipril, amlodipine and Symbicort inhaler. Her exercise tolerance is limited by fatigue after roughly 300 meters, indicating a moderate level of physical activity. She last had a chest infection 3 months ago, requiring oral steroids and nebuliser treatment. Her lung function tests show FVC 2.71, FEV1 1.46 (65% predicted), and FEV$_1$/FVC 54% (69% predicted). ECG shows sinus rhythm with right bundle branch block. Blood tests reveal a haemoglobin of 110 g L^{-1} and mild renal impairment, but are otherwise unremarkable.

1. **What are the key patient-related issues?**

This patient, despite having multiple risk factors for undergoing surgery, also demonstrates resilience and a strong will to overcome these challenges.

   1. Recent chest infection on a background of moderate COPD, suggesting potential for significant perioperative respiratory impairment.

A. Pal (✉)
Wexham Park Hospital, Frimley Health NHS
Foundation Trust, Slough, UK

   2. Ischaemic heart disease with decreased functional capacity, indicative of limited physiological reserve

   3. Raised BMI with a risk of undiagnosed obstructive sleep apnoea, which can complicate the patient's respiratory function during and after surgery.

   4. Previous cerebrovascular accident, and so at increased risk of perioperative cerebral ischaemic event

   5. Anaemia

2. **What are the surgical and anaesthetic considerations relating to this case?**

   1. Beach chair positioning for arthroscopic surgery
   - Risk of compromising hemodynamic and cerebral function
   - Risk of air embolus

   2. Surgical preference for intraoperative blood pressure control, which may conflict with the patient's co-morbidities such as ischaemic heart disease and the risk of cerebral hypoperfusion.

   3. Rotator cuff surgery is associated with significant post-operative pain

3. **Describe the innervation of the shoulder.**

The shoulder receives innervation from nerves arising from cervical (C3,4) and brachial (C5,6) plexuses (Table 1.1). The predominant nerves involved in the motor and sensory innervation of the shoulder are the suprascapular and axillary nerves. Minor innervation is derived from the lat-

Table 1.1 Innervation of the Shoulder Joint

Nerve	Origin	Innervation
Suprascapular	Brachial plexus (superior trunk)	1. Joints: Glenohumeral joint—superior and posterior capsule Acromioclavicular joint 2. Bone: posterior scapula 3. Muscle: supraspinatus, infraspinatus, teres minor
Axillary	Brachial plexus (posterior cord)	1. Cutaneous: over deltoid (= *superior lateral cutaneous branch of the axillary nerve*) 2. Joint: inferior capsule of the glenohumeral joint 3. Bone: humeral head and neck 4. Muscle: deltoid, teres minor
Lateral pectoral	Brachial plexus (lateral cord)	1. Joint: anterior capsule of the glenohumeral joint 2. Muscle: lateral portion of the pectoralis major
Musculocutaneous	Brachial plexus (lateral cord)	1. Joint: anterior capsule of the glenohumeral joint 2. Muscle: long head of biceps brachii
Subscapular	Brachial plexus (posterior cord)	1. Joint: anterior capsule of the glenohumeral joint 2. Bone: anterior scapula 3. Muscle: subscapularis
Supraclavicular	Cervical plexus (C3,4)	1. Cutaneous: cape of the shoulder and upper thoracic region

eral pectoral, musculocutaneous, and subscapular nerves (Figs. 1.1, 1.2, 1.3, and 1.4).

4. **What would be your anaesthetic strategy?**

Two options:
   1. General anaesthesia plus regional anaesthesia for postoperative analgesia
   2. Regional anaesthesia for surgical anaesthesia and postoperative analgesia

5. **What would be your analgesia strategy?**

In line with PROSPECT recommendations [1], multimodal analgesia should be employed, incorporating the following:
   1. Systemic analgesia with paracetamol and non-steroidal anti-inflammatory drugs (NSAIDs), administered pre-operatively or intra-operatively and continued postoperatively.
   2. A single dose of intravenous (i.v) dexamethasone is recommended because it can increase the analgesic duration of peripheral nerve blocks, decrease the need for analgesics, and have anti-emetic effects.
   3. Regional analgesia
   4. Opioids: should be reserved as rescue analgesia in the postoperative period

Options for regional analgesia include (Figs. 1.5 and 1.6):
   1. Interscalene brachial plexus block, single shot
   2. Interscalene brachial plexus block, continuous
   3. Suprascapular nerve block, with or without axillary nerve block (but not as first choice)

Interventions that have **not** been recommended due to the lack of procedure-specific evidence are outlined below:

Pre-operative
- Gabapentin
- Subacromial or intra-articular injection
- Stellate ganglion block
- Cervical epidural block
- Perineural adjuncts added to the local anaesthetic solution:
  - Opioid (buprenorphine, tramadol)
  - Glucocorticoid (dexamethasone, betamethasone)
  - α_2-adrenoreceptor agonist (clonidine)*Post-operative*
- Early motion protocols vs delayed motion protocols
- Specific postoperative shoulder immobilisation device

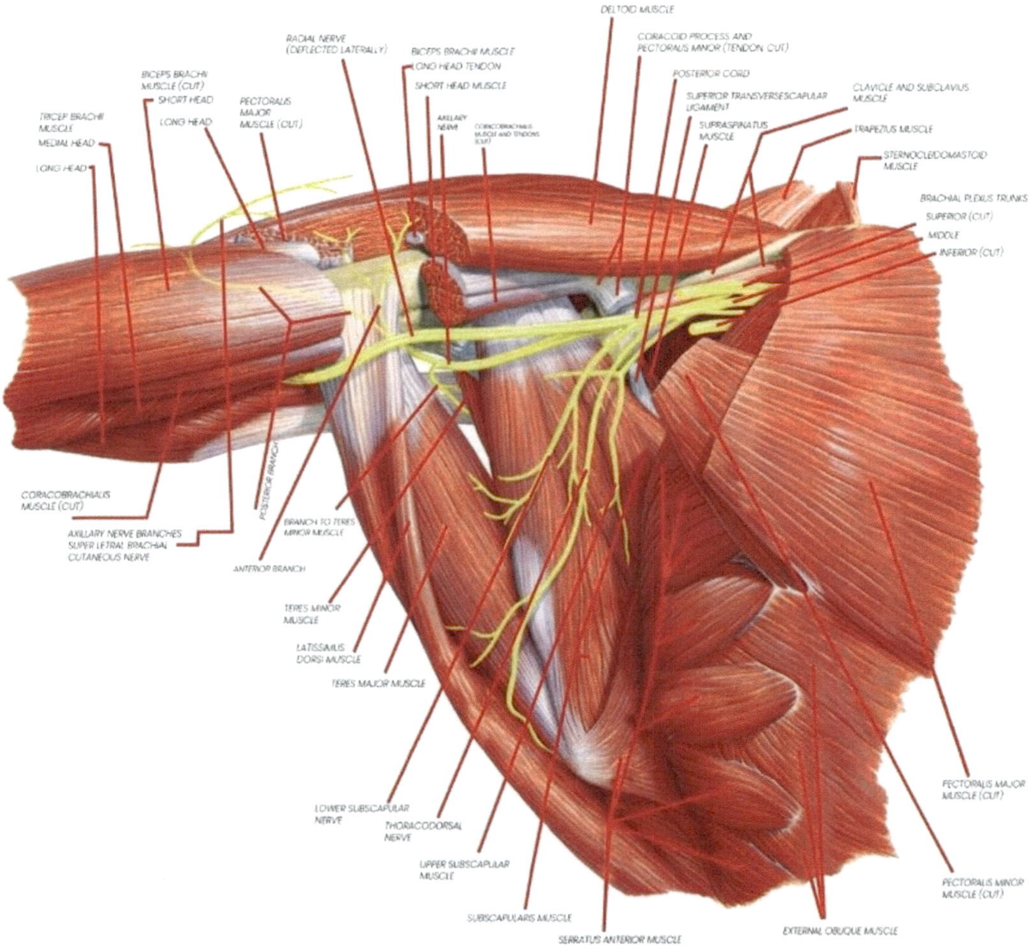

Fig. 1.1 Innervation of the shoulder joint

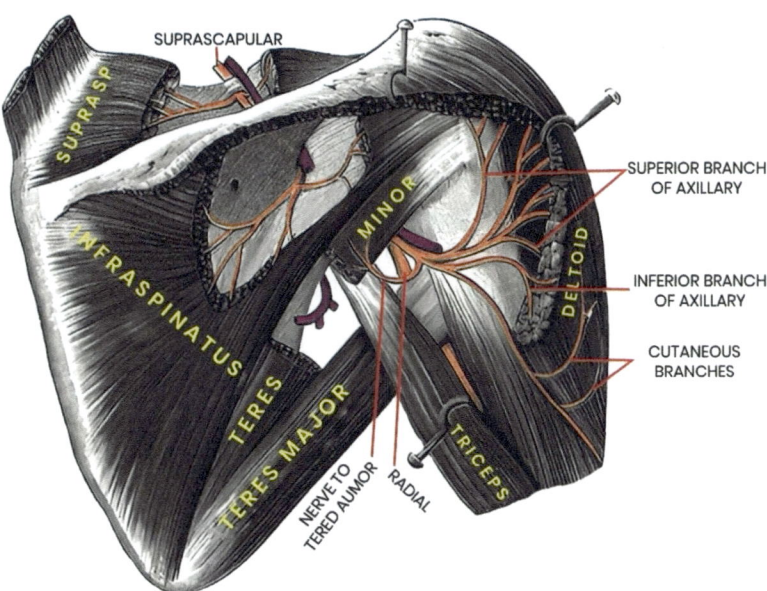

Fig. 1.2 Nerve innervation and muscle anatomy of the posterior shoulder

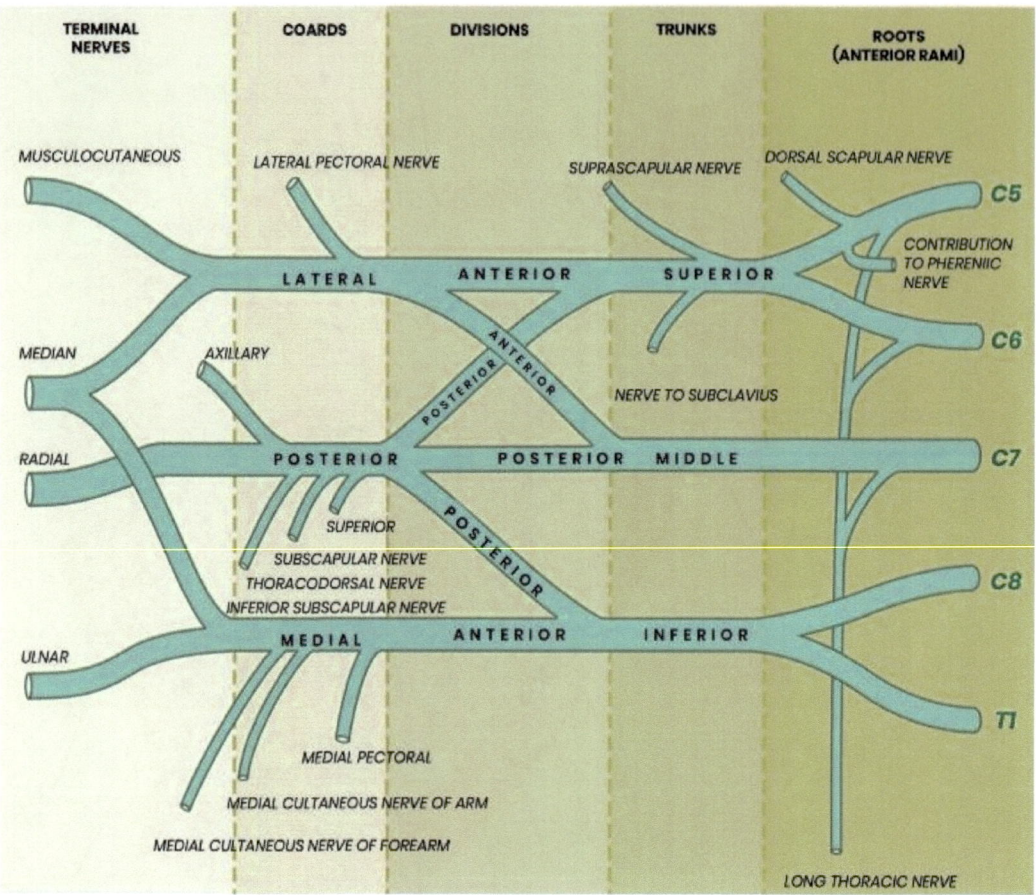

| TERMINAL NERVES | COARDS | DIVISIONS | TRUNKS | ROOTS (ANTERIOR RAMI) |

Fig. 1.3 Schematic showing branches of the brachial plexus

- TENS
- Compressive cryotherapy or ice wrapping
- Zolpidem as a sleep aid

6. **What are the advantages and disadvantages of interscalene brachial plexus block?**

Advantages

1. Provides reliable, reproducible anaesthesia and analgesia for both open and arthroscopic procedures involving the shoulder joint, lateral two-thirds of the clavicle and proximal humerus
   - Effectively blocks the required nerve roots and crucial nerves (i.e. suprascapular nerve, which exits relatively proximally from the plexus).
2. Represents the best option for conducting surgery under regional anaesthesia alone

Disadvantages

1. Phrenic nerve blockade
   - The phrenic nerve lies on the superficial surface of the anterior scalene muscle, near the C5 and C6 nerve roots, before moving away from the plexus over the muscle surface more distally
   - A randomised controlled trial comparing low-volume (5 ml) vs high-volume (20 ml) interscalene block showed that even with 5 ml, the incidence of phrenic nerve palsy is approximately 25–50% (although this is still significantly less than 100% with 20 ml) [2].
   - FEV_1 may be reduced by up to 40%, leading to significant respiratory embarrassment in patients with rele-

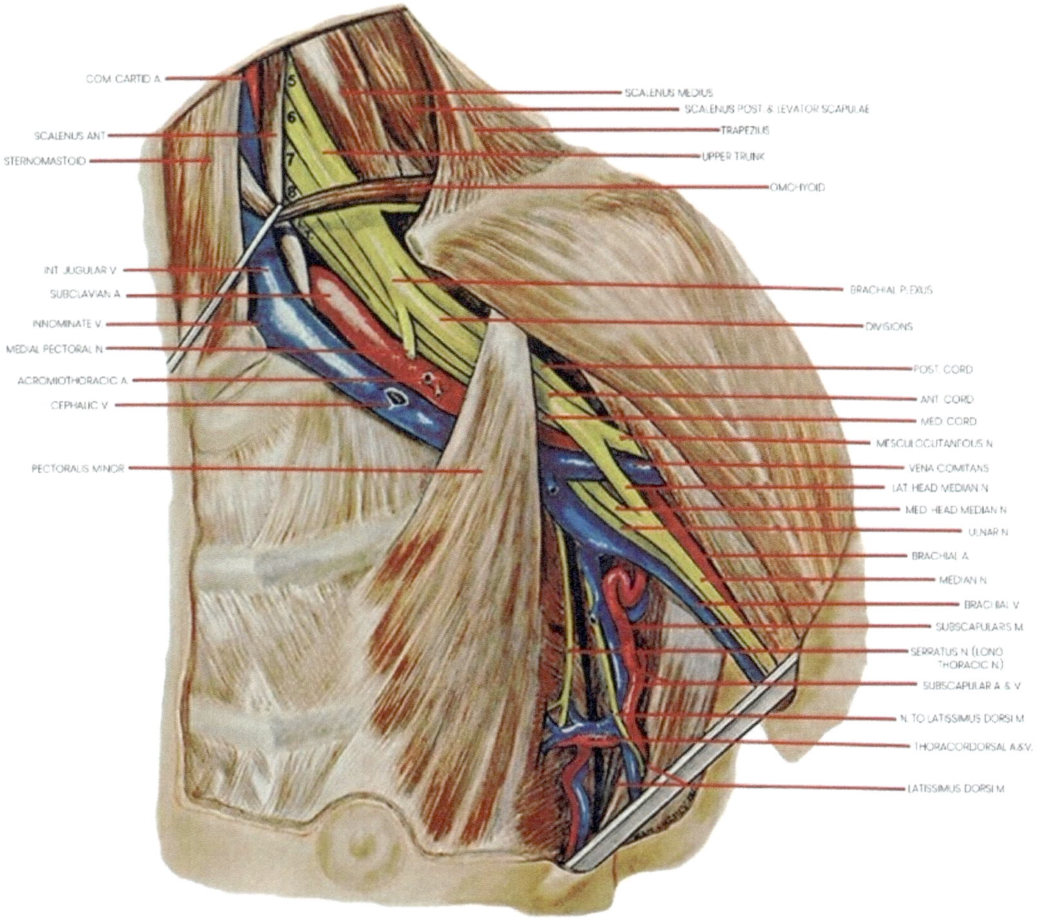

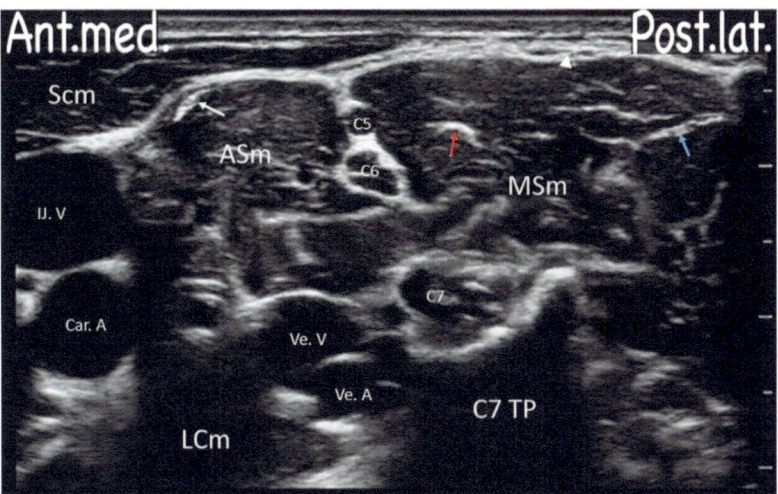

Fig. 1.4 Anatomy of the brachial plexus and surrounding structures in the shoulder region

Fig. 1.5 Interscalene Nerve Block (Ultrasound Cross-Section of Neck Anatomy Depicting Sternocleidomastoid (Scm), Anterior Scalene Muscle (ASm), Internal Jugular Vein (IJ. V), Carotid Artery (Car. A), Vertebral Vein (Ve. V), Vertebral Artery (Ve. A), Longus Colli Muscle (LCm), Middle Scalene Muscle (MSm), and Cervical Nerve Roots (C5, C6, C7) Red arrow – long thoracic nerve, blue arrow – dorsal scapular nerve, white arrow – phrenic nerve. C7 TP = C7 Transverse process

Fig. 1.6 Ultrasound Anatomy for Anterior Suprascapular Nerve Block: Anterior Scalene (ASm), Subclavian Artery (Sa), Omohyoid (OHm), Middle Scalene (MSm), Serratus Anterior (SAm), Suprascapular Nerve (SSn), Intercostal Muscle (ICm), 1st and 2nd Ribs, arrowheads (pleura)

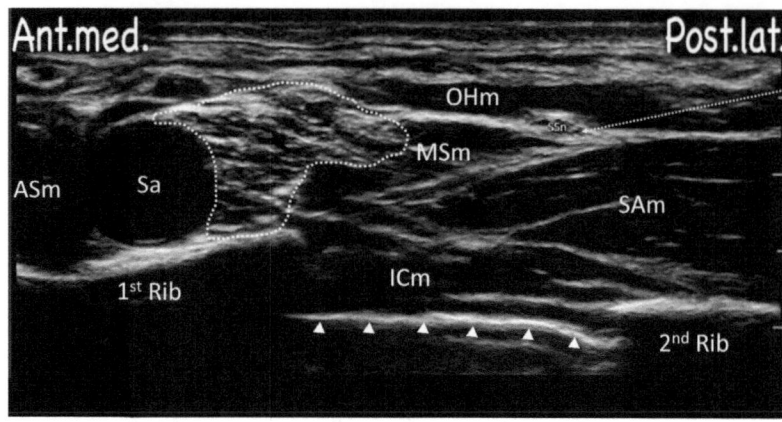

vant co-morbidities, particularly respiratory disease and obesity [3].

2. Neurological injury
   - Interscalene block has been reported to be associated with a higher incidence of neurological dysfunction than other peripheral blocks (up to 14% at 10 days) [4].
   - Neurological injury from cervical cord trauma has also been described
3. Spread to surrounding structures
   - Recurrent laryngeal nerve palsy—transient hoarseness usually of no clinical significance. Due to local anaesthetic spread over anterior scalene muscle
   - Horner's syndrome—generally resolves spontaneously as the block wears off.
4. Local anaesthetic systemic toxicity (LAST)
   - Proximity of vessels to the plexus, especially the vertebral artery near the C7 root
   - Rapid delivery of local anaesthetic from the vertebral artery to the brain can result in central nervous system adverse effects and convulsions

7. **What measures could you take to mitigate the perioperative risk of pulmonary complications in this patient?**
   1. Pre-operative identification of this patient as a high-risk patient and appropriate optimisation

   - Optimisation of COPD medication
   - Ensuring resolution of effects of chest infection before proceeding with elective surgery
   - Smoking cessation intervention, if required
   - Plan for possible post-operative respiratory support in high dependency unit
   2. Use intra-operative high-flow nasal oxygenation (Optiflow) or CPAP to treat symptomatic dyspnea or desaturation (if surgery is under regional anaesthesia) [5].
   3. Modification of anaesthetic technique:
      - Use of short-acting agents if using sedation or general anaesthesia
      - Reducing the dose of local anaesthetic to the minimum possible for interscalene block
      - Use short-acting local anaesthetic for interscalene block to minimise the impact of phrenic nerve blockade
      - Consideration of alternative, potentially phrenic-sparing regional anaesthetic techniques
   4. Use of a perineural catheter for postoperative analgesia to minimise opioid use

8. **Discuss the alternative regional anaesthesia strategies to the interscalene block for rotator cuff repair**
   1. Superior Trunk Block
      - C5 and C6 nerve roots are tracked distally in the interscalene groove, where they fuse to form the superior trunk

- 10–15 ml of local anaesthetic around here (**before** the suprascapular nerve leaves the superior trunk) will effectively block the major innervation to the shoulder joint
- Case report evidence indicates effective analgesia and absence of phrenic nerve blockade because of the more distal approach
- However, there is no prospectively randomised data to support this technique

2. Supraclavicular brachial plexus block
   - Can produce similar analgesic efficacy for shoulder surgery to interscalene block, with a reduction in certain adverse effects, e.g. Horner's syndrome
   - No appreciable reduction in risk of phrenic nerve blockade [6].
   - Risk of missing suprascapular nerve as it departs relatively proximally from the superior trunk
   - Not mentioned in PROSPECT guidelines for rotator cuff repair surgery

3. Suprascapular nerve block (+/− axillary nerve block)
   - As all nerves innervating the shoulder are not blocked, this technique is only suitable in combination with general anaesthesia (i.e. not as a sole regional anaesthetic technique)
   - Suprascapular nerve can be blocked either
     - Anteriorly: as it departs the superior trunk and travels laterally, deep to the omohyoid muscle
     - Posteriorly: in the supraspinatus fossa
   - Suprascapular nerve block provides analgesia that is superior to just intra-articular infiltration. This is further enhanced by the addition of an axillary nerve block
   - Combined suprascapular and axillary nerve block has been shown to reduce pain scores and opioid use after surgery, with non-inferior analgesia to interscalene block at 6–24 h post-op, whilst preventing phrenic nerve blockade.
   - However, compared to interscalene block, there is increased pain in the immediate post-operative phase up until 6 h [9].
   - Furthermore, up to 40% of patients may fail to demonstrate sensory or motor block after combined suprascapular and axillary nerve block [3].
   - Evidence is primarily limited to case reports

9. **What are the advantages of conducting arthroscopic rotator cuff repair with regional anaesthesia as a sole anaesthetic technique?**
   1. Minimising effects of anaesthesia on this patient's multiple risk factors, i.e. avoidance of potential airway, respiratory, and cardiovascular complications of general anaesthesia
   2. Reduced adverse effects of general anaesthesia such as postoperative nausea, vomiting and cognitive dysfunction, and reduced risk of need for overnight stay.
   3. Quicker return to postoperative drinking, eating and mobilising ("DrEaMing").
   4. Efficiency savings for the health system through reduction in recovery and discharge time
   5. Increased engagement of patients in their care (patients able to see their pathology and observe their treatment on the monitor in real-time)

10. **Aside from the nerve block, what are the key considerations when planning awake shoulder surgery?**

Pre-operative

In addition to a thorough routine pre-operative assessment incorporating meticulous systemic review and optimisation, specific considerations to awake shoulder surgery include:

- Appropriate patient selection
  - Need to ensure that adequate, effective co-operation and communication will be possible with the patient throughout surgery

- Need to ensure the absence of other patient factors that would make awake surgery not amenable, e.g. movement disorders
- Detailed, consistent counselling and written information about the regional anaesthetic technique and conduct of surgery whilst conscious
- Ensuring adequate awareness amongst the theatre team regarding necessary logistics for this case, including:
  - Adequate time built in to list planning for nerve block conduct and testing
  - Team awareness of awake patient in theatre throughout surgery
  - Senior surgeon involvement in conducting timely, meticulous surgery
  - Contingency plans for failure
- Plan for anticipated recovery and postoperative pain management

Intra-operative

Positioning considerations

- Draping
  - Allow to self-position
  - Avoid lying on the patient's face
  - Needs to allow an option for the patient to view the operation via surgical monitor
- Pillow under knees—reduces stretch on the hamstrings and increases comfort

Sedation

- Carefully titrated use of desired sedative agent, e.g. midazolam, propofol target-controlled infusion
- Supplemental oxygen and capnography monitoring

Management of intra-operative pain—10–20% of patients will experience intra-operative pain at some point.

- Titration of alfentanil i.v. will allow surgery to continue in virtually all patients by providing analgesia without disinhibition

*Post-*operative

Limb care

- All patients should be instructed to protect the insensate limb from accidental damage until the nerve block has worn off

Ongoing systemic analgesia—one-fifth of patients report their postoperative pain after shoulder surgery as 'the worst pain imaginable' once the block has worn off .

- Ensure the patient receives multimodal systemic analgesia **before** the block has worn off
- Strong opioids are often required in the first 48 h after block resolution

Suggested Reading

1. Toma O, Persoons B, Pogatzki-Zahn E, Van de Velde M, Joshi GP, PROSPECT Working Group collaborators. PROSPECT guideline for rotator cuff repair surgery: systematic review and procedure-specific postoperative pain management recommendations. Anaesthesia. 2019;74(10):1320–31.
2. Riazi S, Carmichael N, Awad I, Holtby RM, McCartney CJL. Effect of local anaesthetic volume (20 vs 5 ml) on the efficacy and respiratory consequences of ultrasound-guided interscalene brachial plexus block. Br J Anaesth. 2008;101:549–56.
3. Hewson DW, Oldman M, Bedforth NM. Regional anaesthesia for shoulder surgery. BJA Education. 2019;19(4):98–104.
4. Borgeat A, Ekatodramis G, Kalberer F, Benz C. Acute and nonacute complications associated with interscalene block and shoulder surgery: a prospective study. Anesthesiology. 2001;95(4):875–80.
5. Ferré F, Cugnin N, Martin C, Marty P, Bonnevialle N, Kurrek M, Minville V. Regional anesthesia with non-invasive ventilation for shoulder surgery in a patient with severe chronic obstructive pulmonary disease: a case report. A&A Case Reports. 2017;8(10):261–4.
6. Guo CW, Ma JX, Ma XL, Lu B, Wang Y, Tian AX, Sun L, Wang Y, Dong BC, Teng YB. Supraclavicular block versus interscalene brachial plexus block for shoulder surgery: a meta-analysis of clinical control trials. Int J Surg. 2017;45:85–91.
7. Shukla B, Chaddock M, Price D. The shoulder block. ATOTW Tutorial 453. 2021. https://resources.wfsahq.org/atotw/the-shoulder-block/.
8. Price D, Abeysekera A, Chaddock M. A randomised comparison of combined suprascapular and axillary (circumflex) nerve block with interscalene block for postoperative analgesia following arthroscopic shoulder surgery. Anaesth Intensive Care. 2012;40(1):183–4.
9. Hussain N, Goldar G, Ragina N, Banfield L, Laffey JG, Abdallah FW. Suprascapular and interscalene nerve block for shoulder surgery: a systematic review and meta-analysis. Anesthesiology. 2017;127(6):998–1013.
10. Wilson AT, Nicholson E, Burton L, Wild C. Analgesia for day-case shoulder surgery. Br J Anaesth. 2004;92(3):414–5.

Jonathan Major

Case Scenario

A 6-year-old girl presents with left arm pain, having fallen from a climbing frame onto her outstretched left hand with hyperextension of the elbow. She remains in considerable discomfort despite oral analgesia and is refusing to move her arm. On examination, there is evident swelling, ecchymosis around the elbow and altered sensation distally over the volar aspect of the index finger. She is unable to make the "A-OK" sign. An x-ray demonstrates a posteriorly displaced supracondylar fracture; she is listed for theatre later today. She has a history of sleep-disordered breathing and is awaiting elective adenotonsillectomy; a recent sleep study was consistent with severe obstructive sleep apnoea.

1. **What is meant by a supracondylar fracture?**

The distal humerus features readily palpable extracapsular projections of bone, the lateral and medial epicondyles. Distally, the trochlea articulates with the ulna; lateral to this, the capitellum articulates with the radial head. A supracondylar fracture occurs through the distal humerus's thin part above the level of the epicondyles; this is proximal to the growth plate (epiphysis).

Supracondylar fractures are the most common type of elbow fracture in children, especially in the first decade of life, with a peak incidence between 5 and 7 years. Most are extension-type injuries. They are rarely seen in adults. The Gartland classification is based on the degree of displacement seen on lateral x-ray and helps inform the management decision: conservative vs. closed reduction vs. open reduction.

2. **What are the potential patterns of neurovascular compromise with this injury?**

A meticulous neurovascular examination and an urgent orthopaedic opinion are imperative for all patients with a supracondylar fracture, particularly if there is any sign of compromise. Nerve palsies are a common occurrence with supracondylar fractures, with neuropraxia rates around 11% [1], although these rarely lead to a permanent deficit. This was a decent sized systematic review (5148 patients).

However, we could instead quote a range as the incidence does vary from study to study. I think it would be most reasonable, if we want to give a ball park figure, to quote a range of 10–15%.

- **Anterior interosseous nerve** (AIN)

  This is a deep motor branch of the median nerve and most commonly affected by the initial injury. It supplies flexor pollicus longus, pronator quadratus, and the lateral half of flexor digitorum profundus (responsible for flexion of the index and sometimes middle fingers). Classically, injury results in an inability to make the "A-OK" sign.

J. Major (✉)
St George's Hospital, London, UK
e-mail: jonathan.major@nhs.net

- **Median nerve**

  The median nerve itself is also at risk, especially with postero-lateral displacement of the distal fragment. Weakness of forearm pronation, flexion of the hand and wrist, and loss of flexion of the lateral digits (thumb, index, and middle fingers) may occur. A sensory deficit may be evident over the lateral 3½ fingers and palm.

- **Radial nerve**

  This nerve is at highest risk with postero-medial displacement of the distal fragment, and injury may result in weakness of wrist and finger extension. The anatomical snuffbox should be examined for evidence of a sensory deficit.

- **Ulnar nerve**

  Ulnar nerve injury is associated with flexion-type supracondylar fractures and is also the most common postoperative neurological complication, the ulnar nerve being particularly vulnerable during the insertion of a medial K-wire. This can result in a claw-hand deformity.

Signs of vascular compromise include pallor, coldness to touch, prolonged capillary refill time, and reduced or absent distal pulses. The brachial artery is at risk with displacement of the distal fragment, although a rich collateral circulation may maintain perfusion despite arterial injury.

3. **What is the innervation of the elbow?**

Innervation of the elbow joint is complex and principally involves the following nerves and their articular branches:

- Radial (C5–T1 via the posterior cord); this is also responsible for innervating the extensor muscles of the posterior compartment of the arm
- Musculocutaneous (C5–7 via the lateral cord); this is also responsible for innervating the flexor muscles of the anterior compartment of the arm
- Median (C5–T1 via lateral and medial cords)

In addition, the following nerves are responsible for some of the overlying cutaneous innervation:

- Medial cutaneous nerve of the arm and medial antebrachial cutaneous nerve (both C8-T1 via medial cord) supply the anterior and medial aspects
- Posterior and lateral cutaneous innervation is via sensory branches of the radial and musculocutaneous nerves, respectively.

Considering the origin and course of these nerves will facilitate the selection of an appropriate block (see below). It is important to remember that innervation of the upper extremity is often variable and overlapping and does not always conform to the neat pictures depicted in textbooks.

4. **What are the options for regional anaesthesia in this case?**

Various approaches to the brachial plexus may be employed to provide adjunctive analgesia or surgical anaesthesia. In this case, a combination with general anaesthesia is almost certainly necessary if a block is to be performed.

- A supraclavicular approach, targeting the three trunks of the plexus as they split into their respective anterior and posterior divisions.
- An infraclavicular block targeting the lateral, posterior, and medial cords. The traditional paracoracoid approach or an alternative, such as the costoclavicular approach, would be reasonable.
- An axillary approach, individually identifying and targeting the radial, musculocutaneous, median, and ulnar nerves. Although this approach may miss the medial cutaneous branches as they arise directly from the medial cord, they remain near the axilla. If missed, local (surgical) infiltration should be adequate (Figs. 2.1, 2.2, and 2.3).

5. **What are some of the important considerations when performing regional anaesthesia in paediatric patients?**

Awake vs. asleep

Fortunately, serious adverse events after regional anaesthesia (RA) in children are rare. For reasons related to anxiety and communication/understanding, performing RA in an awake child may not be practical. However, potential advantages include early detection of systemic toxicity (see

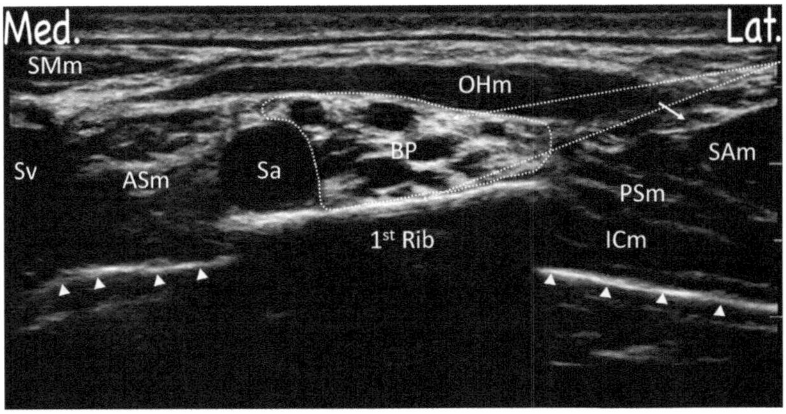

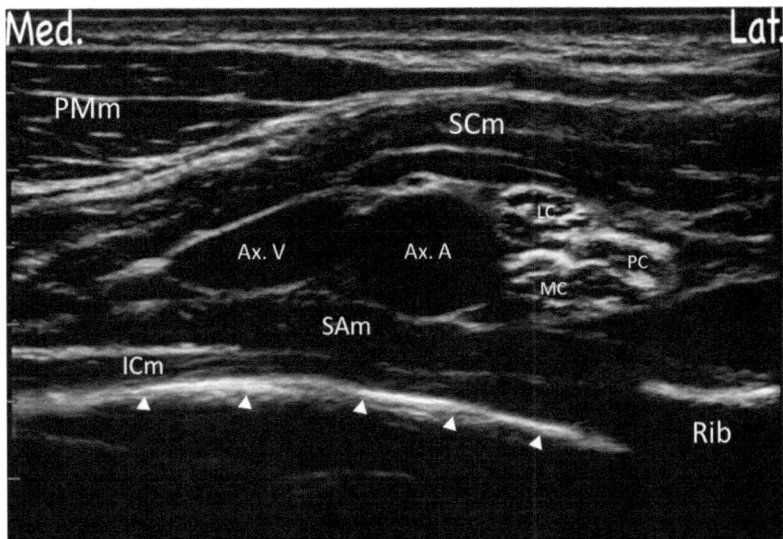

Fig. 2.1 Ultrasound image of the supraclavicular region for supraclavicular brachial plexus block. Med. (Medial), Lat. (Lateral), SMm (Sternocleidomastoid Muscle), Sv (Subclavian Vein), ASm (Anterior Scalene Muscle), Sa (Subclavian Artery), BP (Brachial Plexus), OHm (Omohyoid Muscle), 1st Rib (First Rib), SAm (Serratus Anterior Muscle), PSm (Posterior Scalene Muscle), ICm (Intercostal Muscle). The small white triangles indicate the lung pleura with its underlying acoustic artefact. The white arrow indicates the suprascapular nerve

Fig. 2.2 Ultrasound image of the infraclavicular region for the costoclavicular approach to the brachial plexus. Med. (Medial), Lat. (Lateral), PMm (Pectoralis Major Muscle), SCm (Subclavius Muscle), Ax. V (Axillary Vein), Ax. A (Axillary Artery), SAm (Serratus Anterior Muscle), ICm (Intercostal Muscle), Rib (Rib), LC (Lateral Cord of the brachial plexus), MC (Medial Cord of the brachial plexus), PC (Posterior Cord of the brachial plexus). The small white triangles indicate the lung pleura with its underlying acoustic artefact

below) and reduced risk of intraneural injection. Data from the Paediatric Regional Anaesthesia Network (PRAN) demonstrate a higher incidence of postoperative neurologic symptoms when blocks are performed in awake or lightly sedated children. ESRA-ASRA firmly support the performance of RA in children under general anaesthesia or deep sedation based on acceptable safety, and indeed, this should be viewed as the standard of care.

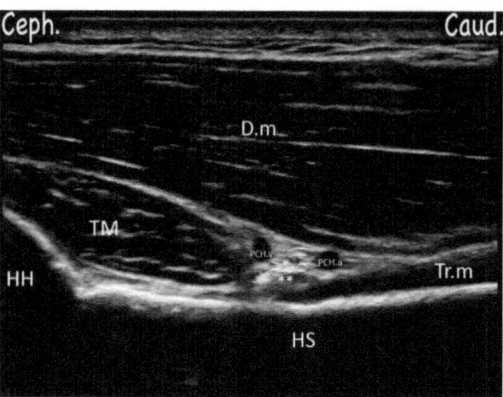

Fig. 2.3 Ultrasound Image for Axillary Block: Ceph. (Cephalad), Caud. (Caudad), D.m (Deltoid Muscle), TM (Teres Minor Muscle), Tr.m (Teres Major Muscle), HH (Humeral Head), HS (Humeral Shaft), PCH.v (Posterior Circumflex Humeral Vein), PCH.a (Posterior Circumflex Humeral Artery)

Compartment syndrome

Concern that RA may mask the signs of ischaemic pain that accompany acute compartment syndrome (ACS) is sometimes cited as a reason for avoiding such techniques in at-risk patients. Furthermore, timely diagnosis may be more difficult in pre-verbal children. However, a delay in the diagnosis of ACS is most usually due to inadequate identification of at-risk individuals and insufficient post-operative monitoring. There is no evidence that RA in paediatric patients increases the risk of a delayed ACS diagnosis [3]. Nevertheless, the following are recommended:

- Thorough pre-operative discussion with the surgical team and the child's family, informing them of this rare but potentially severe complication.
- Single-shot peripheral nerve blocks with 0-1-0.25% bupivacaine, levobupivacaine, or ropivacaine are less likely to mask ischaemic pain.
- For continuous infusions, low concentrations of bupivacaine, levobupivacaine, or ropivacaine should be used.
- High-risk patients should be identified and receive appropriate follow-up.
- If ACS is suspected, urgent assessment, including measurement of compartment pressures, must occur.

Dosing and systemic toxicity

Pharmacokinetic and pharmacodynamic differences in the paediatric population warrant careful attention to dosing. However, data are scarce. Fortunately, the incidence of local anaesthetic systemic toxicity (LAST) in children is infrequent, although infants appear to represent a higher-risk group. Vigilance and a high index of suspicion are vital, especially as most children will be either anaesthetised or heavily sedated. Therefore, the detection of CNS symptoms may not be possible. ECG changes and cardiovascular collapse may represent the first symptoms. ESRA-ASRA recommendations suggest a dose of 0.5–1.5 mg/kg of bupivacaine, levobupivacaine or ropivacaine for upper (and lower) extremity blocks performed under ultrasound guidance in children [3].

Adjuncts

Evidence supports the use of adjuvant clonidine for peripheral nerve blocks in children [3], although the optimum dose is unclear. No other adjuncts have consistently been shown to improve postoperative analgesia in this context.

6. **Why might a regional technique be of particular benefit in this case?**

Given the history of severe obstructive sleep apnoea, an opioid-sparing anaesthetic is desirable. This is eminently achievable if a successful brachial plexus block is performed. If opioids are required, shorter-acting agents (e.g. fentanyl) should be used in preference to longer-acting agents (e.g. morphine), and a monitored bed should be considered for overnight oxygen saturation monitoring.

Suggested Reading

1. Babal JC, Mehlman CT, Klein G. Nerve injuries associated with pediatric supracondylar humeral fractures: a meta-analysis. J Pediatr Orthop. 2010;30(3):253–63.
2. Walker BJ, Long JB, Sathyamoorthy M, et al. Complications in pediatric regional anesthesia: an analysis of more than 100,000 blocks from the pediatric regional anesthesia network. Anesthesiology.

2018;129(4):721–32. https://doi.org/10.1097/ALN.0000000000002372.

3. Lönnqvist PA, Ecoffey C, Bosenberg A, et al. The European society of regional anesthesia and pain therapy and the American society of regional anesthesia and pain medicine joint committee practice advisory on controversial topics in pediatric regional anesthesia I and II: what do they tell us? Curr Opin Anaesthesiol. 2017;30(5):613–20.

4. Merella F, Canchi-Murali N, Mossetti V. General principles of regional anaesthesia in children. BJA Educ. 2019;19(10):342–8.

Analgesia for Surgery of the Clavicle

3

Jonathan Major

Case Scenario

A 54-year-old, right-handed man presents following a bicycle crash during a triathlon event. He has suffered multiple superficial lacerations and is complaining of right shoulder pain. X-ray imaging demonstrates a severely displaced midshaft clavicle fracture. SpO2 is 96% on air, and there is no evidence of pneumothorax on chest x-ray. The surgeons are keen to proceed with an internal fixation on tomorrow's trauma list.

1. **What is the relevant anatomy and innervation of the clavicle?**

We must consider:

1. Overlying **cutaneous innervation**. The supraclavicular nerves (which divide into medial, intermediate and lateral branches) are derived from the C3 and C4 roots of the cervical plexus). These nerves also have some osseous innervation, especially superiorly and anteriorly.

2. **Osseous innervation** of the clavicle. This is complex, and it is best to consider the clavicle's muscular attachments (see Fig. 3.1), the innervation of which will also supply that region of bone.

    Lateral anterior—*deltoid* muscle: axillary nerve (C5, C6)

J. Major (✉)
St George's Hospital, London, UK
e-mail: jonathan.major@nhs.net

Lateral posterior—*trapezius* muscle: sensation C3, C4 spinal nerves; NB motor supply is from the spinal accessory nerve CN XI

Medial anterior—clavicular head of *pectoralis major*: C5, C6, C7 nerve roots via the lateral pectoral nerve; NB the medial pectoral nerve (C8, T1) supplies the sternal head of pectoralis major.

Posterior medial—*sternocleidomastoid* muscle: sensation C2, C3, spinal nerves; NB motor supply is from the spinal accessory nerve CN XI

Inferior—*subclavius* muscle: nerve to subclavius (C5, C6) via the superior trunk of the brachial plexus

Additionally, the following nerves usually account for some sensory innervation:

Long thoracic nerve via C5, C6, C7 nerve roots

Suprascapular nerve (C5, C6) from the superior trunk

In summary, the osseous innervation is complicated, but much of the sensory supply of the clavicle is via the C5 and C6 nerve roots. Cadaveric dissection has demonstrated the most consistent contribution from the supraclavicular, lateral pectoral and subclavius nerves [1].

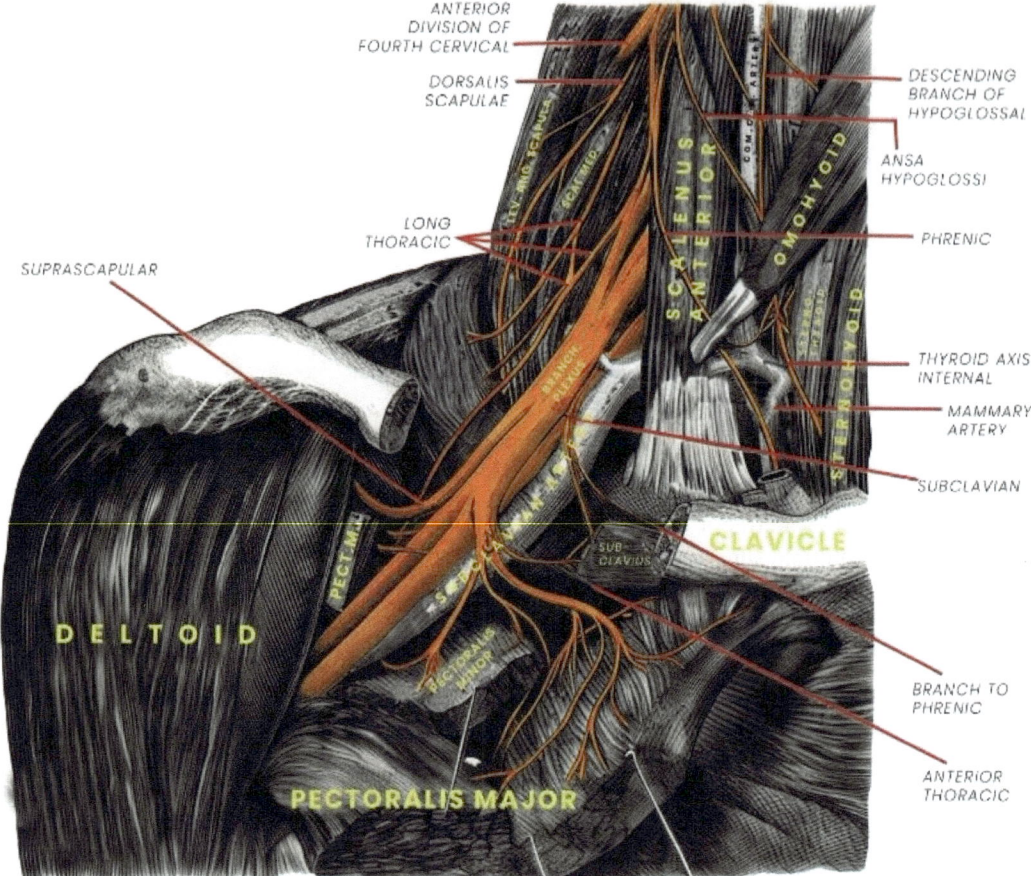

Fig. 3.1 Anatomical illustration showing the clavicle, brachial plexus and associated nerves. (Reproduced from Leurcharusmee et al. [1])

3. The **clavipectoral fascia** encloses the clavicle, and its limits provide a more localised target for regional analgesia/anaesthesia (see Fig. 3.3).

Superiorly, its anterior and posterior layers encircle the clavicle and become continuous with the investing layer of the deep cervical fascia.

Inferiorly, these layers enclose the subclavius muscle before fusing and continuing down to the pectoralis minor muscle. Again, they split to enclose pectoralis minor before fusing and continuing down into the axilla.

Medially, it is attached to the first two costochondral joints.

Laterally, it is attached to the coracoid process of the scapula.

2. **How might you provide intraoperative analgesia?**

A multimodal analgesia strategy is recommended. The following would be advisable:

- Paracetamol
- NSAID or COX-2 selective inhibitor
- A regional anaesthetic technique (see below)
- Dexamethasone if regional anaesthesia performed
- Rescue opioids

3. **What are the regional anaesthesia options?**

It is not practical to target all the terminal nerves as described above. Regional options to consider are (Figs. 3.2 and 3.3):

- **Interscalene** brachial plexus block—targeting the C5 and C6 nerve roots

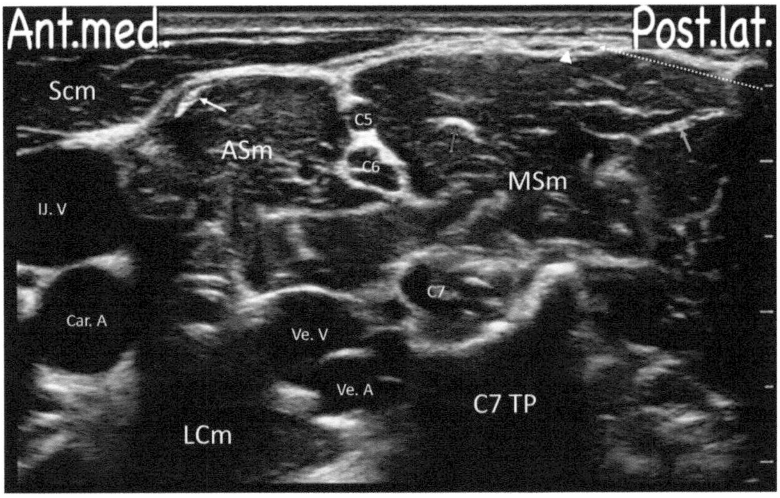

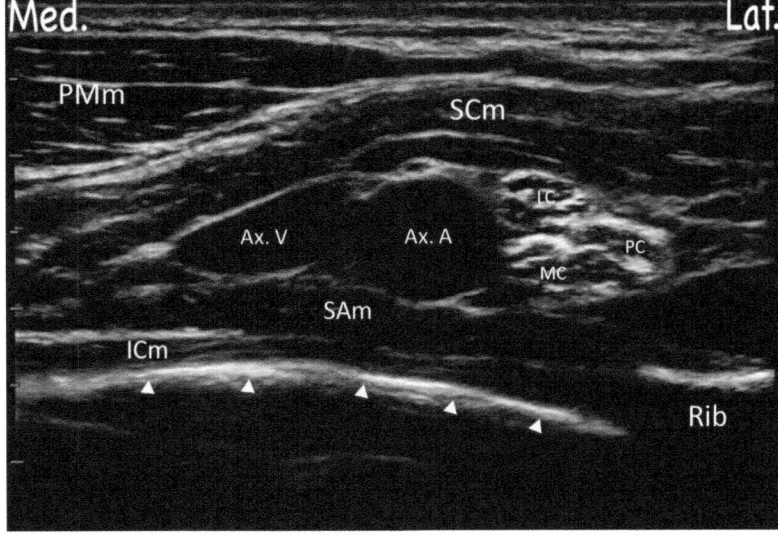

Fig. 3.2 Ultrasound image of the neck for selective supraclavicular nerve block from anteromedial (Ant. med.) to posterolateral (Post. lat.) view, showing sternocleidomastoid muscle (Scm), anterior scalene muscle (ASm), middle scalene muscle (MSm), lateral scalene muscle (LCm), internal jugular vein (IJ. V), carotid artery (Car. A), vertebral vein (Ve. V), vertebral artery (Ve. A), and C5, C6, C7 cervical nerve roots with C7 transverse process (C7 TP). The white, red and blue arrows indicate the phrenic, long thoracic and dorsal scapular nerves respectively. The target, the supraclavicular nerves, are indicated by the white triangle with the needle trajectory indicated by the dashed white arrow.

Fig. 3.3 Ultrasound image demonstrating the anatomy for the costoclavicular block from medial (Med.) to lateral (Lat.) view, showing pectoralis major muscle (PMm), subclavius muscle (SCm), axillary vein (Ax. V), axillary artery (Ax. A), lateral cord (LC), posterior cord (PC), medial cord (MC), serratus anterior muscle (SAm), intercostal muscle (ICm), and the underlying rib

- **Superior trunk** brachial plexus block—potentially 'phrenic-sparing'
- **Clavipectoral fascial plane** block, a motor-sparing approach

The blocks above may result in cutaneous coverage due to the spread of local anaesthetic, especially if larger volumes are used. If not, the skin overlying the clavicle can be blocked in various ways:

- **Cervical plexus** block (superficial or intermediate)
- Selective **supraclavicular nerve** block
- **Subcutaneous infiltration**

4. **What are the advantages of the clavipectoral fascia plane block over more proximal brachial plexus blocks?**

Avoidance of the risks and complications associated with the interscalene block, namely:

- Phrenic nerve blockade—especially relevant in the presence of pre-existing respiratory compromise and other chest injuries such as rib fractures, pulmonary contusions, or pneumothorax
- Horner's syndrome
- Vascular injury or intravascular injection
- Neuraxial injection or spread

The clavipectoral fascial plane block is a more targeted block for clavicle surgery. Due to the lack of phrenic nerve involvement, it is perfectly acceptable to perform bilateral blocks if indicated, although care must be taken not to exceed local anaesthetic dosing limits.

5. **How would you perform a clavipectoral fascial plane block?**

Scan in a parasagittal plane from the medial end of the clavicle using a linear probe. Identify the hyperechoic bony clavicle and the pectoralis major muscle inferiorly. An in-plane, caudal-to-cephalad approach should be used with the local anaesthetic deposited just superficially to the body of the clavicle itself. Making contact with the bone and then withdrawing 1–2 mm before injection is reasonable. A successful injection will result in the separation of the clavipectoral fascia from the clavicle.

Following clavicle trauma, it should be possible to identify the fracture on ultrasound. Local anaesthetic should be deposited medial and lateral to this point as the fracture and its associated haematoma may otherwise prevent adequate spread. A volume of 10–15 ml on each side of the fracture is recommended.

6. **Which clavicle fractures would be less suited to a clavipectoral fascial plane block?**

Medial fractures, especially those extending to the sternoclavicular joint, are less well covered by this block as the relevant nerve fibres run outside this fascial plane. It is generally appropriate for mid-shaft and lateral clavicle fractures.

7. **Are there any additional considerations regarding this block for subsequent surgery?**

If metalwork is being removed, the clavipectoral fascia may have been sufficiently disrupted during the original surgery to result in a patchy or incomplete block due to compromised spread of local anaesthetic. A brachial plexus block (interscalene or superior trunk) may be considered in this situation, either as the primary technique or as a rescue if the clavipectoral block proves insufficiently effective.

8. **What technique could you use to block the supraclavicular nerves?**

Either a **superficial or intermediate cervical plexus block** or a **selective supraclavicular nerve block**.

The cervical plexus's cutaneous branches emerge from the sternocleidomastoid muscle's (SCM) posterior border at the level of the thyroid notch (C4). These are:

- Supraclavicular (of interest for clavicle surgery)
- Transverse cervical
- Greater auricular
- Lesser occipital

Intermediate cervical plexus block

This will block all four cutaneous branches.

Start scanning at the level of the thyroid cartilage (C4/5) with the probe in a transverse orientation and slide it laterally. Identify the vascular contents of the carotid sheath, namely the carotid artery and internal jugular vein, and the SCM superficially. Keep scanning laterally until the posterior border of the muscle is reached. Immediately beneath this is the deep cervical fascia's superficial (investing) layer. Deeper, the pre- or perivertebral fascia can be seen surrounding the anterior and middle scalene muscles and their interscalene groove, and more posteriorly, the posterior scalene and levator scapulae muscles.

The entry point should be at or just lateral to the posterior border of SCM, using an in-plane, lateral to-medial approach, with the local anaesthetic injected between the superficial (investing) and prevertebral fascial layers. Technically, the block described should be considered an 'intermediate' cervical plexus block, while a true 'superficial' cervical plexus block is superficial to the superficial (investing) layer of deep cervical fascia. The intermediate block should provide better spread and more reliable cutaneous coverage. While a landmark technique is acceptable, ultrasound will significantly facilitate the deposition of local anaesthetic in the desired fascial plane.

Selective supraclavicular nerve block

The supraclavicular nerve emerges at the posterior border of SCM and divides into its medial, intermediate and lateral branches. These supply the skin from the second rib anteriorly to the spine of the scapula posteriorly and from the midline to the tip of the shoulder. They travel in the fascial plane, superficial to the middle scalene muscle, before rising to pierce the deep cervical fascia's superficial (investing) layer. These branches may be identifiable on ultrasound and can be seen moving laterally as the probe is moved caudally; if identified, they can be selectively targeted with the advantage of needing a reduced volume of local anaesthetic.

9. **Are there any additional considerations for a medial surgical entry point?**

The skin overlying the medial aspect of the clavicle may be partially cross-innervated by the medial branch of the contralateral supraclavicular nerve. Local subcutaneous infiltration should be sufficient to cover this.

10. **What are the advantages and disadvantages of a nerve catheter technique for post-operative analgesia?**

Advantages include:

- Extension of analgesia with an option for continuous infusion, PCRA or PIB of local anaesthetic.
- Ambulatory regional anaesthesia via an elastomeric pump may be possible.

Disadvantages include:

- May be difficult to anchor the catheter in sufficient muscle, risking dislodgement and consequent failure.
- Risk of infection.

Suggested Reading

1. Leurcharusmee P, Maikong N, Kantakam P, Navic P, Mahakkanukrauh P, Tran Q. Innervation of the clavicle: a cadaveric investigation. Reg Anesth Pain Med. 2021;46(12):1076–9.

Wrist Surgery

4

Matthew Sinnott

Case Scenario

A 44-year-old, right-handed man presents following a bicycle crash. He has suffered multiple superficial lacerations and is complaining of right wrist pain. X-ray imaging demonstrates a distal radius fracture. SpO2 is 96% on air, and there is no evidence of pneumothorax on chest x-ray. The surgeons want to proceed with an internal fixation.

1. *Describe the dermatomal innervation of the forearm, wrist and hand*

The forearm, wrist and hand are covered by dermatomes C5—T1. The radial/lateral aspect of the forearm and wrist is C5/6. The medial/ulnar aspect of the forearm is C8/T1. The dorsal aspect of the forearm and wrist is C6/7. In the hand, the thumb and lateral aspect is C6, the second and third digits are C7 and the fourth and fifth digits and medial aspect of the hand is C8. Note there is considerable overlap (Fig. 4.1).

2. *Describe the cutaneous innervation of the forearm, wrist and hand*

- Lateral cutaneous nerve of the forearm/lateral antebrachial cutaneous nerve (a branch of the musculocutaneous nerve) supplies the radial/lateral aspect of the forearm

- Medial cutaneous nerve of forearm/median antebrachial cutaneous nerve (a branch directly from the medial cord of the brachial plexus) supplies the medial/ulnar aspect of the forearm

- Posterior cutaneous nerve of the forearm/posterior antebrachial cutaneous nerve (a branch of the radial nerve) supplies the dorsal aspect of the forearm

- The radial nerve supplies the lateral aspect of the thumb and dorsal hand across the lateral/radial 3 ½ digits

- The median nerve supplies the palmar surface of lateral 3 ½ digits (and their dorsal tips) and lateral palm and wrist

- Ulnar nerve supplies the palmar and dorsal aspects of the median 1 ½ digits and medial palm and wrist

3. *Describe the osteotomal innervation of the forearm, wrist and hand.*

Osteotomal innervation is not as clearly defined as cutaneous. The median nerve supplies the ventral/volar aspect of the radius and ulna. The dorsal aspect of the radius and ulna is largely supplied by the radial nerve (except at the elbow when innervation comes from the ulnar nerve). Both ulnar and median nerves supply the ventral/volar aspect of the carpal bones. The radial nerve supplies the dorsal aspect of the carpal bones. The innervation of the metacarpals and phalanges

M. Sinnott (✉)
Anaesthetic Department, Ashford and St Peter's Hospitals NHS Foundation Trust, Chertsey, UK
e-mail: matthewsinnott@doctors.org.uk

S. Phillips et al. (eds.), *Regional Anaesthesia*, https://doi.org/10.1007/978-3-032-05165-3_4

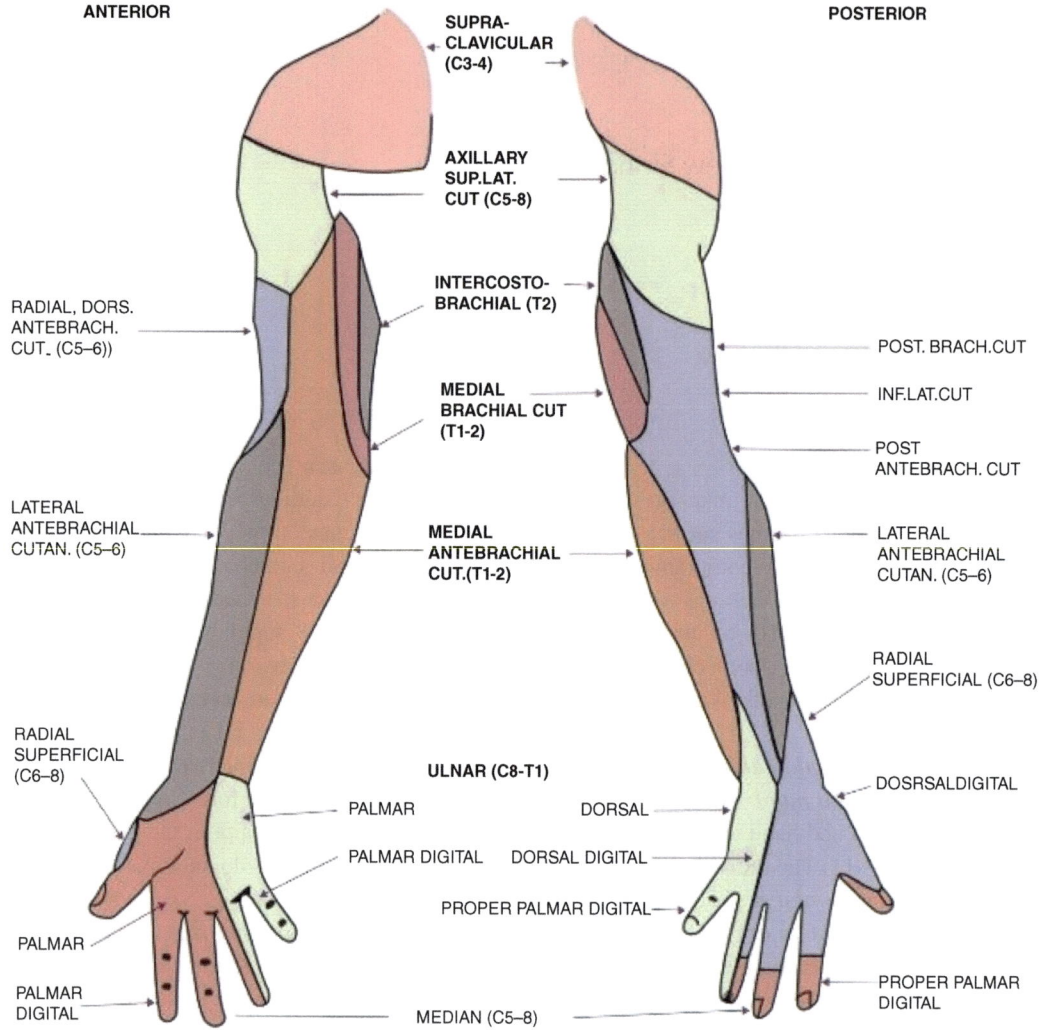

Fig. 4.1 Cutaneous nerve distribution of the upper limb: anterior and posterior views

follows the same pattern as the cutaneous innervation—the volar aspect of the lateral 3 ½ digits is supplied by the median, the radial supplies the dorsal aspect of the same digits, and the medial 1 ½ digits is supplied by the ulnar nerve.

4. *List some of the common operative procedures on the hand and wrist which may take place under regional block*

Procedures which may commonly be performed under regional block include:
- ORIF distal radius/ulna
- Trigger finger or carpal tunnel release
- Dupytren's contracture release
- Metacarpophalangeal joint replacement (usually performed for rheumatoid arthritis)
- Tendon grafts
- Ulnar head excision or trapeziectomy (usually performed for rheumatoid arthritis)

5. *What brachial plexus blocks are appropriate for hand and wrist procedures? Please describe local anaesthetic choices and doses*

Commonly performed brachial plexus blocks for hand and wrist procedures include the supraclavicular, infraclavicular, and axillary plexus blocks. For these blocks, 10–30 ml

LA is typically used. The choice of LA depends on the desired block characteristics. Commonly used agents include lidocaine, bupivacaine and ropivacaine, which may be used individually or in combination and with or without adjuncts.

6. *What is the role of distal nerve blocks in the upper limb?*

Distal nerve blocks can be performed as the sole anaesthetic technique for minor hand or wrist procedures, which do not require a tourniquet. They can also be used in combination with a brachial plexus block. Using long-acting LA distally may provide prolonged analgesia and facilitate the use of a shorter-acting LA more proximally, allowing an earlier return of upper limb motor function. They can also be used as a rescue technique if the patient were to experience pain intra- or post-operatively.

7. *What are the advantages of distal nerve blocks in the upper limb?*

Distal nerve blocks avoid critical structures potentially at risk from brachial plexus blocks, including the pleura, subclavian, and axillary vessels. They also avoid blocking the phrenic nerve, so they are beneficial in patients with pre-existing respiratory disease. Preserving motor function improves patient satisfaction and may facilitate some surgical procedures where structural integrity needs to be assessed intra-operatively.

When used in combination with brachial plexus blocks, they can hasten block onset time, which may facilitate the timely running of lists. They also allow improved post-operative analgesia while limiting post-operative motor weakness when a short—and long-acting LA agent is used at the brachial plexus and distally, respectively.

8. *What are the disadvantages of distal nerve blocks in the upper limb?*

Distal nerve blocks will miss nerves, which arise more proximally. The lateral cutaneous nerve of the forearm (which arises from the musculocutaneous nerve) will not be blocked, nor will the medial cutaneous nerve of the forearm (which arises directly from the brachial plexus). If muscle relaxation is required for the procedure, the radial and median nerves must be blocked high enough to ensure the posterior and anterior interosseous nerve anaesthesia, respectively, are anaesthetised.

If distal nerves are being blocked after a brachial plexus block, adequate monitoring to minimise the risk of intra-neural injection is required since the patient may well not feel any pain or paraesthesia from iatrogenic trauma.

Distal blocks will not prevent tourniquet pain. They require multiple injection sites, which can be unpleasant for the patient. Due to their significant anisotropy, identifying the peripheral nerves can be challenging for less experienced practitioners.

9. *How would you anaesthetise for an ORIF distal radius fracture?*

I would pre-assess the patient, asking about the mode of injury and any other injuries sustained. I would ask about prior anaesthetics, past medical and surgical history, and drug history and check for allergies. As the history indicates, I would perform a routine airway assessment and check blood results, ECG and other investigations. Provided there are no contra-indications, my preferred technique would be to perform a supraclavicular block with 15–20 ml 1% lidocaine with 1:200,000 adrenaline, which I would also infiltrate subcutaneously along the axillary crease to aim to block the intercostobrachial nerve to mitigate tourniquet pain. I would add distal blocks of the radial, ulnar and median nerves with around 3 ml 0.5% bupivacaine each (Figs. 4.2, 4.3, 4.4, and 4.5). The patient can remain completely awake, however I would discuss this with the patient and consider their preferences. Sedation and/or GA could be offered. I would ensure the patient is fully consented for these procedures based on a risk/benefit discussion and taking into account the patient's wishes.

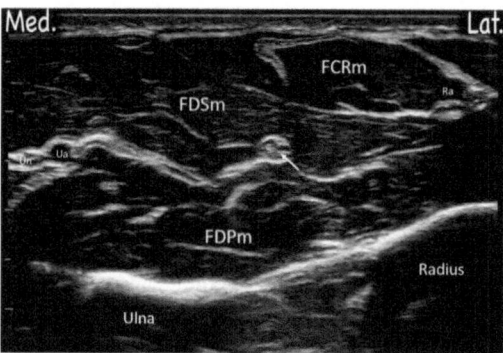

Fig. 4.2 Ultrasound image of the forearm showing the median nerve anatomy, including the ulnar nerve (Un), ulnar artery (Ua), flexor digitorum superficialis muscle (FDSm), flexor digitorum profundus muscle (FDPm), flexor carpi radialis muscle (FCRm), radial artery (Ra), with the radius and ulna bones labeled. White arrow indicates median nerve

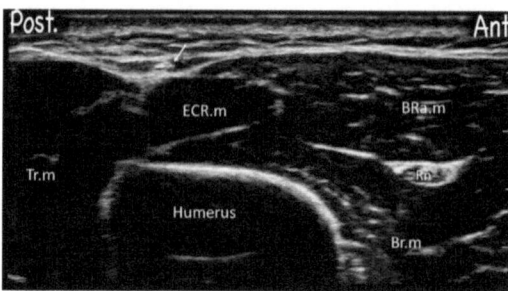

Fig. 4.4 Ultrasound image of the distal arm highlighting the radial nerve from posterior (Post.) to anterior (Ant.) view, showing the extensor carpi radialis muscle (ECR.m), brachioradialis muscle (BRa.m), radial nerve (Rn), brachialis muscle (Br.m), triceps muscle (Tr.m), and the humerus bone. Arrow indicates posterior cutaneous nerve of forearm

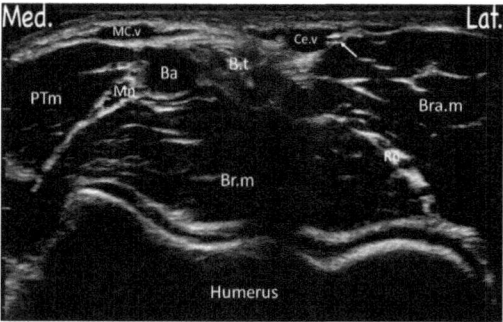

Fig. 4.3 Ultrasound image of the antecubital fossa (ACF) highlighting the radial nerve anatomy from medial (Med.) to lateral (Lat.) view, showing median cubital vein (MC.v), brachial artery (Ba), biceps tendon (B.t), cephalic vein (Ce.v), median nerve (Mn), pronator teres muscle (PTm), brachialis muscle (Br.m), brachioradialis muscle (Bra.m), radial nerve (Rn), and humerus bone

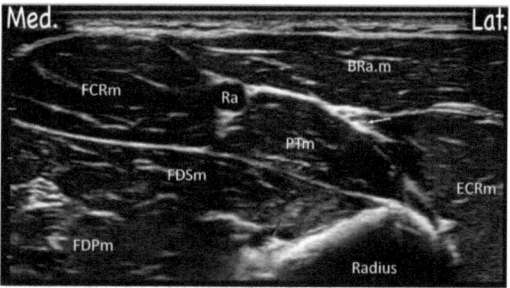

Fig. 4.5 Ultrasound image showing the superficial branch of the radial nerve from medial (Med.) to lateral (Lat.) view, including flexor carpi radialis muscle (FCRm), radial artery (Ra), brachioradialis muscle (BRa.m), pronator teres muscle (PTm), extensor carpi radialis muscle (ECRm), flexor digitorum superficialis muscle (FDSm), flexor digitorum profundus muscle (FDPm), and the radius bone. White arrow indicates the superficial branch of radial nerve and red arrow indicates the anterior interosseous nerve and vessels

10. *What are the limitations of an interscalane brachial plexus block for this surgery?*

The interscalene block will usually miss the lower roots of the brachial plexus (C8—T1) and, subsequently, the inferior trunk and ulnar nerve. The patient would likely experience pain in the medial/ ulnar aspect of the forearm and hand.

11. *How would you test for block success before surgery starts?*

Motor block can be easily assessed before commencement. Weakness of elbow flexion assesses the musculocutaneous nerve, weakness of elbow extension assesses the radial nerve, while the median and ulnar nerves can be evaluated via flexion of the 2nd and 5th digits respectively.

12. *What are some of the practicalities which must be considered when performing this procedure under regional anaesthesia?*

Local anaesthetic should be administered subcutaneously before block performance. An awake patient often needs reassurance. Their comfort must be considered, including positioning on the operating table, avoiding excessive IV fluids and allowing emptying of the bladder before surgery commences. The timing for block performance and onset must be factored in to minimise delays to the list. A clear backup plan must be in place in case of block failure.

13. *What nerves mediate tourniquet pain and how can it be prevented in an awake patient?*

Tourniquet pain is mediated via several nerves from the brachial plexus—including the musculocutaneous nerve, and medial and posterior cutaneous nerves of the arm. Distal blocks will miss these but can be blocked via proximal brachial plexus approaches. The intercostobrachial nerve arises from the lateral cutaneous branch of T2 and will be missed by brachial plexus blocks. It can be anaesthetised via subcutaneous infiltration of LA along the axillary crease.

14. *Please describe the role of haematoma blocks for managing distal radius fractures*

Haematoma blocks involve injecting LA into the fracture cavity to allow manual reduction. They are mostly performed in the emergency department as they do not require an anaesthetist or patient fasting and are thus less resource-intensive than other regional anaesthetic techniques. However, the analgesia provided may be unreliable, particularly if time has passed since the original injury and the haematoma has had time to organise. The lack of muscle relaxation makes reduction more technically challenging and patients may require subsequent procedures under a more formal anaesthetic technique.

15. *Please describe the role of IV regional anaesthesia for managing distal radius fractures*

IV regional anaesthesia is technically easy to perform and can provide good conditions for manual reduction of distal fractures. However, the risk of LA toxicity requires

careful consideration of tourniquet protocols, and practitioners must have adequate training to minimise risk. Patients can experience pain from limb exsanguination and tourniquet use, even when a 2-tourniquet technique is used.

16. *What are the purported benefits of WALANT?*

The WALANT technique is another method for providing anaesthesia for distal upper limb surgery. There is no need for an anaesthetist, and the risks associated with sedation or GA are avoided. Patients do not need to be fasted and there is no requirement for an IV cannula or tourniquet. This can potentially provide benefits in terms of patient experience and resource requirements. Patients retain motor function which can facilitate assessment of adequacy of surgical repair in some procedures.

Suggested Reading

1. Capek A, Dolan J. Ultrasound-guided peripheral nerve blocks of the upper limb. BJA Educ. 2015;15(3):160–5.
2. Carrera A, Lopez AM, Sala-Blanch X, Kapur E, Hasanbegovic I, Hadzic A. Functional regional anaesthesia anatomy. https://www.nysora.com/topics/anatomy/functional-regional-anesthesia-anatomy. Accessed 2/3/22.
3. Farag E, Mounir-Soliman L, Brown D. Atlas of regional anesthesia. 5th ed. Elsevier; 2017.
4. Griffiths R, Leighton R. Orthopaedic surgery. In: Oxford handbook of anaesthesia. 3rd ed. OUP; 2014.
5. Handoll H, Madhok R, Dodds C. Anaesthesia for treating distal radial fracture in adults. Cochrane Database Syst Rev. 2002;2002(3):CD003320.
6. Shembi H, Madjdpour C, Shah UJ, Chin KJ. Ultrasound guided distal peripheral nerve block of the upper limb: a technical review. J Anaesthesiol Clin Pharmacol. 2015;31(3):296–307.
7. Steiner MM, Calandruccio JH. Use of wide-awake local anaesthesia no tourniquet in hand and wrist surgery. Orthop Clin N Am. 2018;49:63–8.
8. Tonwsley P, Bedforth N, Nicholls B, Wilkinson D. A pocket guide to ultrasound-guided regional anaesthesia. 2nd ed. Regional Anaesthesia-UK; 2019.

Anaesthesia for Arteriovenous Fistula [AVF] Creation

5

Sangeetha Selvaraj, Zhu Jiasi,
and Ashokka Balakrishnan

Case Scenario

A 65-year-old male patient with end-stage kidney disease [ESKD] is listed for the creation of an AV fistula. His significant past medical history includes diabetes mellitus on insulin therapy, ischaemic heart disease [IHD] post percutaneous cardiac intervention and stent insertion 4 years ago, COPD on chronic bronchodilator therapy and ESKD on peritoneal dialysis. The patient was admitted 1 month ago for fluid overload and was managed with transient haemodialysis through temporary central venous access.

1. **What are your concerns?**

Patient

- ESKD patients may have multiple associated comorbidities, which should be optimised before elective surgery.

Surgical

- The AVF creation site would determine the choice of regional anaesthesia [RA] and assist in planning the type of RA. The patient's history of previous AVF surgeries may indicate a potential lengthy surgery and significant blood loss.

Anaesthesia

- Persistent coagulopathy/inadequately suspended antiplatelet/anticoagulant therapy may preclude deep, non-compressible blocks. ESKD can have peripheral neuropathies and are prone to local anaesthetic toxicity.

2. **What is the indication for creating an AVF?**

AV fistula serves as a vascular access for dialysis in ESKD patients requiring long-term haemodialysis. Vascular access aims to provide reliable, repeated circulatory access with minimal complications and achieve a minimal flow rate of 600 ml/min to facilitate effective haemodialysis.

3. **What types of anaesthesia can be given for AVF creation?**

AVF can be created under general, regional, or local anaesthesia [LA] with or without sedation. The choice of operative anaesthesia is based on the patient's comorbidities, contraindications to regional anaesthesia, the location of the AVF creation, anaesthetic expertise, familiarity, and feasibility. ESKD patients have multiple comorbidities, with 30-day post-operative mortality of 2.6%, which may make general anaesthesia unsuitable or

S. Selvaraj (✉)
Singapore General Hospital, Singapore

Z. Jiasi · A. Balakrishnan
National University Hospital Singapore,
Singapore

unsafe. Hence, regional anaesthesia is preferred.

4. **Is Regional anaesthesia beneficial? If yes, why?**

The anaesthetic technique is one of the factors believed to influence AVF maturation and outcome. Unlike local anaesthesia, regional anaesthesia achieves sympathetic blockade and may be associated with a higher success rate secondary to vasodilatation, increased fistula blood flow, and rapid maturation time. Several studies have demonstrated superior short-term patency rates of AVF created under brachial plexus block compared to LA.

5. **What are the sites for the creation of AV fistulas?**

They are typically created in the upper limb but can be placed in the lower limb. AVFs are created by end-to-side anastomosis between the artery and vein. Native fistulas have a high primary failure rate but a low complication rate and offer superior long-term patency. The decision to create an AVG (arterio-venous graft) in the upper extremity is at the opera-tor's discretion and based on best clinical judgement, considering the patient's ESKD life expectancy. There is inadequate evidence to demonstrate any difference in patency or complication (such as infections, hospitalisa-tions, and mortality) between forearm and upperarm AVGs.

The most common sites are as follows:

1. Radiocephalic fistula at wrist; often first choice, preserves proximal locations for use in the future. It has the lowest flows of all.

2. The brachiocephalic fistula at the elbow; more proximal, thus higher flows are attainable. However, it may result in an increased steal effect due to arterial blood diversion through the fistula, leading to distal limb arterial insufficiency and isch-aemia and occasional residual neuro-praxia requiring therapeutic ligation.

3. Transposed brachiobasilic arteriovenous fistula (TBBAVF): Often used after multi-ple failed distal fistulas, but it is more chal-lenging to create.

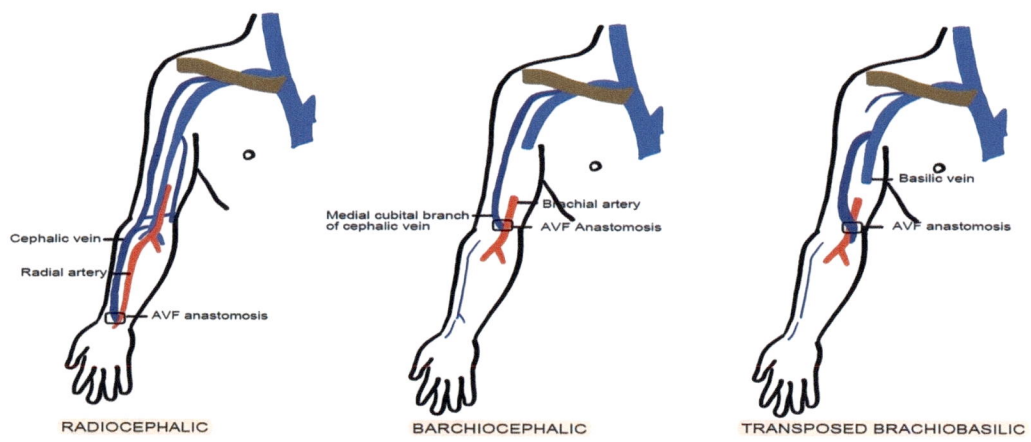

RADIOCEPHALIC   BARCHIOCEPHALIC   TRANSPOSED BRACHIOBASILIC

6. **How do you determine which nerves to block for the procedure?**

The proposed vascular access site governs the choice of regional anaesthetic technique. Supraclavicular, infraclavicular and axillary brachial plexus blocks are all appropriate techniques. The costoclavicular approach to brachial plexus block can also provide appropriate analgesia and surgical anaesthesia. If required, additional supplementation can be provided with a superior trunk block, a superficial cervical plexus block, and a pectoral nerve block (PECS-2). (Table 5.1).

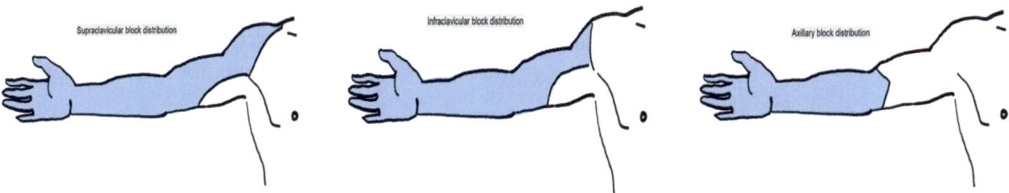

Table 5.1 Regional anaesthesia techniques for AV fistula creation

Surgery/Area	Nerves involved	Type of brachial plexus blocks (standard practice)	Nerves spared/Top-up required
Radiocephalic fistula at the wrist	The lateral cutaneous nerve of forearm (musculocutaneous C5,6) The posterior cutaneous nerve of forearm (radial C5,6,7,8) Median (C6,7,8) Radial (C6,7,8)	Axillary Infraclavicular Supraclavicular	Usually well covered by BPB
Brachiocephalic/ Brachiobasilic fistula at the elbow	The lateral cutaneous nerve of forearm (musculocutaneous C5,6) The medial cutaneous nerve of forearm (medial cord C8, T1) Medial cutaneous nerve of arm (medial cord C8, T1) The inferior lateral cutaneous nerve of arm (radial C5,6)	Axillary Infraclavicular Supraclavicular	The medial cutaneous nerve of the forearm/arm originates from the medial cord, which is missed by the axillary block and requires local anaesthetic supplementation at the surgical site.
Transposed Brachiobasilic fistula AVF	The lateral cutaneous nerve of forearm (musculocutaneous C5,6) The medial cutaneous nerve of forearm (medial cord C8, T1) Medial cutaneous nerve of arm (medial cord C8, T1) The inferior lateral cutaneous nerve of arm (radial C5,6) Intercostobrachial nerve (T2)	Axillary Infraclavicular Supraclavicular	BPB does not block the intercostobrachial nerve and would need a separate injection. Intercostal nerves T2 and T3 also have anterior and posterior branches that anastomoses with the medial cutaneous nerve of the arm to supply the medial arm and floor of the axilla, which will require subcutaneous infiltration, intercostal block [41] or PEC II block [42]

7. **Can you briefly describe supraclavicular, infraclavicular and axillary brachial plexus blocks? Are all appropriate for the creation of brachiocephalic AVF?**

[For a detailed description, refer to the chapter on individual blocks]

Supraclavicular block: [SCB]

Relevant anatomy: Brachial plexus blocked at the level of divisions.

Key landmarks: 1st rib, pleura and subclavian artery

The brachial plexus lies above the 1st rib, lateral and superficial to the subclavian artery

Technique and Target: Place a transverse ultrasound probe just proximal to the clavicle, slightly posterior to its midpoint, and tilt it caudally to visualize the subclavian artery and the brachial plexus. Use Color Doppler imaging to identify any intervening vessels. Infiltrate the skin 1 cm lateral to the probe with 1–2 mL of local anesthetic using a 25–27G needle. Advance the block needle inplane from lateral to medial, initially no deeper than 1 cm. Use hydro-localization before targeting the brachial plexus. Deposit the local anaesthetic around the trunks and divisions of the brachial plexus within the brachial sheath posterior to the subclavian artery.

Needle strategies for conventional supraclavicular blocks consist of sub-epineurium injection (e.g., double injection), intracluster injection (e.g., triple, focused intracluster infusion), or extra-epineurium injection (e.g., corner pocket injection).

Tips: The ulnar nerve lies deep to the plexus and may be missed, and the musculocutaneous nerve may have an early take-off in 10% of patients and would require a supplemental block.

It provides the most intense block, and since the nerve bundles are compactly arranged, a smaller volume is required. It also has a rapid onset of action.

Complications: Pneumothorax, phrenic nerve block and vascular injury are potential complications. The subclavian and dorsal scapular arteries may cross the brachial plexus at this level, making

vascular injury possible. There are concerns of suprascapular nerve sparing. Inferior trunk sparing can occur even with ultrasound-guided inferior pocket injection (4–36%).

Operative anaesthesia: Supraclavicular block provides excellent surgical access to the upper extremity but spares the intercostobrachial nerve. Hence, the intercostobrachial nerve must be additionally blocked to facilitate the creation of transposed brachiobasilic arteriovenous fistulas or brachiobasilic fistulas requiring an extension of the incision towards the medial side of the arm.

Infraclavicular block [ICB]

Relevant anatomy: Brachial plexus at the level of cords

Key landmarks: Axillary artery under the clavicle, pleura, brachial plexus [cords], axillary vein

It provides similar coverage to the supraclavicular block with more distal coverage and a lower risk of pneumothorax. It is a deep block, making it difficult to compress in the event of an accidental vascular puncture.

Technique and Target: Position the transducer in the parasagittal plane to locate the axillary artery, typically found 3 to 5 cm deep. Once identified, try to locate the hyperechoic cords of the brachial plexus relative to the artery. Insert the needle in-plane from the cephalad end of the probe, just below the clavicle, aiming toward posterior aspect of the axillary artery and passing through the pectoralis major and minor muscles. Not required to identify the specific cords; simply deposit the local anaesthetic in a U-shaped pattern around the axillary artery, cephalad, caudal and posterior to the axillary artery.

The infraclavicular region is the best site to place the catheter, as the pectoral muscles hold it in place to prevent displacement. Previous vascular access scars in the infraclavicular area can make this block technically challenging and increase the likelihood of a patchy block. Compared to the SCB, the ICB is associated with a lower incidence of ulnar nerve sparing but a higher incidence of incomplete radial nerve block.

Operative anaesthesia: Blocks at the supraclavicular and infraclavicular region provide similar analgesia, with the former providing better coverage of the shoulder area. The infraclavicular block is an excellent alternative to the supraclavicular block for all types of vascular access surgeries along the upper limb, especially if the patient has a dialysis catheter in the supraclavicular region. Like the supraclavicular block, ICB would need an additional intercostobrachial or pectoral II block to cover the axillary region. Both supraclavicular and infraclavicular approaches to the brachial plexus have been used to provide satisfactory sensory and motor block in patients with ESKD undergoing the creation of AVF of the distal upper extremity. Research indicates that both blocks provided excellent analgesia lasting 6 to 8 hours, with the first supplementary analgesia required 9 to 10 hours later. Patients were satisfied with both blocks, and no complications were reported.

Axillary block

Relevant anatomy: Brachial plexus at the level of branches

Key landmarks: Axillary artery [pulsatile hypoechoic structure], humerus and individual branches [hyperechoic]; radial nerve is usually deep, ulnar, and median nerve encircle the artery, and musculocutaneous nerve lies within the belly of the coracobrachialis muscle.

Technique and Advantages: Place the transducer transversely over the intersection of the pectoralis major and biceps muscle insertion, avoiding a high position in the axillary fossa. Identify the conjoint tendon, axillary artery, neurovascular sheath (containing the median, ulnar, and radial nerves), the biceps, coracobrachialis and latissimus dorsi muscles, and the musculocutaneous nerve. Insert the needle in-plane from lateral to medial toward the axillary artery and inject 20 mL of local anaesthetic (around the axillary artery and the musculocutaneous nerve). Safer block, easy to perform, and can be easily compressed in the event of accidental vascular puncture/bleeding.

Operative anaesthesia: An axillary block provides excellent conditions for vascular access in surgical procedures distal to the elbow. To ensure complete anaesthesia, a separate injection is required to block the musculocutaneous nerve (C6, C7). Additional local anaesthetic infiltration is required for any extension of the incision proximal to the elbow.

8. **Can you describe how to perform a costoclavicular brachial plexus block?**

Costoclavicular nerve block [CCN]:
The costoclavicular space [CCS] is located deep and posterior to the midpoint of the clavicle, where the cords of the brachial plexus are relatively superficial in location, cluster together with each other, lateral to the axillary artery and share a consistent relationship with each other and with the axillary artery. This contrasts with the infraclavicular fossa block, where the cords are located quite deep [3–6 cm], are separated from one another, and are in significantly varied positions relative to the axillary artery. Additionally, all three cords are rarely visualised in a single ultrasound image. Karmaker et al. recently outlined a 5-step process to describe the sononanatomy for performing a CCN block.

Technique and Key landmarks: Place the transducer directly over the midpoint of the clavicle in the transverse orientation, with its orientation marker directed laterally (outward). Gently move the transducer caudally until it slips off the inferior border of the clavicle, alowing visualisation of the axillary artery (first part) and the vein. While maintaining the same transducer position, gently tilt the cephalad to direct the ultrasound beam toward the CCS, which is located between the posterior surface of the clavicle and the second rib. Identify the brachial plexus cords—lateral, medial, and posterior—located lateral to the axillary artery. These cords appear as hyperechoic oval structures arranged in a triangular formation. Insert the needle in-plane from lateral to medial, positioning it between the three cords, ideally between the lateral and posterior cords. Inject 15-20 mL of local anaesthetic.

Target: Needle tip at the centre of the nerve cluster [ideally between the lateral and posterior cord]

Tips: Avoid the cephalic vein or thoracoacromial artery, as this would indicate needle insertion distal to the CCS. Ensure the subclavius muscle is always visualised.

Complications: Inadvertent vascular [cephalic vein and axillary vessels] and pleural puncture.

Operative anaesthesia: The CCN block can provide reliable anaesthesia and analgesia for AVF surgeries, eliminating the need for additional top-up or supplemental blocks.

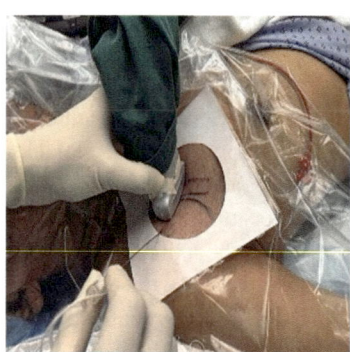 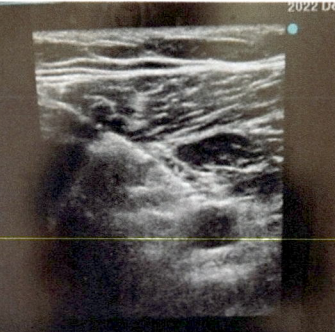 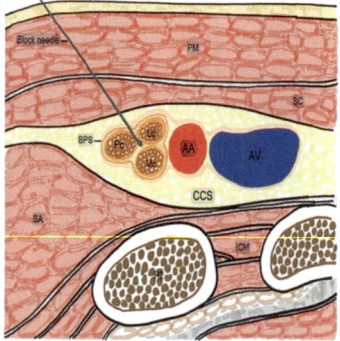

CCS Costoclavicular space; BPS brachial plexus sheath; Pc/Mc/Lc posterior/ medial and lateral cord; PM pectoralis major; SC serratus anterior; ICM intercostal muscles; SA serratus anterior; AA axillary artery; AV axillary vein

9. **What other supplemental blocks might be required in addition to brachial plexus blocks?**

   • Pectoral nerve block

     Pectoral nerve block (Pecs) I and II is a technique for blocking the thoracic nerve, the 3rd to 6th intercostal nerves, the intercostal nerves, and the long thoracic nerve. It is an additional block given for axillary coverage.

     Key landmarks: Identify the pectoralis major muscle, pectoralis minor muscle, serratus anterior, and the thoracoacromial artery (pectoral branch)

     Target: LA placed between the pectoralis major and pectoralis minor, then between the pectoralis minor and serratus anterior

     Complications: They are usually rare as the pleura and the blood vessels are visualised throughout the procedure, but the most common complications are pneumothorax and infection.

   • Intercostobrachial nerve block can be blocked by an additional subcutaneous injection just distal to the axilla.

   • Superior trunk block

   • Superficial cervical plexus block: This is beneficial for subclavicular incision during tunnelled graft placement and can be performed in combination with PECS 1&2 plane blocks to achieve complete surgical anaesthesia.

10. **In which situations is supplementation necessary?**
    - Complicated surgery
    - High upper arm operation
    - Hyper analgesia: neuropathies
    - Tunnelling of the graft brachial basilic/axillary to infraclavicular area

11. **Are you aware of newer regional anaesthesia techniques for upper limb surgeries?**
    - Intertruncal approach: In this approach to the supraclavicular brachial plexus (IA-SCB), the needle tip targets the two inter truncal tissue planes between the 3 trunks, but the biggest challenge is identifying the correct plane. There is also an ongoing trial comparing double injection vs triple injection inter truncal approach in patients undergoing upper limb arteriovenous access surgery
    - Selective truncal block [SeTB]: all-purpose (C5–T1) regional anaesthetic technique for upper extremity surgery is based on the principle that the majority of innervation of the upper extremity arises or passes through the three trunks of brachial plexus: upper, middle, and lower trunks. Local anaesthetic is directed at the individual trunks.

12. **Are you familiar with any Hybrid brachial plexus block [BPB] techniques? What are the limitations?**
    - Axillary-Interscalene BPB (Axis Block)—Urmey described a combined axillary-interscalene (axis) block to achieve complete anaesthesia of the upper limb
    - Interscalene-Axillary BPB (Reverse AXIS Block)—(Axillary-Interscalene) Block can be performed in a patients presenting with Fractures of the Left Shoulder and Elbow
    - Interscalene-Supraclavicular BPB or UGSCIS Block
    - Infraclavicular BPB-Suprascapular nerve block

    Limitation: Requires large volume of local anaesthetic, approximately 30–50 mls

Common debates regarding the local anaesthetics

13. **What is the ideal local anaesthetic concentration and volume needed for the blocks described above?**
    "Regional anaesthesia always works—provided you put the right dose of the right drug in the right place."

    The debate surrounding how the concentration and mass of locan anaesthetic influence both the success and duration of peripheral nerve blocks continues. The correlation between injection volume, local anaesthetic concentration, and duration of conduction block has been studied, and conflicting results have been obtained. Some authors have reported prolonged sensory and motor blockades with higher doses of local anaesthetics and suggested that the additional analgesic effect of sensory block warrants the use of high doses of local anaesthetic. However, other studies find no significant clinically relevant difference in block characteristics.

    Conventionally, LA [Ropivacaine/bupivacaine] concentration as low as 0.3% can be used for analgesia, and 0.5% and above can be used for operative anaesthesia.

14. **Is there a need for dose reduction for ESKD patients? If yes, why?**
    Chronic kidney disease can significantly alter the pharmacokinetics of local anaesthetics. An enhanced initial absorption at the injection site is observed, potentially due to a relative alkalinization of LA in an acidotic patient. This is coupled with an increased blood flow secondary to the hyper-dynamic circulation, resulting in rapid attainment and maintenance of high peak plasma concentration. Clearance of metabolites is also reduced in impaired kidney function. Hence, a 25% dose reduction is recommended in these patients with higher side effect risk profiles. A further reduction may need to be considered in the elderly, as they are more sensitive to LAs due to decreased neural density and slower nerve conduction velocity. The presence of pre-existing uremic peripheral neuropathies could affect the intended anaesthetic plans and warrant LA dose modifications.

Questions

1. An adult patient is scheduled for the formation of an arteriovenous fistula at the wrist.
   (a) Describe the nerve supply relevant to this surgery.
   (b) Discuss the suitability of an interscalene block in this situation.
2. Describe SUIT visualisation of the brachial plexus.
3. What are the disadvantages of axillary block for AVF creation?
4. Which blocks are needed to supplement BCB for AVF surgery?

Suggested Reading

1. Malinzak EB, Gan TJ. Regional anaesthesia for vascular access surgery. Anesth Analg. 2009;109:976–80.
2. Aitken E, Jackson A, Kearns R, et al. Effect of regional versus local anaesthesia on outcome after arteriovenous fistula creation: a randomised controlled trial. Lancet. 2016;388:1067–74.
3. Cerneviciute R, Sahebally SM, Ahmed K, et al. Regional versus local anaesthesia for haemodialysis arteriovenous fistula formation: a systematic review and meta-analysis. Eur J Vasc Endovasc Surg. 2017;53(5):734–42.
4. National Kidney Foundation. KDOQI clinical practice guidelines for vascular access clinical practice guidelines 2019 update.
5. Arab SA, Alharbi MK, Nada EM, et al. Ultrasound-guided supraclavicular brachial plexus block: single versus triple injection technique for upper limb arteriovenous access surgery. Anesth Analg. 2014;118(5):1120–5.
6. Techasuk W, Gonzalez AP, Bernucci F, et al. A randomised comparison between double-injection and targeted intracluster-injection ultrasound-guided supraclavicular brachial plexus block. Anesth Analg. 2014;118(6):1363–9.
7. Luo Q, Yao W, Shu H, et al. Double-injection technique assisted by a nerve stimulator for ultrasound-guided supraclavicular brachial plexus block results in better distal sensory-motor block: a randomised controlled trial. Eur J Anaesthesiol. 2017;34(3):127–34.
8. Dhir S, et al. Infraclavicular and supraclavicular approaches to brachial plexus for ambulatory elbow surgery: a randomised controlled observer-blinded trial. J Clinical anaesthesiology. 2018;48:67–72.
9. Park S-K, et al. Comparison of supraclavicular and infraclavicular brachial plexus block: a systemic review of randomized controlled trials. Anaesthesia analgesia. 2017;124(2):636–44.
10. EI-Sawy A, et al. Ultrasound-guided supraclavicular versus intraclavicular brachial plexus nerve block in chronic renal failure patients undergoing arteriovenous fistula creation. Egypt J Anaesth. 2013;30:161–7. Accepted 08 Nov 2013.
11. Li JW, Songthamwat B, Samy W, Sala-Blanch X, Karmakar MK. Ultrasound-guided costoclavicular brachial plexus block: sonoanatomy, technique, and block dynamics. Reg Anesth Pain Med. 2017;42:233–40.
12. Battista C, Krishnan S. Pectoralis nerve block. In: StatPearls [Internet]. Treasure Island: StatPearls Publishing; 2022. PMID: 31613471.
13. Siddiqui U, Perlas A, Chin K, et al. Intertruncal approach to the supraclavicular brachial plexus, current controversies, and technical update: a daring discourse. Reg Anesth Pain Med. 2020;45(5):377–80.
14. Luo Q, Liu H, Deng L, et al. Effects of double vs triple injection on block dynamics for ultrasound-guided intertruncal approach to the supraclavicular brachial plexus block in patients undergoing upper limb arteriovenous access surgery: study protocol for a double-blinded, randomized controlled trial. Trials. 2022;23:295. https://doi.org/10.1186/s13063-022-06260-6.
15. Sivakumar RK, Areeruk P, Karmakar MK. Selective trunk block (SeTB): a simple alternative to hybrid brachial plexus block techniques for proximal humeral fracture surgery during the COVID-19 pandemic. Reg Anesth Pain Med. 2021;46:376–8.
16. Marhofer P, Eichenberger U, Stöckli S, et al. Ultrasonographic guided axillary plexus blocks with low volumes of local anaesthetics: a crossover volunteer study. Anaesthesia. 2010;65:266–71.
17. Uppal NN, Jhaveri M, Hong S, et al. Local anaesthetics for the nephrologist. Clin Kidney J. 2021;15(2):186–93.
18. Quek KH, Low EY, Tan YR, Ong ASC, Tang TY, Kam JW, et al. Adding a PECS II block for proximal arm arteriovenous access-a randomised study. Acta Anaesthesiol Scand. 2018;62:677–86.

Analgesia for Breast Surgery

6

Arunangshu Chakraborty and Amit Dixit

Case Scenario

A 64-year-old female diagnosed with invasive ductal carcinoma of the breast is scheduled for a modified radical mastectomy with axillary dissection. Her past medical history includes global LV hypokinesia (LVEF 25%) and moderate to severe pulmonary hypertension. She takes ramipril, spironolactone and clopidogrel (stopped 5 days before). She complains of dyspnoea on exertion (NYHA Grade 3). Her oxygen saturation is 96% on room air. Blood investigations are unremarkable.

1. **What are the key issues?**

Patient evaluation: This patient has multiple risk factors:
   1. Low cardiac output state with pulmonary hypertension.
   2. Decreased functional capacity, NYHA −3, suggestive of reduced cardiopulmonary reserve.
   3. Raised creatinine.
   4. Treatment with antiplatelet drugs.

2. **What are the relevant surgical factors?**
   1. Extensive dissection involving muscles of the anterior chest wall.

A. Chakraborty (✉)
Sultan Qaboos Comprehensive Cancer Care and Research Centre, Muscat, Oman

A. Dixit
Department of Anaesthesia, Ruby Hall Hospital, Pune, India

   2. Axillary dissection
   3. With or without breast implantation

3. **Describe the anatomical innervation of the breast.**

The mammary gland receives its innervation from the ventral rami of T2 to T6 spinal nerves (Fig. 6.1).

Dermatome

Breast dermatomal innervation: T2–T6 (anterior and lateral cutaneous branches)

Axillary dissection: T1 and T2 (Intercostobrachial Nerve)

Postop surgical drain: May extend unto T7

Infraclavicular area: Supraclavicular Nerves.

Myotome: (Predominantly by brachial plexus)

Pectoral muscles: Lateral & Medial Pectoral Nerve (Brachial plexus)

Serratus Anterior: Nerve to Serratus Anterior

Latissimus Dorsi: Nerve to Latissimus Dorsi (Thoracodorsal Nerve)

4. **What would be your anaesthesia strategy?**
Either

   GA + Regional Anaesthesia for postoperative analgesia

   Or

   Regional Anaesthesia for surgical anaesthesia and postoperative analgesia

5. **What will be your analgesia strategy?**

As per the recommendation by the PROSPECT group, the analgesia regimen should be that of

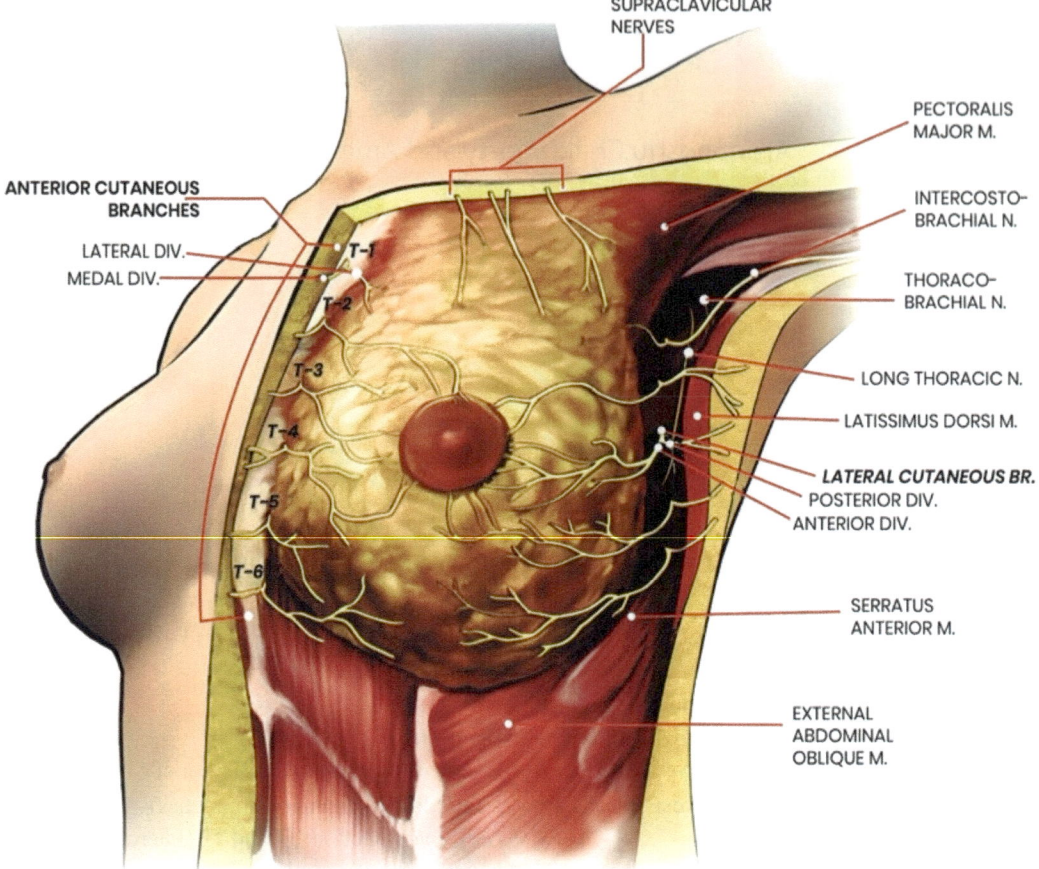

Fig. 6.1 Nerve supply of breast

a multimodal analgesia depending upon whether the surgery is minor or major breast surgery. For minor breast surgery, one can give a combination of the following:

1. Systemic analgesia with paracetamol and non-steroidal anti-inflammatory drugs (NSAIDs) is administered pre-operatively or intraoperatively and continued postoperatively.
2. Pre-operative gabapentinoids
3. A single dose of intravenous (i.v) dexamethasone- is recommended for its ability to increase the analgesic duration of peripheral nerve blocks, decrease the need for analgesics and have anti-emetic effects.
4. LA wound infiltration

For major surgery one of the following regional anaesthesia techniques can be used in addition to pharmacological therapy.

1. TPVB
2. Pectoral nerves block- as an alternative to TPVB
3. Thoracic epidural analgesia

Interventions such as retrolaminar block, erector spinae plane block and perineural adjuncts have not been recommended due to sparsity of evidence. Opioids- should be reserved as rescue analgesia in the postoperative period.

Local anaesthetic infiltration- plain or liposomal- should be performed if no regional block is provided.

Tumescent mastectomy, a technique that employs large volume infiltration of diluted local anaesthetic solution with adrenaline, has been considered effective in selected patients and a safe alternative for performing mastectomy when general anaesthesia is hazardous, with minimal blood loss and long-lasting postoperative analgesia without an additive effect on the operative time, hospital stay, and intraoperative and postoperative complications.

6. **What are the newly introduced regional anaesthesia techniques for analgesia for breast surgery?**

Various ultrasound-guided regional anaesthesia techniques have been introduced recently. Though not substantiated by systematic reviews, they hold promise as more evidence is surfacing. They are-
1. ESPB single shot at T4 with or without catheter.
2. Retrolaminar block,
3. MTP (midpoint transverse process to pleura) block,
4. Rhomboid intercostal block.

Blocks targeting the lateral cutaneous divisions of intercostal nerves
- Interpectoral and Pectoserratus blocks
  In addition to the intercostal nerves, the interpectoral blocks such as pecs 1 and pecs 2 blocks the lateral and medial pectoral nerves which originate from the brachial plexus and innervate the pectoral muscles.
- Serratus anterior plane block (Superficial and Deep)

Blocks targeting the anterior cutaneous divisions of intercostal nerves
- Pecto-intercostal fascial plane block.
- Transverse thoracic muscle plane block.

Blocks targeting other ancillary nerves supplying the breast region
- Selective supraclavicular nerve block
- Superficial cervical plexus block
- Brachial plexus block (e.g., costoclavicular block used to block pectoral N)

Systemic analgesia options
Multimodal analgesia
    IV opioid patient-controlled analgesia (PCA)

7. **What will be your key considerations when regional anaesthesia is chosen as sole technique for surgical anaesthesia (awake breast surgery):**

1. Patient factors- cooperation, reassurance
2. Adequate time to prepare for blocks and testing, meticulous surgery, team to be aware of awake patient, calculated LA dosages for supplementation
3. Plan for failure and rescue plan B techniques.

Sedation strategy: Titrated use of midazolam, fentanyl, dexmedetomidine, propofol infusion or inhalational anaesthetic to achieve Ramsay sedation score 2–3 or BIS reading between 60–80.

Awake breast surgeries exclusively under regional anaesthesia with minimal sedation are being utilised for high-risk breast surgeries and breast aesthetic surgeries.

8. **Enumerate troubleshooting RA strategies**

The mammary gland derives all its nerve supply from the ventral rami of the T2–T6 spinal nerves. Small breast surgeries, such as breast lumpectomy, fibroadenoma excision, or small superficial breast abscess drainage, can be done exclusively under the multilevel paravertebral block.

Surgeries involving dissection or cauterising of anterior chest wall muscles will require blockage of brachial plexus elements. For example, Interpectoral and Pectoserratus blocks can block the lateral and medial pectoral nerve and long thoracic nerve (Fig. 6.2).

Surgeries involving axillary dissection will require an intercostobrachial nerve block. The intercostobrachial nerve (T2) can be blocked using pectoserratus or serratus anterior plane block or targeted TPVB injection at T1 and T2.

Surgeries involving the medial aspect of the breast will require additional blocks like pectointercostal fascial plane block or transverse thoracic muscle plane block for achieving complete surgical anaesthesia.

Surgeries involving dissection near the infra-clavicular area will require either a selective supraclavicular nerve block or a superficial cervical plexus block.

The thoracic paravertebral catheters can be placed at T3 or T4 for postoperative analgesia.

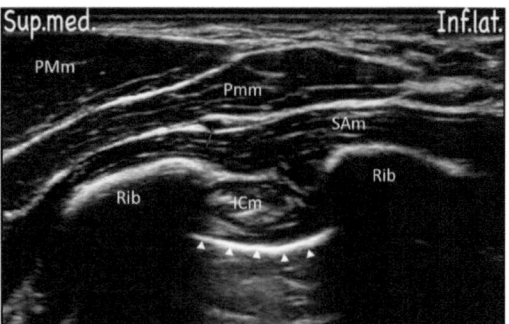

Fig. 6.2 Ultrasound image showing the pectoserratus and interpectoral plane from superior-medial (Sup. med.) to inferior-lateral (Inf. lat.) view, illustrating pectoralis major muscle (PMm), pectoralis minor muscle (Pmm), serratus anterior muscle (SAm), intercostal muscle (ICm), pleura (arrows) and multiple ribs, highlighting the anatomical layers and interfascial planes

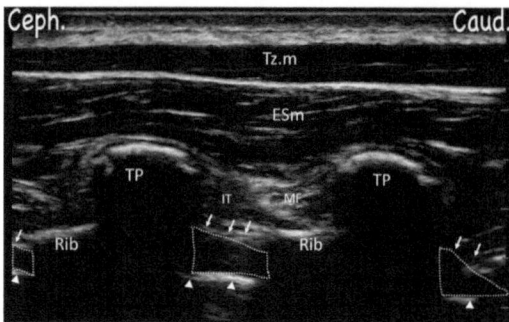

Fig. 6.3 Ultrasound image of the paravertebral sagittal plane from cephalad (Ceph.) to caudal (Caud.) view, showing trapezius muscle (Tz.m), erector spinae muscle (ESm), transverse process (TP), intertransverse ligament (IT), multifidus muscle (MF), ribs, and interfascial space. The white arrows indicate the intertransverse ligament (IT), while the arrowheads mark the interfascial space between the transverse process and ribs

Programmed intermittent boluses and patient-controlled analgesia provide better quality analgesia (more dermatomal coverage) with an LA-sparing effect. 0.1%–0.2% Ropivacaine or 0.125% Levobupivacaine can be used for LA infusion (Figs. 6.3 and 6.4).

Multilevel TPVB with pectoserratus block with or without supraclavicular N block or pecto-intercostal fascial plane block will provide excellent surgical anaesthesia.

0.375% Ropivacaine or 0.3% Levobupivacaine with adrenaline can be used as a stock solution. Usually, 3–5 ml of LA in each TPVB, 10 ml in PECs 1, and 15–20 ml in PECs 2 will provide adequate surgical anaesthesia for most breast cases.

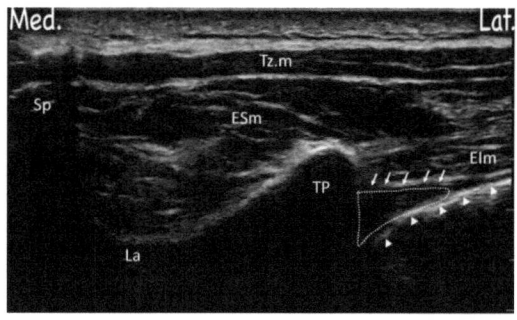

Fig. 6.4 Ultrasound image of the paravertebral transverse plane from medial (Med.) to lateral (Lat.) view, showing spinous process (Sp), trapezius muscle (Tz.m), erector spinae muscle (ESm), transverse process (TP), latissimus dorsi muscle (La), and external intercostal muscle (Elm). The white arrows indicate the intercostal membrane, while the arrowheads mark the interfascial plane between the transverse process and external intercostal muscle

9. **What are the advantages of Thoracic Paravertebral (TPVB) and Thoracic Epidural Analgesia (TEA)?**

These blocks forms the gold standard for surgical anaesthesia and can also be effectively utilised for postoperative analgesia.

TPVB causes sympathetic chain blockade so provides better quality of visceral analgesia as compared to interfacial plane blocks. Sympathetic blockade can also cause some degree of hypotension.

10. **What are the disadvantages of TPVB and thoracic epidural analgesia:**

TPVB and TEA should be avoided in patients with blood clotting disorders due to the risk of hematoma formation in the fixed space of the spinal canal (leading to spinal cord compression).

Thoracic epidural causes more hypotension than TPVB.

TPVB is a level 3 skill set and can cause various complications, including pneumothorax (incidence—0.5%)

Multilevel TPVBs are better than single-level TPVB blocks for surgical anaesthesia (any reference would be good).

TPVB with ultrasound is better than landmark TPVB technique (reference).

11. **What are the advantages/disadvantages of Interfascial Plane Blocks (PECs, SAP, ESPB)?**

Advantages

These superficial blocks can be utilised in patients with minor coagulation issues after the risk and benefit are weighed at the discretion of the concerned anaesthesiologist.

These blocks are easier to perform as compared to TPVB/TEA

Interpectoral and pectoserratus blocks can be performed in hemodynamically labile patients.

Pecs block is considered superior to, or equally efficacious as TPVB for providing postoperative analgesia for radical mastectomy.

ESPB is an effective and safe alternative to TPVB for postoperative analgesia.

Interpectoral and pectoserratus blocks cause paralysis of pectoral muscles. They provide better analgesia than LIA in cases where the pectoral muscles are stretched, such as breast implant surgery.

It is desirable to perform all interfacial plane blocks preoperatively to have a favourable impact on intraoperative hemodynamics and the analgesic requirement. Pectrol blocks are difficult to perform after surgery due to increased air pockets and poor ultrasound visibility.

Disadvantages

These are volume-dependent blocks, and the analgesia efficacy is variable depending on the spread of LA within the interfacial compartment.

The interfascial plane block cannot provide exact and predictable dermatomal coverage like that of TPVB/TEA, so it cannot be utilised solely for surgical anaesthesia.

12. **What is your dosage regimen for Pecto serratus blocks?**

The usual dosage regimen is 0.2%–0.375% Ropivacaine or 0.25%–0.3% Levobupivacaine with or without 4 mg dexamethasone, 20–25 ml (0.3–0.7 ml/kg).

13. **Enumerate the role of blocks in ERAS Pathways**

Site-specific anaesthesia and analgesia.

Loco-regional opioid sparing, motor sparing, and multimodal analgesia are the strategies.

Multimodal Analgesia

Pregabalin 75 mg OD or Gabapentin 200 or 400 mg OD preoperatively.

IV magnesium sulphate 30 mg/kg with or without 10 mg/kg infusion

IV Ketamine 0.2–0.3 mg/kg

IV Paracetamol 20 mg/kg–60 mg/kg in divided doses

IV NSAIDs

LIA (Local Infiltration Analgesia)

Use of regional anaesthesia techniques (vs Morphine IV PCA) for intraoperative pain management may reduce the incidence of chronic pain and cancer recurrence.

Reduction in cancer recurrence needs to be proved with further clinical trials.

Questions

1. ESRA/ASRA anticoagulation guidelines
2. Why is blockade of the lateral or medial pectoral nerves essential and how can they be achieved?
3. Are any adjuvants used in regional anaesthesia that can prolong analgesia?
4. If the patient was on chronic opioids, how would you plan analgesia?
5. What will be your typical LA doses, and how much will you allow the surgeon to give?
6. Tumescent analgesia for breast surgery

Suggested Reading

1. Jacobs A, Lemoine A, Joshi GP, Van de Velde M, Bonnet F. PROSPECT guideline for oncological breast surgery: a systematic review and procedure-specific postoperative pain management recommen-

dations. Anaesthesia. 2020;75:664–73. https://doi.org/10.1111/anae.14964.

2. Khater A, Mazy A, Gad M, Taha Abd Eldayem O, Hegazy M. Tumescent mastectomy: the current indications and operative tips and tricks. Breast Cancer (Dove Med Press). 2017;9:237–43. Published 2017 Mar 30. https://doi.org/10.2147/BCTT.S131398.

3. Kulhari S, Bharti N, Bala I, Arora S, Singh G. Efficacy of pectoral nerve block versus thoracic paravertebral block for postoperative analgesia after radical mastectomy: a randomized controlled trial. Br J Anaesth. 2016;117(3):382–6. https://doi.org/10.1093/bja/aew223.

VATS/Thoracic Surgery

7

Arunangshu Chakraborty and Amit Dixit

Case Scenario

69-year-old female hypertensive patient weighing 35 kgs with a history of 1-month intensive care stay due to pneumonia and complex pleural effusion. Past medical illness includes a history of hypertension and previous COVID-19 infection. During this admission, the patient required non-invasive bilateral positive pressure ventilation (BiPAP) for 2 weeks and was weaned off respiratory support. During her admission, she developed a cardiac arrest, from which she was successfully resuscitated. Her Chest X-ray shows complete right-sided lung collapse with moderate pleural effusion.

2D Echocardiography showed a left ventricular (LV) ejection fraction of 20%, with global left and right ventricular hypokinesia, biatrial dilatation, and grade −1 diastolic dysfunction.

Her present room air Spo2 is 88%, which rises to 94%, with oxygen supplementation via nasal cannula at 2 litres/min.

She is scheduled for a video-assisted thoracoscopic surgery (VATS) pleural biopsy and decortication.

A. Chakraborty (✉)
Sultan Qaboos Comprehensive Cancer Care and Research Centre, Muscat, Oman

A. Dixit
Department of Anaesthesia, Ruby Hall Hospital, Pune, India

1. **What are the key issues (patient-related)?**

Post Cardiac arrest status with poor LV and RV systolic functions

Poor respiratory reserve (room air SPO2–88)

Right lung collapse with complicated pleural effusion on the same side.

Given the patient's poor nutritional status, which is highly likely due to her prolonged bedridden state in the ICU and low body weight of 35 kgs, special considerations need to be made in the surgical and anaesthesia plan to ensure optimal patient outcomes.

2. **What are the surgical factors relevant here?**
   1. Lateral decubitus position
   2. One lung ventilation
   3. Duration of surgery
   4. Number of ports
   5. Dissection around diaphragm
   6. Risk of bleeding
   7. Likelihood of conversion to open thoracotomy

3. **What are the anatomical considerations?**

What is the nerve supply of the chest wall? A comprehensive understanding is crucial for successful surgery.

Dermatomes (Figs. 7.1 and 7.2)

Ventral rami of T1–T7 spinal nerves (anterior and lateral cutaneous branches)

S. Phillips et al. (eds.), *Regional Anaesthesia*, https://doi.org/10.1007/978-3-032-05165-3_7

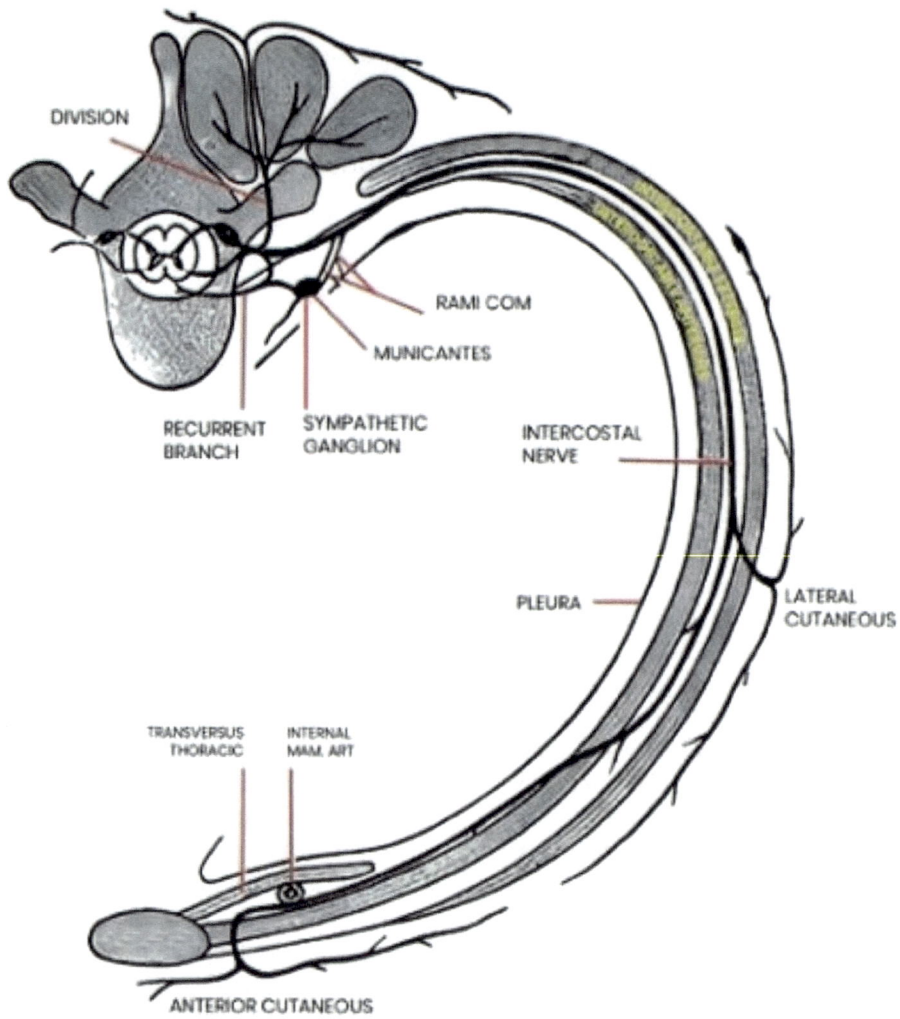

Fig. 7.1 Anatomy of the intercostal nerve and sympathetic chain

Myotomes

Intercostal muscles (Intercostal nerves T1–T7 via anterior and lateral cutaneous branches)

Anterior chest wall muscles

Pectoralis major (C5–T1) and minor (C8–T1) -medial and lateral pectoral nerves

Serratus anterior (C5–C7)—long thoracic nerve.

Posterior chest wall muscles

Trapezius muscle C2–C4 (Spinal Accessory Nerve)

Rhomboid Major C5—(Dorsal Scapular Nerve)

Infraspinatus muscle C5–C6 (Suprascapular Nerve)

Latissimus Dorsi C6–C8 (Thoracodorsal Nerve)

The diaphragm is supplied by the phrenic nerve (C3–C5).

Osteotome: Ribs—intercostal nerves via its sensory and motor branches.

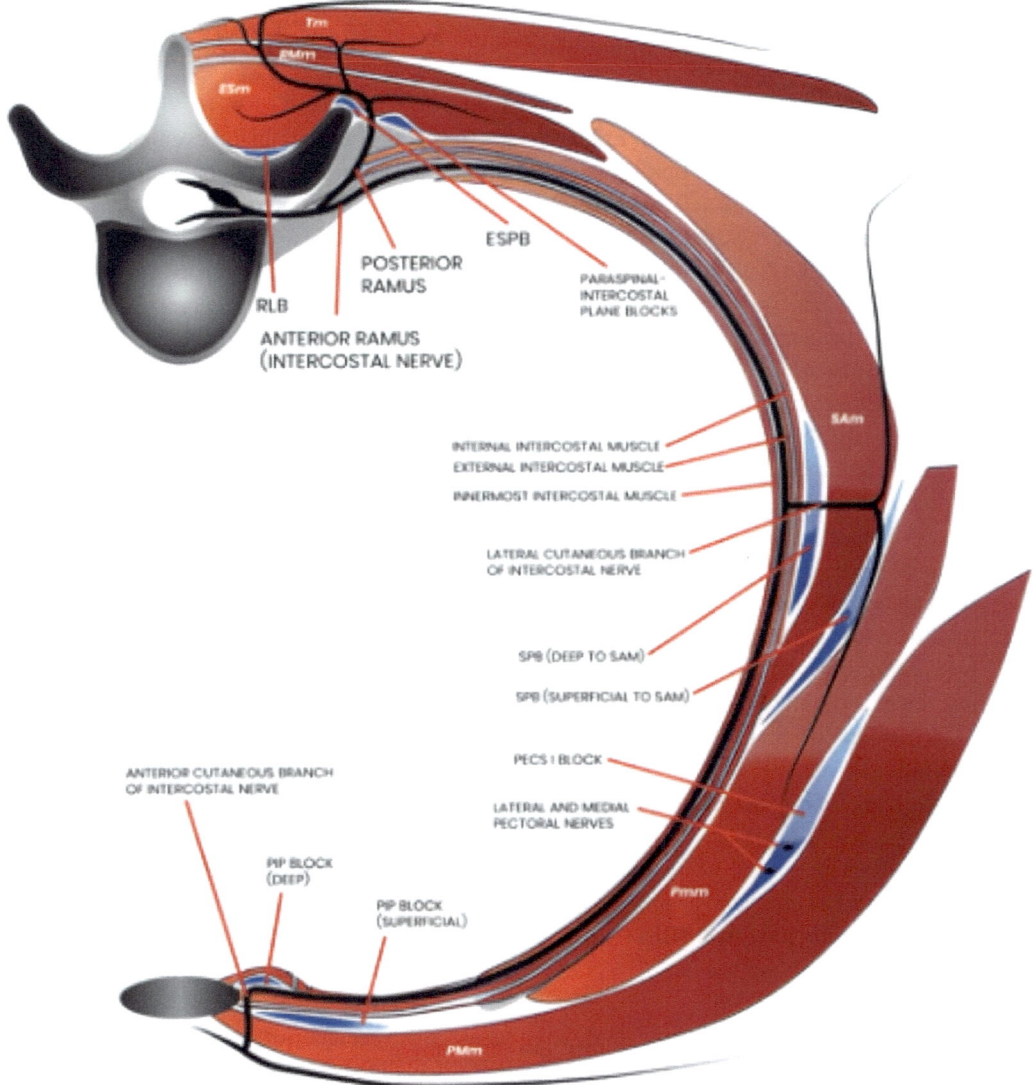

Fig. 7.2 Intercostal nerve in the intercostal space

Visceral component

The intercostal nerves (T1–T11), phrenic nerve (C3–5), and vagus supply the somatic pleura.

Visceral pleura is pain insensitive.

Lungs, heart and aorta, tracheobronchial tree, and mediastinum have rich sympathetic (via thoracic sympathetic chain) and parasympathetic (vagus) innervations.

4. **What would be your anesthesia options**?
   1. General anesthesia for surgery along with regional anaesthesia (single shot block) or a catheter technique for postoperative analgesia
   2. Awake VATS under regional anaesthesia with or without titrated sedation
5. **What will be your analgesia strategy**?

Postoperative analgesia for VATS can be achieved using a variety of options, namely.

Central neuraxial blocks

1. Thoracic epidural analgesia (intermittent boluses or infusion) or Lumbar Epidural with boluses of hydrophilic opioids
2. Single level TPVB at T4 or T5 (surgically congruous)
3. Multilevel TPVB T2, T4, T6 or T3, T5 and T7
4. Intrathecal (segmental spinal using isobaric ropivacaine or isobaric levobupivacaine with or without lipophilic opioids)

As Per prospect guidelines, the thoracic paravertebral block is preferred to the thoracic epidural block given decreased complications in VATS and open thoracotomy surgeries.

Non-neuraxial blocks

1. Intra pleural blocks
2. Erector spinae plane block
3. Newer thoracic wall blocks like retrolaminar block, rhomboid intercostal block, MTP (midpoint transverse process to pleura)
4. Serratus anterior plane block (superficial or deep)
5. A multilevel intercostal nerve block with or without liposomal bupivacaine
6. Local infiltration analgesia (LIA) with or without liposomal bupivacaine

Systemic techniques

1. Intravenous lidocaine infusion (1.5–2.0 mg/kg bolus followed by 1.5 mg/kg/h)

Multimodal analgesia: NSAIDS, Paracetamol, LIA, Opioid PCA (covered below), low-dose ketamine.

6. **What will be your key considerations when regional anaesthesia is chosen as a sole technique for surgical anaesthesia (Awake VATS)**

Awake VATS has the following advantages as compared to GA

• Ventilator-induced lung injury, trauma to the trachea, intubation trauma, bronchial cuff damage and impaction are more familiar with GA
• One lung ventilation predisposes to cardiac arrhythmia, transient hypoxemias, and

cognitive impairment, which can be safely avoided in awake VATS.

Challenges in Awake VATS

1. Cough
2. Sudden diagrammatic excursion
3. Patient movement, cooperation

Regional Anaesthesia Strategy for Awake VATS

1. Patient factors- cooperation, reassurance
2. Adequate time to prepare for blocks and testing, meticulous surgery, team to be aware of awake patient, calculated local anaesthetic dosages for supplementation
3. Plan for failure and rescue plan B techniques.

7. **Troubleshooting RA strategies**

Role of local infiltration anaesthesia (LIA) by surgeon

1. Surgical ports are inserted through muscles supplied by nerves from brachial plexuses (not covered by TPVB or TEA), making the local site skin infiltration (preprocedure) mandatory.
2. The phrenic nerve supplies the diaphragm; isolated phrenic nerve block is rarely practised. Diaphragmatic instillation of local anaesthetic is usually sufficient.
3. Isolated vagal nerve block is a theoretical option but logically improbable.
4. Selective suprascapular nerve block for shoulder pain is rarely required for VATS.
5. Selective suprascapular nerve block (via either an anterior or posterior approach) is usually recommended in long-duration open thoracotomies.

Plan B is conversion to general anaesthesia, and the anaesthesia team should be ready for any such change in the anaesthesia plan.

8. **What are the advantages and disadvantages of Thoracic Paravertebral (TPVB) and Thoracic Spinal & Epidural Analgesia (TEA)?**

1. TPVB and TEA can provide surgical anaesthesia
2. All these blocks can cause hemodynamic changes (hypotension), which are detrimental to patients with low cardiac output. Spinal>Epidural>TPVB

3. TPVB and TEA should be avoided in patients with blood clotting disorders due to the risk of hematoma formation in the fixed space of the spinal canal (leading to spinal cord compression).

4. Segmental epidural assessment for high thoracic epidural is as follows:

ESSAM (Epidural Scoring Scale for Arm Movements)

Four grades (0–3) based on number of absent movements

1. Handgrip (C8-T1)
2. Wrist flexion (C7-C8)
3. Elbow flexion (C5-C6)

5. Thoracic segmental spinal anaesthesia is usually half of the dose used for lumbar spinal anaesthesia. Isobaric 1% chloroprocaine 2.5–3.5 ml with 10 mcg of dexemetomidine provides excellent surgical anaesthesia for 40–60 min. Isobaric ropivacaine 0.5%–0.75% 1.5–2 ml or isobaric levobupivacaine 0.5% 1.5–2 ml with or without adjuvants like fentanyl or alpha two agonists can provide adequate segmental anaesthesia.

9. **What would be a typical dose regime for TPVB or TEA?**

Intraoperative/Surgical anaesthesia

TPVB: 0.375%–0.75% Ropivacaine or 0.25%–0.5% Levobupivacaine with adrenaline can be used as a stock solution. Usually, 3–5 ml of local anaesthetic in each TPVB level

If a single level is chosen, 10–15mls via single shot or a catheter covers 3–5 segments.

Postoperative analgesia regimes

Continuous infusion

Epidural: 0.1%–0.2% Ropivacaine or 0.1% Bupivacaine with 2mcg/ml fentanyl, usual range 5–10 mls/h

TPVB: 0.1%–0.2% Ropivacaine or 0.1%–0.125% Bupivacaine LA infusions without opioids at 5–10 mls/h

PCEA (patient-controlled epidural analgesia) & PIB (programmed intermittent bolus) with no background infusion. It provides better dermatomal coverage, less motor blockade, and LA sparing.

10. **What are the advantages and disadvantages of interfacial plane blocks (IFPB)?**

Advantages

1. IFPB are easier to learn and perform, are effective, carry lesser complication rates and can be performed with less stringent relative contraindications
   - ESPB and serratus anterior plane blocks are superficial and can be utilized in patients with minor coagulation issues. They have a lower risk of causing pneumothorax and can be performed by less skilled personnel.

2. IFPB causes less hemodynamic disturbances and motor blockade can be a part of early ambulation and enhanced recovery protocols

Disadvantages

1. Multilevel blocks or combination blocks may be needed
   - Some interfascial plane blocks, like the serratus anterior plane block, will not cover the visceral component of pain relief and only cover the lateral divisions of the intercostal nerves
   - ESPB is better than serratus anterior plane block as it covers the visceral component of pain relief via its indirect paravertebral action as the involvement of the sympathetic chain in the TPVB provides better quality of analgesia than serratus anterior plane block

2. Higher failure rates
3. Long-term data is needed.

11. **What would be the typical dosages for IFPB?**

Interfascial Plane block:

0.2%–0.375% Ropivacaine or 0.25%–0.3% Levobupivacaine with or without 4 mg dexamethasone, 20–25ml (0.3–0.7ml/kg) is the usual dosage regimen for most of the IFPB

12. **Why would this patient need LA dosage adjustments?**

With this clinical scenario, the RA societies highlight the importance of dose adjustment in cardiac disease, renal disease, frailty, and reduced muscle mass.

In this particular scenario with cardiac—post CPCR status and low cardiac output state. Body weight-based LA dose for an interfascial plane block is fraught with dangers of LAST.

13. **Intercostal blocks: Describe the anatomy of the intercostal nerves.**

Spinal nerves from T2 to T12 supply the thorax and abdomen.

T1 predominantly contributes to the brachial plexuses. T2 and T3 join to form the intercostobrachial nerve, which supplies skin in the upper arm and axilla. T12 is the subcostal nerve and does not run along the rib cage.

Each nerve root divides into dorsal and ventral rami. Dorsal rami supplies the skin and muscles in the paravertebral area.

At the midaxillary line, the intercostal nerve gives rise to the lateral intercostal nerve.

Each intercostal nerve terminates as the anterior intercostal nerve near the midline of the chest and abdomen, supplying skin and muscles in the parasternal and rectus abdominis area. Each ventral rami continue as intercostal nerve. It passes through the subcostal groove of the rib.

14. **What are the approaches to performing an intercostal nerve block?**

    Medial approach: This is usually 4–5 cm lateral from the spinous process. The intercostal nerve is deep to internal and external intercostal muscles just above the pleura and endothoracic fascia.

    Lateral approach: This point is lateral to the costal angle. The intercostal nerve is in the subcostal groove between the innermost and internal intercostal muscles.

    The lateral approach is desirable as there is less chance of pneumothorax.

    The intercostal nerve is accompanied by intercostal vessels so ultrasound can reduce vascular puncture.

What would be the LA dosage for an intercostal block?

Local anaesthetic: 3–5 ml of 0.25%–0.5% of levobupivacaine with or without adrenaline.

Or 0.2%–0.5% ropivacaine with or without adrenaline. Analgesia duration is 6–12 h.

Liposomal bupivacaine can be utilised for a prolonged duration of analgesia.

15. **What are the disadvantages of the intercostal block?**
    1. Multiple-level injections needed
    2. The risk of pneumothorax is compounded due to the need for multiple injections
    3. Rapid plasma concentrations due to vascularity (Higher risk of local anaesthetic systemic toxicity)
    4. It may not provide visceral analgesia
    5. Shorter duration of analgesia
    6. Cannot place catheters to extend the analgesic duration

16. **Discuss ERAS Pathways and Multimodal Analgesia relevant to this patient**

Strategy: Site-specific anaesthesia and analgesia

Pre-emptive loco-regional opioid sparing, motor sparing multimodal analgesia.

Multimodal strategy
1. Gabapentinoid
2. Alpha 2 agonist -Dexemetomidine
3. Dexamethasone
4. NSAIDS and COX2 inhibitors.
5. Paracetamol
6. Ketamine
7. Magnesium
8. Opioids: IV PCA
9. LIA (Local infiltration anaesthesia) -wound infiltration
10. Intravenous lidocaine
11. TENS

IV Opioid PCA is beneficial if no regional technique is utilised or in the case of a backup for accidental catheter dislodgments (for epidurals or TPVB catheters) in case of open thoracotomies. The use of regional anaesthesia techniques along with multimodal analgesia prevents the development of chronic pain and thereby decreases the incidence of post-thoracotomy chronic pain syndrome.

17. **What are the PROSPECT recommendations for VATS (2021)?**

The PROSPECT guidelines for VATS recommend-[1]

1. Systemic analgesia should include paracetamol and non-steroidal anti-inflammatory drugs or cyclo-oxygenase-2-specific inhibitors administered pre-operatively or intra-operatively and continued postoperatively.
2. Intraoperative administration of intravenous dexmedetomidine is recommended when basic analgesics cannot be given.
3. Regional analgesic techniques such as paravertebral block and erector spinae plane block are recommended. Serratus anterior plane block can be used as a second choice.
4. Opioids should be used as rescue analgesics postoperatively.
5. Thoracic epidural analgesia is not recommended for postoperative analgesia as per PROSPECT guidelines.

18. **What are techniques not recommended by PROSPECT for pain management in patients undergoing VATS?**

Some commonly used techniques are not recommended by PROSPECT due to inconsistent evidence, a lack of procedure-specific evidence, or better, less invasive techniques available.

These include gabapentinoids, corticosteroids, magnesium sulfate, intravenous lignocaine, transcutaneous electric nerve stimulation, wound infiltration, intrapleural analgesia and thoracic epidural.

19. **What are the recommendations for analgesia for thoracotomy?**

The preferred technique for analgesia in thoracotomy is continuous infusion of LA with/without opioids through thoracic epidural or TPVB in addition to NSAID/COX-2 (or paracetamol if these are contraindicated). If these blocks are contraindicated, then a combination of pharmacological drugs like NSAID/COX-2 (or paracetamol if these are contraindicated) in combination with opioids may be used. For post-thoracotomy shoulder pain, a suprascapular nerve block can be used, and topical LA can be used for the removal of chest drains.

Questions

1. Prevention of LAST in intercostal blocks
2. Prevention and management of pneumothorax in TPVB
3. Complications of TPVB block
4. Complications of thoracic spinal and epidural
5. What is your opinion about the use of cervical epidural for surgical anaesthesia?
6. What is your opinion about unilateral spinal for thoracic surgery?
7. What Role does a combination of isobaric and heavy bupivacaine for thoracic spinal anaesthesia?
8. Complications of thoracic epidural placement and prevention.
9. Epidural infection—how will you detect it? Most common organism? Prevention and management?
10. Is thoracic spinal safe? What is the difference in the dural sac (cross-sectional) arrangement at the lumbar and thoracic levels?
11. Prevention of PDPH after thoracic spinal?
12. What are the curves in the vertebral column, and what is their significance?
13. How will you identify that your thoracic or TPVB is congruous?
14. What are the different ways to confirm thoracic spinal interspace level with and without ultrasound?
15. Incidence, prevention and management of post-thoracotomy chronic pain syndrome?

Suggested Reading

1. Feray S, Lubach J, Joshi GP, Bonnet F, Van de Velde M, PROSPECT Working Group *of the European Society of Regional Anaesthesia and Pain Therapy. PROSPECT guidelines for video-assisted thoracoscopic surgery: a systematic review and procedure-specific postoperative pain management recommendations. Anaesthesia. 2022;77(3):311–25. https://doi.org/10.1111/anae.15609. Epub 2021 Nov 5. PMID: 34739134.

Cardiac Surgery: Open Heart Surgery Through Median Sternotomy

8

Arunangshu Chakraborty and Archana Areti

Case Scenario

A 25-year-old female patient with rheumatic heart disease, complaints of progressive breathlessness for the last 2 years and has a diagnosis of mitral stenosis. She takes Metoprolol 25 mg twice daily and Furosemide 40 mg once daily.

The patient weighs 57 kg, and her blood tests were within normal limits. A 2D ECHO revealed the mitral valve area to be 1.8 cm^2, a left ventricular ejection fraction of 67%, pulmonary artery pressure of 50 mmHg, mild mitral regurgitation in sinus rhythm and no regional wall motion abnormality.

She is scheduled to undergo mitral valve replacement via median sternotomy.

1. **What are the key considerations here?**
   1. Patient-related-
      - Fixed cardiac output state
      - Poor cardiopulmonary reserve
      - Pulmonary artery hypertension
   2. Anaesthetic considerations: (as for any cardiac surgery)
2. **What factors should be considered when performing regional anaesthesia for cardiac surgery?**

A. Chakraborty
Sultan Qaboos Comprehensive Cancer Care and Research Centre, Muscat, Oman

A. Areti (✉)
KMCH Institute of Health Sciences and Research, Coimbatore, Tamil Nadu, India

- Systemic anticoagulation (complicates the performance of central neuraxial techniques due to the high risk of hematoma)
- Hemodynamic disturbances- patients may be on vasopressors (central neuraxial techniques may complicate by causing hypotension)
- Organ dysfunction is predominantly renal, so dosage adjustments to LA may be needed.

3. **Describe the somatic and visceral nerve supply for open cardiac surgery.**

Dermatome
- For the surgical incision—Bilateral Ventral Rami of the T2—T6 Intercostal nerves (anterior cutaneous branches)
- For post-surgical drains
  – Mediastinal (Midline)—Bilateral ventral rami of T6—T8 Intercostal nerves (anterior cutaneous branches)
  – Intercostal (Lateral)—Ventral Rami of the T5—T6 Intercostal nerve on the side of the drain (anterior and lateral cutaneous nerve)

Myotome
- Pectoralis Major Muscle from both sides—Lateral and Medial Pectoral Nerves (Branches of the brachial plexus.
- Second to sixth Intercostal muscles from both sides—corresponding ventral rami of the

intercostal nerve (Anterior and lateral cutaneous branches of the intercostal nerve)

- Transversus thoracis muscle on either side of the sternum—supplied by the ventral rami off the T2—T6 intercostal nerve (anterior cutaneous branch)
- Diaphragm—Phrenic Nerve (C3–5)

Osteotome

- Sternum supplied by the ventral rami off the T2—T6 intercostal nerve (anterior cutaneous branch) from both sides.
- 2nd to 7th ribs—corresponding ventral rami of the intercostal nerve (Anterior and lateral cutaneous branches of the intercostal nerve)

Visceral component

- The T1–T11 Intercostal Nerves, phrenic nerve (C3–5) and vagus nerve are supplied to the somatic pleura.
- Visceral pleura is pain insensitive.
- The heart, pericardium, pleura, lungs, and mediastinum have a sympathetic supply via the thoracic sympathetic chain and a parasympathetic supply via the vagus nerve.

4. **What would be your anesthesia option?**

General Anaesthesia with controlled endotracheal mechanical ventilation and regional block, either a single shot or continuous catheter technique for postoperative analgesia.

5. **What are the regional analgesia options?**

Regional strategies used for postoperative analgesia following a median sternotomy include either central neuraxial or peripheral regional chest wall blocks.

Central Neuraxial Blocks (CNB)

1. Thoracic Epidural—as intermittent boluses
2. Thoracic Paravertebral—single shot or catheter technique performed bilaterally at the T4–T5 level.
3. Intrathecal Morphine

Peripheral Regional Blocks for Median Sternotomy

Either single shot or continuous catheter techniques

1. T2–T6 Intercostal nerve blocks any approach (see intercostal block chapter)
2. Superficial parasternal intercostal plane block (previously Pecto-intercostal plane block)
3. Deep parasternal intercostal plane block (previously Transversus Thoracis Muscle Plane Block)
4. Interpectoral plane block (previously PECS I) and Pectoserratus plane block (previously PECs II Block)
5. Serratus anterior plane blocks (superficial and deep)
6. Erector Spinae Block at the level of the T5

6. **What are the advantages and disadvantages of central neuraxial blocks?**

Advantages

- The thoracic epidural and paravertebral blocks can also provide surgical anaesthesia.
- The sympathetic blockade conferred by these blocks can cause vasodilation of the coronary vessels, thereby enhancing blood supply to the myocardium.
- Intrathecal morphine can provide postoperative analgesia for up to 24 h with a single dosage.
- Provide better analgesia, especially at the drain sites—medial or lateral.

Disadvantages

- CNB's can produce hypotension, which may be undesirable, especially in fixed or low cardiac output states.
- Due to anticoagulation during surgery, there is a potential risk for hematoma formation in the spin,e causing spinal cord compression.
- Intrathecal morphine can cause nausea, vomiting, pruritus, respiratory depression and prolonged sedation.

- It can be technically challenging to perform.
- The paravertebral technique requires bilateral performance and placement of catheters.
- Increased local anaesthetic absorption following thoracic paravertebral injections, increasing the risk for local anaesthetic systemic toxicity.
- There is a risk of causing a pleural puncture during paravertebral performance, leading to pneumothorax.

7. **How would you perform central neuraxial blocks?**

CNB's must be performed preoperatively and timed at least 1 h before administering heparin for anticoagulation. A meticulous technique must be followed, and the best possible attempt must be made to avoid multiple needle passes. In case of a bloody tap or vascular puncture, the procedure must be abandoned and the surgery postponed for at least 24 h. Due to these constraints & with enhanced recovery after surgery (ERAS) protocols, CNB's are a less preferred modality of postoperative analgesia.

8. **How would you administer intrathecal morphine?**

Following a strict aseptic technique, a 27G Whitacre needle should be used to perform a lumbar puncture at the L2–3 space. Whitacre needle is preferred as it may be less traumatising than the Quincke tip needle, which is a cutting type. After achieving free-flowing and clear CSF, 10 to 20 mcg/Kg of morphine (drawn and diluted with normal saline to a total volume of 2 ml), must be injected at a rate of 0.2 ml/s.

9. **What post-operative regimens can be used for analgesia via the CNB's?**

Epidurals or Paravertebral catheters may be activated at least 1 h before heparin administration. Still, no further dosing will be done until anticoagulation has been reversed and the patient is hemodynamically stable following surgery.

Postoperatively Intermittent bolus or continuous infusions may be used, with 0.1%–0.2%

of Ropivacaine or 0.125% Levobupivacaine, which are more cardiac stable local anaesthetics.

- **Thoracic epidural**—intermittent boluses—5 ml 6th—8th hourly or infusion rate of 3–5 ml/h, and watch for hypotension stop immediately if there is a significant drop in BP.
- **Paravertebral Catheter**—Intermittent bolus with 15 ml 0.2% Ropivacaine given in 5 ml increments, bilaterally for 15 min, to avoid significant BP drop in case of epidural spread of local anaesthetic.

10. **What are the advantages and disadvantages of Peripheral Regional Blocks for cardiac surgery?**

Advantages

- Easier to learn and perform when compared to CNB's
- There is no risk of spinal hematoma in the background of anticoagulation.
- These blocks have lower incidences of complications.
- These blocks cause fewer hemodynamic disturbances (No sympathetic block) and less motor blockade.
- There is less likelihood of pneumothorax or vascular punctures with the fascial plane blocks, except for the intercostal nerve block and deep parasternal intercostal plane block.

Disadvantages

- Need to perform bilaterally
- Larger volumes of local anaesthetic are required, creating a risk of local anaesthetic toxicity.
- Do not provide surgical anaesthesia—less potent blockade
- Do not provide analgesia for the visceral component
- They provide inadequate coverage to the drain sites.
- High failure rates
- More long-term studies are required to investigate the efficacy.

Various peripheral blocks are described in Table 8.1 (Figs. 8.1, 8.2, and 8.3)

11. **What are the problems associated with traditional opioid analgesia in cardiac surgery?**

Intravenous or oral opioids were the cornerstone of pain management in cardiac surgery. Side effects of opioids include nausea, vomiting, constipation, ileus, urinary retention, constipation, pruritus, sedation, delirium and respiratory depression. They can also prolong recovery, increase costs and delay discharge.

Opioids can also cause vasodilatation, decreased blood pressure and heart rate, which may complicate recovery following cardiac surgery.

Perioperative opioids can also lead to both central and peripheral neuronal hyperexcitability that may amplify and prolong pain, leading to chronic pain and the requirement of even more opioids to manage pain. This can contribute significantly to long-term opioid use.

Table 8.1 Comparison of the peripheral blocks

Regional block	Plane of injection	Nerves blocked	Advantages	Side effects
Erector spinae block	Para spinal region ventral to the erector spinae muscles	Dorsal rami and occasionally the ventral rami of the spinal nerves T2—T9	Efficacy like epidural and paravertebral analgesia without major complications; Analgesia includes the upper sternal area: Continuous block through catheter possible.	Mechanism not fully understood. Requires lateral position to perform; Occasional pneumothorax
Serratus anterior plane block	Between serratus anterior and latissimus dorsi, with intercostal muscles	Lateral cutaneous branches of the intercostal nerves (T3-T9), long thoracic nerve and thoracodorsal nerve	Vascular injury & rare. More efficacious for external area	Can cause winged scapula; Needs supplementation, Continuous block through the catheter It is not possible.
(PECs 1) Pectoserratus(PECs II) block	PECS-I- between pectoralis major and minor muscles. PECS-2-between pectoralis minor and serratus anterior muscles	Fourth, fifth, and sixth intercostal nerves	Simple to perform: More reliable chest wall analgesia; Pose a minimal risk of injuries to Pleura and blood vessels:	Injury to thoracodorsal artery Local anaesthesia absorption and toxicity Infra clavicular areas spread
Superficial parasternal Intercostal plane block	Between the pectoralis major and external intercostal muscles at the lateral border of the sternum	Anterior cutaneous branches at their origin from intercostal nerves	Opioid sparing for sternotomy; More efficacious than other anterior chest wall blocks: Catheter option to prolong block.	Local anaesthesia toxicity is possible. Multiple injections required
Deep parasternal Intercostal plane block	Between internal intercostal and transversus thoracis muscles	Anterior intercostal nerves	Efficacious for unilateral rib fractures and CRT device implantation.	Internal mammary artery injury can occur
Intercostal nerve block	Subcostal groove at the angle of the ribs	Individual intercostal nerve	Useful for chest drain placement and minimally invasive surgeries	Caution due to pneumothorax and local anaesthetic toxicity

12. **What is the fast-track/ enhanced recovery approach for cardiac surgery?**

The fast-track approach involves an opioid-sparing, multimodal analgesic strategy to facilitate early extubation, prophylactic medications for gastrointestinal complications, accelerated rehabilitation, early discharge, and nonopioid pain management.

Current multimodal pain management builds on the "Fast Track" concept. By using multiple agents and techniques that each target a different pain pathway, modern multimodal cardiac surgical protocols hope to create a synergy to improve pain control and decrease opioid dependence using multiple agents and techniques that target a different pain pathway.

13. **What are the options for multimodal analgesia for ERAS in cardiac surgery?**

Enhanced Recovery After Surgery (ERAS) is a multimodal, transdisciplinary care that promotes the recovery of patients undergoing surgery throughout their perioperative journey. These programs aim to reduce complications and promote an earlier return to regular activity.

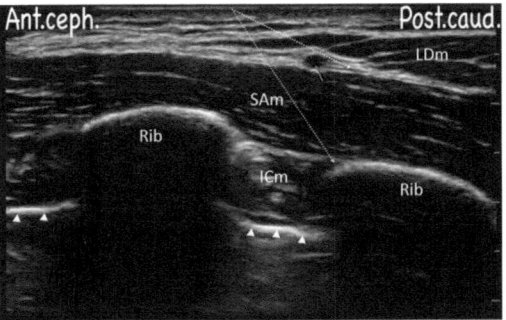

Fig. 8.1 Ultrasound image of the serratus plane block from anterocephalad (Ant. ceph.) to posterocaudal (Post. caud.) view, showing serratus anterior muscle (SAm), latissimus dorsi muscle (LDm), intercostal muscle (ICm), and ribs. White arrow heads are the pleural, red arrow is the thoracodorsal nerve, white arrow the superficial serratus plane and the yellow arrow needle path to the deep serratus plane

Multimodal options

- Regional motor sparing techniques (preemptive performance is preferred but may not always be possible with the chest wall blocks due to interference with the surgical field).
- Acetaminophen 1gm every 8 h
- Tramadol 50 mg every 8 h
- Pregabalin 300 mg given 1–2 h before surgery and 150 mg twice a day continued postoperatively or Gabapentin 1200 mg PO once 21 h before incision and postop—300 mg PO TID

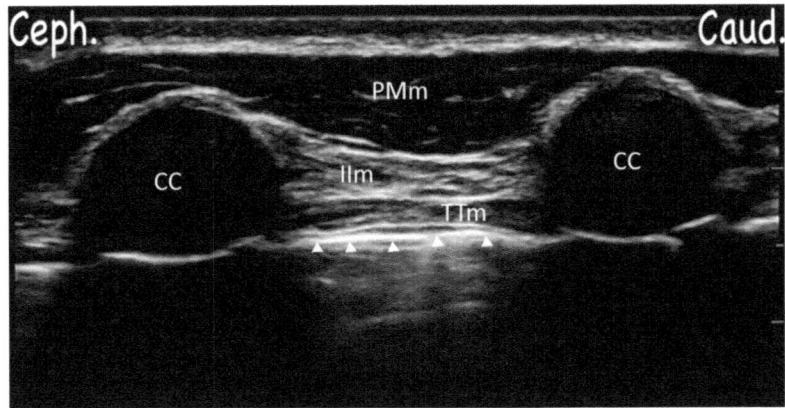

Fig. 8.2 Ultrasound image of the parasternal intercostal plane in a superficial view from cephalad (Ceph.) to caudal (Caud.) orientation, showing pectoralis major muscle (PMm), internal intercostal muscle (IIm), transversus thoracis muscle (TTm), and costal cartilage (CC). The white arrowheads indicate the interfascial plane between the internal intercostal and transversus thoracis muscles

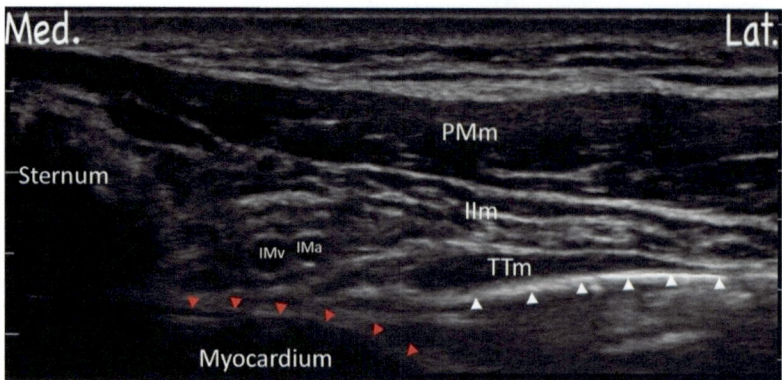

Fig. 8.3 Ultrasound image of the deep parasternal intercostal plane from medial (Med.) to lateral (Lat.) view, showing pectoralis major muscle (PMm), internal intercostal muscle (IIm), transversus thoracis muscle (TTm), sternum, internal mammary vein (IMv), internal mammary artery (IMa), and myocardium. The red arrowheads indicate the myocardium layer

- Dexmedetomidine 0.5–1 mcg/kg over 10 min (loading dose after cardiopulmonary bypass), Followed by 0.4–1.5 mcg/kg/h infusion through extubation
- Ketamine infusion
- Lidocaine
- Magnesium
- Ketorolac/NSAID—reduced or limited dosing due to decreased renal function or coagulation interaction risk.

Recommendations
- Regional anaesthesia can provide intense analgesia and plays an essential role in the management of patients with cardiovascular disease undergoing surgery as part of the multimodal regimen.
- The proposed method should consider surgical issues and the combination of the problems in the individual patient.
- Caution is required in these patients, as a sudden or excessive reduction in peripheral vascular resistance, particularly with central neuraxial block, may precipitate a drop in myocardial perfusion and/or a drop in preload and cardiac output with severe consequences.
- The decision to utilise regional anaesthesia should be cautiously undertaken with appropriate monitoring.
- Attention should be paid to anticoagulation, weighing the potential risks vs benefits.

Preoperatively—Thoracic epidural, paravertebral or intrathecal morphine, pregabalin, gabapentin

Intraoperative—Only intravenous medications ketamine, dexmedetomidine, and magnesium no activation or top-ups during surgery due to anticoagulation for cardiopulmonary bypass and surgery.

Postoperatively—Chest wall blocks, IV acetaminophen, Gabapentin or pregabalin, dexmedetomidine.

Top-up may be initiated at least 6 h after anticoagulation has been reversed, provided the coagulation parameters are within acceptable range.

Questions

1. What risk benefits would you discuss with the patients regarding regional techniques for cardiac surgery?
2. Will the preoperative blocks be performed after or before the placement of invasive lines? What precautions need to be taken?
3. Will the regional block be performed before or after general anaesthesia or surgery? What are the challenges for both?
4. Which blocks can be performed before surgery, and which ones can be performed after?
5. What would be the timing of the removal of catheters and what advice following the removal of catheters?
6. If the thoracic epidural is effective only on one side, how will you manage it?
7. If the thoracic epidural has given a motor block in the legs and the patient couldn't be mobilised, what would you do?
8. The patient has a thoracic epidural in situ on day 3 postoperatively and develops a sudden onset of new back pain and dense motor block in the legs; how would you manage?
9. How would you troubleshoot if your primary regional analgesia strategy fails?
10. How do we prevent, identify and manage LAST?
11. What are the complications of each regional technique?
12. How do we identify the level for performing the chest wall blocks with landmarks and ultrasound?
13. How can the regional technique's pain and success in post-op cardiac patients be assessed?
14. What are the incidence and factors contributing to chronic pain following cardiac surgery?
15. How can chronic pain be prevented following cardiac surgery?

Suggested Reading

1. Jiang T, Ting A, Leclerc M, Calkins K, Huang J. Regional anesthesia in cardiac surgery: a review of the literature. Cureus. 2021;13(10):e18808. https://doi.org/10.7759/cureus.18808.
2. Enhanced recovery for cardiac surgery, Noss C, Prusinkiewicz C, Nelson G, Patel PA, Augoustides JG, Gregory AJ. Enhanced recovery for cardiac surgery. J Cardiothorac Vasc Anesth. 2018;32:2760–70.
3. El Shora HA, El Beleehy AA, Abdelwahab AA, Ali GA, Omran TE, Hassan EA, Arafat AA. Bilateral paravertebral block versus thoracic epidural analgesia for pain control post-cardiac surgery: a randomized controlled trial. Thorac Cardiovasc Surg. 2020;68:410–6.

Fractured Ribs

9

Arunangshu Chakraborty and Amit Dixit

Case Scenario

A 70-year-old male chronic smoker fell from a bike. Head injury and abdominal injuries have been ruled out. He complains of pain in deep breathing. Chest X-ray reveals fractured ribs 5 and 7 on the anterolateral right side of the chest. The fifth rib is broken in two places on the right side.

1. **What are the key issues (patient-related)?**
   (a) Anterolateral rib fractures of the fifth and seventh rib.
   (b) Geriatric and smoker
   (c) Associated brain and spinal cord injury to be ruled out.
   (d) Is the patient on any blood thinner for any reason?
   (e) Associated pneumothorax or haemothorax
   (f) Flail chest or lung contusion assessment
   (g) Pain assessment and documentation: Static and dynamic
2. **What surgical factors are relevant here?**

Surgical fixation is usually required in case of severe thoracic injury, flail chest, complex pain management, un-intubated patient with deterio-

A. Chakraborty (✉)
Sultan Qaboos Comprehensive Cancer Care and Research Centre, Muscat, Oman

A. Dixit
Department of Anaesthesia, Ruby Hall Hospital, Pune, India

rating pulmonary functions and inability to wean from the ventilator.

When left untreated for pain, these patients subsequently develop atelectasis due to poor respiratory effort and retained secretions. Respiratory complications, including pneumonia, are the most common cause of mortality (31%).

Adequate and timely pain relief can save the lives of patients with fractured ribs.

3. **What anatomical considerations are relevant to managing rib fractures?**

There are 12 pairs of ribs. Ribs 1 to 7 are attached anteriorly to the sternum. Ribs 8 to 10 are not directly attached to the sternum, so they are called false ribs. Ribs 11th and 12th are not attached anteriorly, so-called floating ribs. A groove on the inferior aspect of each rib accommodates the neurovascular bundle, namely the intercostal nerve, vein and artery.

Rib fractures of the first three are rare as they are protected by scapula. Rib fractures of the 11th and 12th rib are also rare as they are floating and flexible.

Surgery of rib fracture in the posterior aspect requires dissection of the back muscle for rib localisation and is more painful.

Dermatomes: Ventral and dorsal rami of T1 to T12 spinal nerves.

Myotomes: Anterior and posterior chest wall muscles.

Osteotomes: T1 to T12 intercostal nerves via its sensory and muscular branches.

4. What would be your analgesia strategy?

Central neuraxial
1. Thoracic epidural (whenever fracture is bilateral)
2. Thoracic Paravertebral (single or multi-level with or without catheter)

Non-neuraxial block strategy
1. Posterior or posterolateral rib fractures: Erector spinae plane block (ESPB), retrolaminar, rhomboid intercostal block, midpoint of the transverse process to pleura (MTP) block
2. Lateral or anterolateral rib fractures: Serratus anterior plane block (superficial or deep)
3. Anterior or parasternal rib fractures: Petco intercostal interfascial plane block or transversus thoracis plane block (TTP)
4. Intercostal nerve block—multilevel with or without liposomal bupivacaine.

Multimodal analgesia strategy
Intravenous opioids (PCA)
Ketamine: 0.2–0.3 mg/kg followed by 0.15–0.2 mg/kg/hr
Lidocaine: 1.5 mg/kg/hr. followed by – 1.5 mg/kg/hr
Magnesium: 30 mg/kg bolus followed by 10 mg/kg/hr
Gabapentinoids: T. Pregabalin 75 mg or T. Gabapentin 200–400 mg
Dexmedetomidine: 1 mcg/kg bolus over 10 min followed by 0.2–0.7 mcg/kg/hr
NSAIDS and COX 2 inhibitors
Paracetamol
LIA with or without liposomal bupivacaine

5. What are the advantages and disadvantages of Thoracic Paravertebral (TPVB) and Thoracic Epidural Analgesia (TEA)?
    1. TEA and TPVB provide excellent quality analgesia covering both somatic and visceral components of pain.
    2. They should be avoided in patients with-

    (a) associated head injury or raised intracranial pressure (ICP)
    (b) patients on blood thinners or anticoagulants

6. What are the advantages and disadvantages of interfacial plane blocks

Interfascial plane blocks like ESPB and Serratus, anterior plane blocks, are superficial blocks and can be administered in patients with head injury or mild to moderate coagulopathy.

Ultrasound utilisation has reduced LAST incidence due to decreased incidence of inadvertent vascular punctures.

7. Describe the pain pathways for rib fractures.

Intercostal nerve: The dorsal ramus supplies the skin and muscles in the paraspinal area. In contrast, the ventral ramus gives lateral branches in the midaxillary line and an anterior branch near the sternum. Based on this, the following are a few recommendations:

    (a) For all bilateral fractures, epidural is a preferred choice.
    (b) Posterior or posterolateral rib fractures are commonly treated with TPVB or ESPB block.
    (c) The superficial and deep serratus anterior plane block best manages lateral and anterolateral rib fractures.
    (d) Parasternal rib fractures can be treated with pecto intercostal interfascial nerve block and transversus thoracis plane (TTP) block.
    (e) Intercostal nerve block is indicated in anterolateral and lateral rib fractures.

8. Enumerate the ERAS Pathways and Multimodal Analgesia

Analgesia strategy can be divided depending on the severity of pain, which can be mild, moderate, or severe.
Mild pain: Multimodal analgesics (NSAIDS, PCM, Gabapentin).

Moderate pain: Multimodal analgesia including opioid single shot (morphine) or opioid PCA.

Severe pain: Multimodal analgesia including i.v. opioids with continuous regional blocks such as SAP, ESPB, TPVB, and TEA.

Inability to treat pain, especially in geriatric patients with pre-existing respiratory morbidities and with a history of use of anticoagulants or blood thinners, have a higher chance of mortality. Inadequate pain relief often leads to the retention of secretions, thereby causing atelectasis and pneumonia. Pneumonia is the most common cause of mortality in fracture rib patients, as mentioned earlier.

Adequate analgesia helps in chest physiotherapy and deep breathing exercises, enhancing recovery, early mobilisation, early enteral feeding, and faster hospital discharge.

Early involvement of the acute pain management team and aggressive pain management can change outcomes positively in this group of patients.

STUMBL chest scoring system is a good predictor of morbidity and mortality. **STUMBL chest scoring system:** (Score 1–10 mild, 10–30 moderate, and > 30 severe).

+1 for every 10 years over 10 years.

+2 per 5% reduction in oxygen saturation while breathing room air.

+3 for every fracture (2 fractures on one rib = 6).

+4 anticoagulant or antiplatelets.

+5 chronic lung disease.

Thoracic epidurals used to be the Gold standard. With the advent of ultrasound-guided regional anaesthesia techniques, serratus anterior plane block, ESPB, and TPVB have emerged as equally potent but safer alternatives.

Questions

1. Which block will you choose for placing an intercostal drain (ICD)?
2. Pain management strategy for ICD?
3. How will you assess block action for ESPB and SAP blocks?
4. Which blocks can cause pneumothorax?
5. Prevention and management of pneumothorax
6. ASRA guidelines for patients on clopidogrel or dabigatran?
7. Prevention and management of LAST?
8. Morphine PCA and its role in fracture ribs?

Suggested Reading

1. May L, et al. rib fracture management. BJA Educ. 2016;16(1):26–31.
2. Thiruvenkatarajan V, et al. Regional Analgesia for rib fracture. Curr Opin Anesthesiol. 2018;31:601–7.
3. Adhikary SD, et al. The effects of erector spinae plane block on respiratory and analgesic outcomes in multiple rib fractures: a retrospective cohort study. Anaesthesia. 2019 May;74(5):585–93.
4. Camacho F c d O, et al. Continuous serratus anterior plane block provides analgesia in multiple rib fractures; a case report. Rev. Bras Anestesiol. 2019;69(1):87–90.
5. Williams A, et al. Anaesthetic and surgical management of rib fracture. BJA Edu. 2020;20(10):332–40.

Matthew Sinnott

Case Scenario

A 35-year primigravida underwent emergency caesarean section. Her vitals are stable. What would be your plan for analgesia in this patient?

1. Significance of postoperative analgesia following Caesarean section:

Caesarean delivery is associated with moderate to severe postoperative pain. Increased postoperative pain is associated with a slower return to mobility, increased venous thromboembolism (VTE) risk, and prolonged hospital length of stay. It impacts maternal-neonatal bonding, may delay the establishment of breastfeeding, and has even been implicated in post-natal depression risk. Greater postoperative pain also increases the risk of chronic post-surgical pain and long-term opioid use.

2. Enumerate the strategies to minimise postoperative pain following Caesarean delivery

Multi-modal analgesic regimens are recommended. Central neuraxial block is the gold standard both for anaesthesia and to optimise post operative analgesia. Combinations of further agents allow for optimising the analgesic benefit

while minimising drug side effects. Surgical techniques, such as the incision site and the use of abdominal binders, are also important.

3. Commonly used neuraxial opioids and doses

Opioids can be administered intrathecally or epidurally, depending on the anaesthetic technique for Caesarean delivery. Diamorphine is usually used in isolation, whereas the slower-onset of morphine is offset by combination with the more lipid-soluble fentanyl.

Diamorphine is usually administered at a dose of 300 mcg intrathecally or 2–3 mg epidurally. Morphine is given at a dose of 50–150 mcg intrathecally and 1–3 mg epidurally, while fentanyl is 15 mcg intrathecally and 50–100 mcg epidurally. The doses used are a balance between optimising analgesic benefits whilst minimising side effects such as pruritis, nausea, and delayed respiratory depression [1].

4. What is the mechanism of morphine-induced delayed respiratory depression?

Morphine is the least soluble agent and has the least affinity for non-receptor sites as such it remains in the CSF for the most significant duration of the commonly used agents. The Society of Obstetric Anesthesia and Perinatology recommends 2 hourly respiratory rate monitoring and sedation for 12 h following standard doses of

M. Sinnott (✉)
Anaesthetic Department, Ashford and St Peter's Hospitals NHS Foundation Trust, Chertsey, Surrey, UK
e-mail: matthewsinnott@doctors.org.uk

neuraxial morphine. If higher doses are used, or the patient has additional risk factors, for example, cardiorespiratory disease, obstructive sleep apnoea, or general anaesthesia or additional IV opioids are used, respiration and sedation should be monitored every hour for 12 h, and 2 hourly for a further 12–24 h. Additional monitoring of capnography and pulse oximetry should also be considered.

5. What are the regional anaesthesia options are available for patients who undergo caesarean section

The most commonly performed regional techniques are the transversus abdominis plane (TAP) and quadratus lumborum (QL) blocks. (Figs. 10.1, 10.2, and 10.3) Both have been shown to provide similar analgesic benefits in the absence of long-acting neuraxial opioids, although the benefit is not seen when neuraxial opioids are used. This suggests they are best employed when central neuraxial block has not been possible, for example, if clinical urgency mandates a GA or there are contraindications to CNB. Alternatively, they may be used as a rescue technique for severe breakthrough pain postoperatively. Several factors influence the choice of block in addition to proceduralist experience. (Table 10.1) Since these blocks are often performed in an emergent GA when full informed consent is not possible, they

should be performed only if felt to be in the patient's best interests, with a complete discussion and explanation as soon as possible.

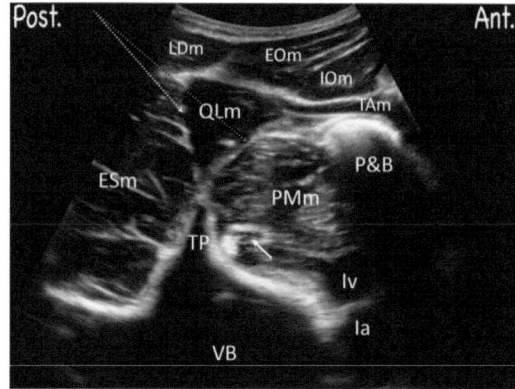

Fig. 10.2 Ultrasound image showing the anatomy for an anterior quadratus lumborum (QL) block from posterior (Post.) to anterior (Ant.) view, including latissimus dorsi muscle (LDm), external oblique muscle (EOm), internal oblique muscle (IOm), transversus abdominis muscle (TAm), quadratus lumborum muscle (QLm), erector spinae muscle (ESm), psoas major muscle (PMm), transverse process (TP), vertebral body (VB), peritoneum and bowel (P&B), iliac vessels (Iv), and iliac artery (Ia). The red dotted line indicates the needle path and end point for an anterior QL block (between QLm and PMm) and the white dotted line for the posterior QL block (between QLm and ESm). The white arrow in the body of the PMm points to the lumbar plexus

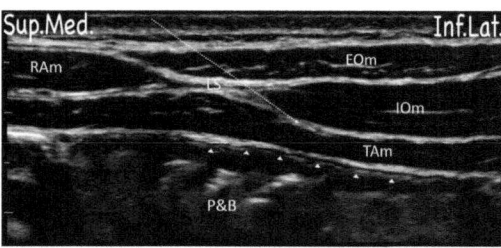

Fig. 10.1 Ultrasound image showing the anatomy for a transverse abdominis plane (TAP) block from superior-medial (Sup. Med.) to inferior-lateral (Inf. Lat.) view, including rectus abdominis muscle (RAm), external oblique muscle (EOm), internal oblique muscle (IOm), transversus abdominis muscle (TAm), and peritoneum and bowel (P&B). The white arrow heads represent the peritoneum. Dotted arrow is the needle trajectory

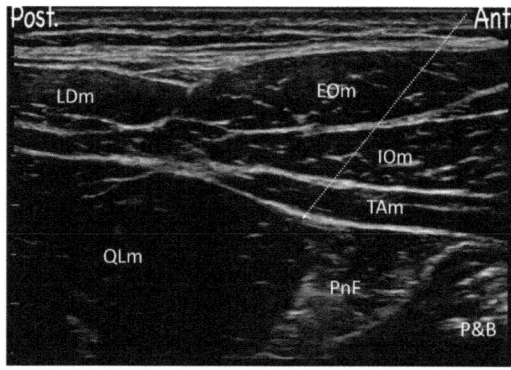

Fig. 10.3 Ultrasound image showing the anatomy for a lateral quadratus lumborum (QL) block from posterior (Post.) to anterior (Ant.) view, including latissimus dorsi muscle (LDm), external oblique muscle (EOm), internal oblique muscle (IOm), transversus abdominis muscle (TAm), quadratus lumborum muscle (QLm), perinephric fat (PnF), and peritoneum and bowel (P&B). The dotted white line indicates the needle path

Table 10.1 Key features of TAP and QL blocks for Caesarean delivery

TAP blocks	QL blocks
Most used and studied	The patient usually
Easy to perform in the supine position	needs to be rolled into a lateral
Surgical insertion under direct vision is faster than the US-guided technique and has the equivalent analgesic benefit	position The optimal approach (lateral, anterior, posterior) is not yet known
Concerns over LAST due to high LA volumes	Can cause leg weakness if LA spreads to the lumbar plexus Area of much on-going research

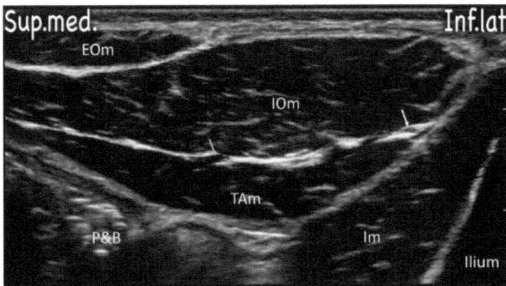

Fig. 10.4 Ultrasound image showing the anatomy for the ilioinguinal nerve block from superior-medial (Sup. med.) to inferior-lateral (Inf. lat.) view, illustrating external oblique muscle (EOm), internal oblique muscle (IOm), transversus abdominis muscle (TAm), iliacus muscle (Im), peritoneum and bowel (P&B), and ilium. The white arrow marks the ilioinguinal nerve, while the yellow arrow indicates the neurovascular bundle

Other regional techniques studied for Caesarean delivery include ilioinguinal and ilio-hypogastric nerve blocks, erector spinae plane blocks, surgical wound infiltration and catheter insertion. (Fig. 10.4) All appear to confer benefit over placebo. However, evidence supporting their use is more limited. Many questions remain as to their role in a multimodal analgesic regimen, the benefits conferred in the presence of neuraxial opioids, and the superiority of one technique over another.

6. **What are the factors which must be considered when prescribing a postoperative analgesic regimen:**

The principle of multimodal analgesia is key, as it optimises the benefits of different agents while minimising side effects. Paracetamol and non-steroidal anti-inflammatory (NSAID) agents are synergistic, and scheduled use should be routine unless contra-indicated. Oral morphine should be used for breakthrough pain only, typically at a dose of 10–20 mg 2 to 4-hourly. Laxatives, antiemetics, and antipruritic drugs should be available if required. Codeine is not recommended in breast-feeding patients due to concerns about the variability in metabolism rates and unpredictable plasma concentrations, which may pose a danger to the neonate. Dihydrocodeine is a commonly used alternative for patients with, or at risk of, increased postoperative pain, provided the neonate is appropriately monitored [1].

7. **What are the PROSPECT pain management recommendations for elective Caesarean section?**

These are as follows:

- Implementation of strategies to minimise opioid consumption after elective caesarean section
- Intrathecal morphine 50–100 mcg or diamorphine 300 mcg, or in the presence of an epidural catheter, epidural morphine 2–3 mg or diamorphine 2–3 mg
- Paracetamol and non-steroidal anti-inflammatory post-delivery and regularly post-operatively
- Single IV dexamethasone dose post-delivery
- Consideration of single injection of LA infiltration, continuous wound LA infusion +/− fascial plane blocks if intrathecal morphine is not used

- Surgical technique to include Joel-Cohen incision (straight incision rather than Pfannenstiel), non-closure of peritoneum and abdominal binders
- Consider TENS as an analgesic adjunct

Questions

Q.1: *What is the innervation of the abdominal wall in relevance to regional anesthesia following caesarean section?*

Q.2: *What strategies exist to minimise postoperative pain following Caesarean delivery?*

Q.3: *Describe commonly used neuraxial opioids and doses.*

Q.4: *Why does morphine pose the greatest risk of delayed respiratory depression? How should this be monitored?*

Q. 5 *What regional anaesthesia options are available for postoperative analgesia for patients who undergo caesarean section?*

Q.7: *What is the role of ilioinguinal/iliohypogastric nerve blocks for analgesia following caesarean section?*

Q.6: *What are the PROSPECT pain management recommendations for elective CD?*

Suggested Reading

1. Neall G, Bampoe S, Sultan P. Analgesia for Caesarean section. BJA Educ. 2022;22(5):197–203.
2. Roofthooft E, Joshi GP, Van de Velde M, and on behalf of the PROSPECT Working Group of the European Society of Regional Anaesthesia and Pain Therapy and supported by the Obstetric Anaesthetists' Association. PROSPECT guideline for elective caesarean section: updated systematic review and procedure-specific postoperative pain management recommendations. Anaesthesia. 2021;76:665–80.
3. Bauchat JR, Weiniger CF, Sultan P, Habib AS, Ando K, Kowalczyk JJ, Kato R, George RB, Palmer CM, Carvalho B. Society for obstetric anaesthesia and perinatology consensus statement: monitoring recommendation for prevention and detection of respiratory depression associated with administration of neuraxial morphine for caesarean delivery analgesia. Anesth Analg. 2019;129(2):458–74.
4. El-Boghdadly K, Desai N, Halpern S, Blake L, Odor PM, Bampoe S, Carvalho B, Sultan P. Quadratus lumborum block vs transversus abdominis plane block for caesarean delivery: a systematic review and network meta-analysis. Anaesthesia. 2021;76:393–403.
5. Sultan P, Sultan E, Carvalho B. Regional anaesthesia for labour, operative vaginal delivery and caesarean delivery: a narrative review. Anaesthesia. 2021;76(Suppl. 1):136–47.
6. Singh NP, Monks D, Makkar JK, Palanisamy A, Sultan P, Singh PM. Efficacy of regional blocks or local anaesthetic infiltration for analgesia after caesarean delivery: a network meta-analysis of randomised controlled trials. Anaesthesia. 2022;77:463–74.

Analgesia for Upper Abdominal Surgery with Midline Incision

11

Arunangshu Chakraborty and Srimanta Halder

Case scenario

A 68-year-old female diagnosed with cancer of the stomach is posted for emergency gastrectomy for upper gastrointestinal bleeding. Medical history reveals ischemic heart disease. She is on Tab Aspirin 75 mg and Atorvastatin 10 mg. Preoperative investigation reports are unremarkable except for Hb-7.8 g/dl (normal range 12–15) and sinus tachycardia with a rate of 105 bpm; 2d echo showed an ejection fraction of 64% with no significant abnormalities. On examination, her BP was 96/50 mm Hg without any vasopressor support.

1. What are the anatomical considerations for nerve blocks of the abdominal wall?

The lateral part of the abdominal wall is made up of three muscles with their fascial sheath: the external oblique, internal oblique, and transversus abdominis muscles, along with paired rectus abdominis muscles on either side of the midline separated by the linea alba. (Fig. 11.1).

The anterior abdominal wall runs superiorly from the sternum's costal margin and xiphoid process to the inguinal ligament and pelvic bone inferiorly and the mid-axillary line laterally.

The anterior rami of the lower six thoracic nerves (T7 to T12) and the first lumbar nerve (L1) supplying the skin, muscles, and parietal peritoneum run in the plane between the internal oblique and transversus abdominis muscle. The thoracic nerves T7 to T11 enter and travel along this neurovascular plane at the costal margins, piercing the posterior wall of the rectus sheath as anterior cutaneous branches that supply the overlying skin. T7 to T9 nerves emerge to supply the skin above the umbilicus. T11, the cutaneous branch of the subcostal T12, the iliohypogastric nerve, and the ilioinguinal nerve supply the skin inferior to the umbilicus, whereas T12, the iliohypogastric nerve, and the ilioinguinal nerve supply the skin superior to the umbilicus.

2. What are the key considerations in this patient?

(a) Emergency laparotomy is associated with a 30-day mortality approaching 15%, increasing to 25% in those aged >80 years.

(b) Rapid sequence induction of anaesthesia, minimises the risks of pulmonary aspiration.

(c) Haemodynamic stability throughout the perioperative period

(d) Goal-directed fluid management

(e) Protective lung ventilation strategies

(f) Adequate postoperative analgesia: Poorly managed pain after laparotomy may lead to an increased risk of postoperative pul-

A. Chakraborty (✉)
Sultan Qaboos Comprehensive Cancer Care and Research Centre, Muscat, Oman

S. Halder
Tata Medical Center, Kolkata, India

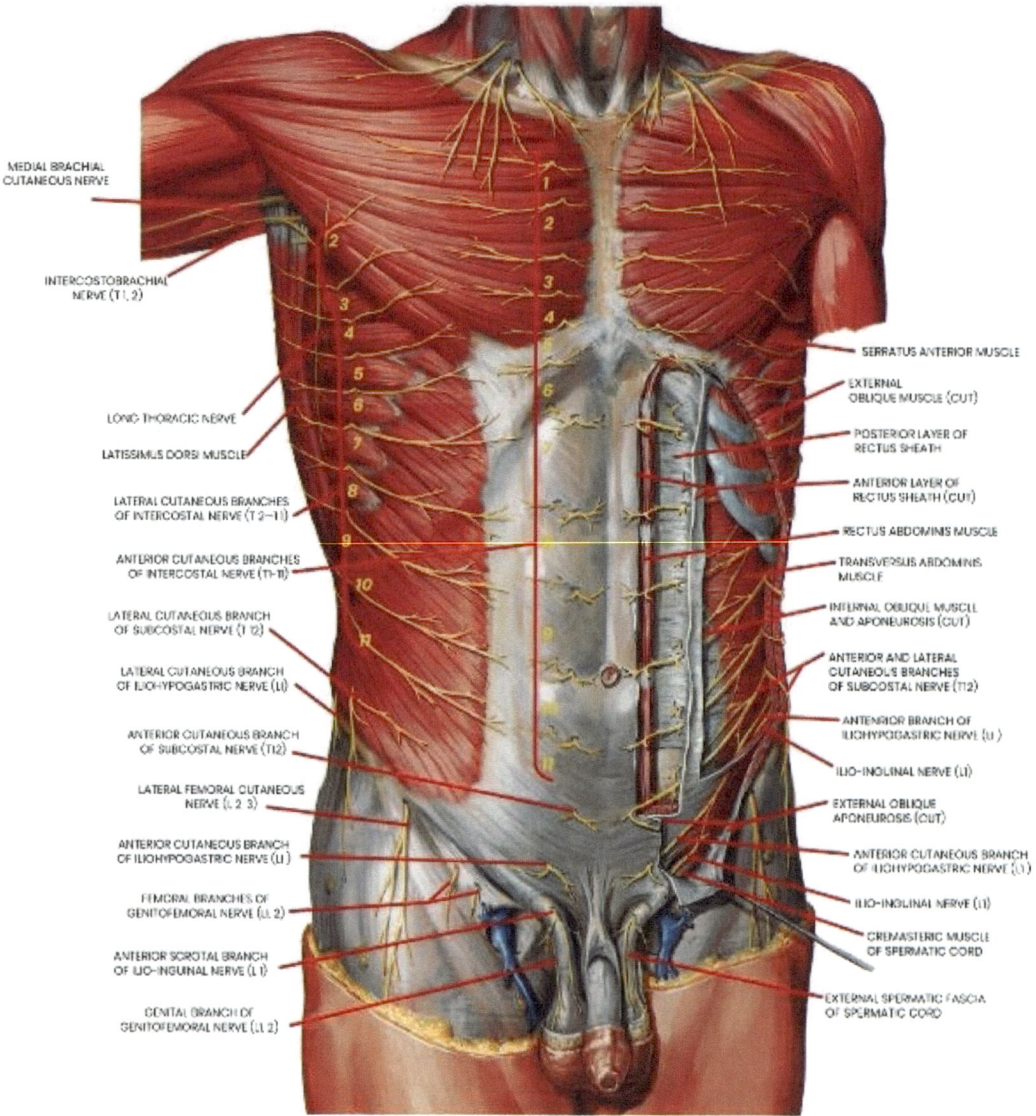

Fig. 11.1 Muscles of the abdominal wall and Cutaneous innervation of the anterolateral abdominal wall

monary complications such as pneumonia and atelectasis, cardiac complications such as myocardial ischaemia, thrombo-embolic events, and a greater stress response.

(g) Postoperative intensive care considerations.

3. **What are the options for intraoperative and postoperative analgesia**

Multimodal opioid-sparing analgesia is recommended for this patient. The options are:

- COX-2-selective inhibitors (only for patients who do not receive epidural analgesia or with the cessation of epidural analgesia)
- Conventional NSAIDs (only for patients who do not receive epidural analgesia or with cessation of epidural analgesia).
- IV lidocaine (when epidural is not feasible or contra-indicated).
- Opioids as a rescue if non-opioid analgesia is insufficient or contra-indicated (Caution with opioids and renal function and in the elderly).

- Paracetamol for moderate- or low-intensity pain.
- Other adjuncts- Alpha-2 agonists (Clonidine, Dexmedetomidine)
- Thoracic epidural analgesia at a level appropriate to the site of incision with patient-controlled epidural analgesia
- Other adjuncts- Alpha-2 agonists (Clonidine, Dexmedetomidine)
- Continuous wound infiltration catheter with local anaesthetics by the surgical team at the end of surgery.
- Bilateral paravertebral block
- Fascial Plane Blocks (FPB) at the end of surgery- B/L Tap block, B/L Rectus sheath block, B/L Quadratus Lumborum block
- IV patient controlled analgesia.

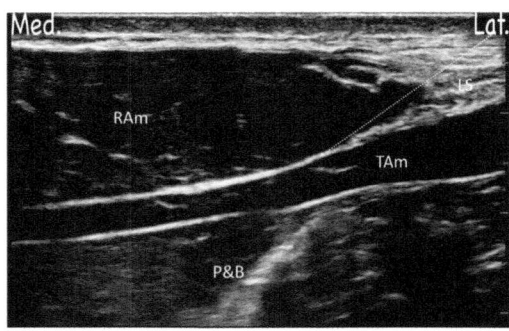

Fig. 11.2 Ultrasound image showing the anatomy for an upper subcostal TAP (Transversus Abdominis Plane) block from medial (Med.) to lateral (Lat.) view, including rectus abdominis muscle (RAm), transversus abdominis muscle (TAm), and peritoneum and bowel (P&B). The dotted white line (LS) indicates the needle path for the TAP block targeting the interfascial plane between the rectus abdominis and transversus abdominis muscles

4. **Describe different approaches to perform transversus abdominis plane blocks.**

The transversus abdominis plane is the fascial plane superficial to the transversus abdominis muscle. In this plane, the intercostal, subcostal, and L1 segmental nerves communicate to form the upper and lower TAP plexuses, which innervate the anterolateral abdominal wall, including the parietal peritoneum. TAP blocks provide somatic abdominal wall analgesia, including the parietal peritoneum. For midline surgeries, the block has to be repeated on both sides.

There are four described approaches to TAP block (Figs. 11.2, 11.3, and 11.4)

1. Posterior TAP: Injection in the lumbar triangle of Petit. Here, the linear transducer is placed in the axial plane in the midaxillary line and moved posteriorly to the posterior limit of the TAP between the internal oblique and fascia transversalis.
2. Lateral TAP: LA is injected in the neurovascular plane between the IOM and TAM, and the ultrasound transducer (UST) is placed transversely in the anterior axillary line between the subcostal margin and the iliac crest.
3. Anterior TAP: The ultrasound transducer is held transversely in the midclavicular line and

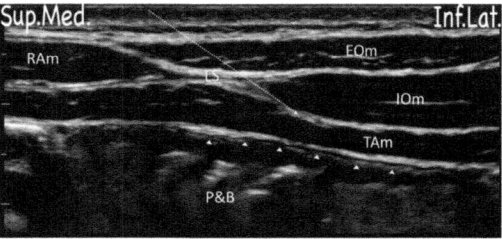

Fig. 11.3 Ultrasound image showing the anatomy for a lower subcostal TAP (Transversus Abdominis Plane) block from superior-medial (Sup. Med.) to inferior-lateral (Inf. Lat.) view, including rectus abdominis muscle (RAm), external oblique muscle (EOm), internal oblique muscle (IOm), transversus abdominis muscle (TAm), and peritoneum and bowel (P&B). Dotted white line is the needle trajectory and infiltration site. Arrow heads are the peritoneum

scanned laterally until the three abdominal muscles are seen. The needle is inserted from medial to lateral, and the drug is deposited in the TAP plane.
4. Oblique subcostal TAP: A linear transducer is placed alongside the lower margin of the rib cage. Local anaesthetic is injected in the fascial plane between the posterior rectus sheath and the anterior margin of the transversus

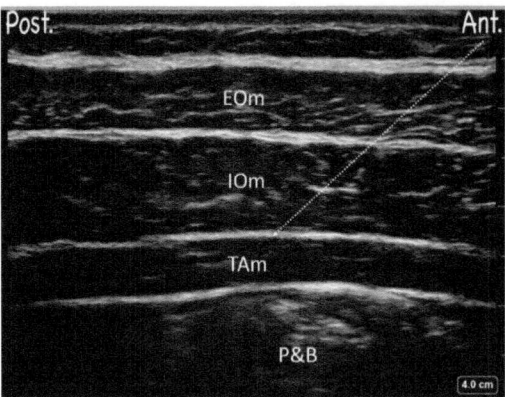

Fig. 11.4 Ultrasound image showing the anatomy for a midaxillary TAP (Transversus Abdominis Plane) block from posterior (Post.) to anterior (Ant.) view, including external oblique muscle (EOm), internal oblique muscle (IOm), transversus abdominis muscle (TAm), and peritoneum and bowel (P&B). The dotted white line indicates the needle path for the TAP block, targeting the interfascial plane between the internal oblique muscle and transversus abdominis muscle

abdominis muscle. Oblique subcostal TAP (OSTAP) is called the 'upper TAP' block.

The term 'Dual TAP' means the administration of TAP block in both 'lower', i.e. lateral approach and 'upper' area. Bilateral administration of dual TAP block (BDTAP) is required to provide complete analgesia to the anterior abdominal wall. This method is also known as the 'four quadrant' TAP block.

5. **Enumerate the indications and possible complications associated with TAP block**

   Unilateral TAP block: For one-sided procedures, such as appendectomy, cholecystectomy, nephrectomy, and renal transplant.

   Bilateral TAP blocks: Midline abdominal surgeries involving the T6 to L1 distribution, surgeries with transverse abdominal incisions, and laparoscopic surgeries.

   An 'upper' TAP block is more effective in upper abdominal surgeries, while pain relief for sub umbilical surgeries is well addressed by a 'lower' TAP block. Four quadrant TAP block has been used for postoperative analgesia in laparotomies using a larger incision.

   A combination of Rectus sheath block and Subcostal TAP block or B/L subcostal TAP blocks can be used for upper abdominal surgeries

with inverted "L-shaped" incisions, like Whipple's procedure.

Complications associated with TAP block are rare, but some reported complications are:

1. Bowel perforation
2. Hematoma
3. visceral trauma, including liver trauma due to needle injury
4. Intraperitoneal injection of local anaesthetic
5. Retroperitoneal hematoma due to vascular injury
6. Transient femoral nerve blockage (LA injected during TAP block may trail on the fascia illiaca below the inguinal ligament, producing an inadvertent blockage of the femoral nerve)
7. Local infection
8. Intravascular injection (In TAP block, LA is injected within an interfacial plane that is well vascularized, the reason why the operator should perform careful aspiration before injecting an LA to avoid an accidental vascular puncture and intravascular injection)
9. Local Anaesthetic systemic toxicity

6. **Describe Rectus sheath block (RSB)**

The rectus sheath is formed from the aponeuroses of the fascial sheaths of EOM, IOM and TAM to form the lateral border of the RAM, termed the linea semilunaris. At the medial border of the RAM, the anterior and posterior portions of the rectus sheath come together, forming the midline linea alba. The anterior rectus sheath extends along the entire vertical length of the RAM, but the posterior rectus sheath extends only along the upper two-thirds of the RAM.

The ventral rami of the T7-L1 thoracolumbar nerves supply the sensorimotor innervation of the anterior abdominal wall. The thoracolumbar nerves course along the anterolateral wall within the transversus abdominis plane (TAP) and continue anteromedial within the TAP, eventually encroaching upon the lateral aspect of the rectus sheath. The nerves then enter the lateral aspect of RAM and form a nerve plexus that runs craniocaudal within the RAM in close relation to the lateral branch of the deep epigastric artery.

Notably, the branches of the thoracolumbar nerves do not cross the midline.

In this case, B/L RSBs with a continuous catheter technique can be given in the immediate postoperative setting as part of a multimodal analgesic approach, along with paracetamol and IV-PCA.

Ultrasound Technique In a supine position, a high-frequency linear array US transducer is positioned transversely over the rectus abdominis muscle (RAM). The layers of the anterior abdominal wall, from superficial to deep, are identified.

Subcutaneous tissue → anterior rectus sheath → RAM (relatively hypoechoic about the rectus sheath) → posterior rectus sheath → deep superior (above the umbilicus) and inferior (below the umbilicus) epigastric arteries (Colour Doppler to confirm) → transversalis fascia → peritoneal cavity (identified by the presence of peristaltic movements of the bowel loops).

A 22G Tuohy needle is inserted into the plane between RAM and the posterior rectus sheath (PRS), and 10–15 mL of LA is injected. A catheter may be placed for a continuous block. The catheter is advanced 5–6 cm into space. The bilateral catheter is required for midline surgery. The mechanism of action of RSB is a "compartment block", as the terminal thoracolumbar nerves are too small to be visualised as discrete structures.

For B/L TAP blocks or RSBs, 15–20 ml ropivacaine 0.2% with 1:400,000 epinephrine or bupivacaine 0.25% with 1:400,000 epinephrine per side will be preferred. Epinephrine decreases the local anaesthetic peak plasma concentration (Cmax), as the spread of local anaesthetic will encompass a relatively large surface area for vascular absorption into the systemic circulation. Based on initial pharmacokinetic studies, the peak plasma concentration (Tmax) is approximately 45 min.

For a continuous catheter technique, a continuous infusion of 2–3 ml/h. along with intermittent bolus injection of 10–20 ml ropivacaine 0.25% per side every 6–10 h is recommended to maintain postoperative analgesia.

7. **Enumerate the concerns related to central neuraxial analgesia in this patient**

Though thoracic epidural analgesia can provide superior analgesia for upper abdominal surgeries, it includes hazardous concerns in emergency laparotomies, including hypotension caused by vasodilatation in a patient with sepsis or hypovolaemia and the presence of contraindicating factors such as coagulopathy or systemic sepsis that increase the risks of epidural haematoma or abscess formation.

Blocking visceral pain conduction with a TAP or rectus sheath block is impossible. Epidural and paravertebral blocks are proven to provide visceral analgesia. Quadratus Lumborum block offers high dermatomal coverage (up to T7), blocks subcostal (T12) and iliohypogastric (L1) nerves, and provides visceral analgesia due to thoracic paravertebral spread with the anterior approach.

So, we should consider giving other modes of opioid-sparing analgesia for visceral coverage along side TAP block or Rectus sheath block.

Transient femoral nerve palsy has been noticed in some patients and is attributed to the spread of local anaesthetic on the fascia iliaca below the inguinal ligament, which inadvertently blocks the femoral nerve.

Suggested Reading

1. Hammi C, Ahn K. Transversus Abdominis Plane Block. [Updated 2021 Oct 9]. In: StatPearls [Internet]. Treasure Island: StatPearls Publishing; 2022. Available from: https://www.ncbi.nlm.nih.gov/books/NBK547730/.
2. Saunders DI, Murray D, Peden CJ. Variations in mortality after emergency laparotomy: the first report of the UK Emergency Laparotomy Network. Br J Anaesth. 2012;109:368–75.
3. Ilyas C, et al. Management of the patient presenting for emergency laparotomy. BJA Educ. 2019;19(4):113–8.
4. Carney J, Finnerty O, Rauf J, Bergin D, Laffey JG, Mc Donnell JG. Studies on the spread of LA solution in TAM plane blocks. Anaesthesia. 2011;66:1023–30.
5. Abdallah FW, Chan VW, Brull R. TAM plane block: the effects of surgery, dosing, technique, and timing on analgesic outcomes. A systematic review. Reg Anesth Pain Med. 2012;37:193–209.

6. Abdallah FW, Laffey JG, Halpern SH, Brull R. Duration of analgesic effectiveness after the posterior and lateral TAM plane block techniques for transverse lower abdominal incisions: a meta-analysis. Br J Anaesth. 2013;111:721–35.

7. Hebbard PD, Barrington MJ, Vasey C. Ultrasound-guided continuous oblique subcostal TAM plane blockade: description of anatomy and clinical technique. Reg Anesth Pain Med. 2010;35:436–41.

8. Niraj G, Kelkar A, Hart E, Horst C, Malik D, Yeow C, et al. Comparison of analgesic efficacy of four-quadrant TAM plane (TAP) block and continuous posterior TAP analgesia with epidural analgesia in patients undergoing laparoscopic colorectal surgery: an open-label, randomised, non-inferiority trial. Anaesthesia. 2014;69:348–53.

9. Dieu A, Huynen P, Lavand'homme P, et al Pain management after open liver resection: procedure-specific postoperative pain management (PROSPECT) recommendations regional anesthesia & pain medicine Published Online First: 12 January 2021.

10. Farooq M, Carey M. A case of liver trauma with a blunt regional anesthesia needle while performing transversus abdominis plane block. Reg Anesth Pain Med. 2008;33(3):274–5.

11. Salaria ON, et al. A rare complication of a TAP block performed after caesarean delivery. Case Rep Anesthesiol. 2017;2017:1072576.

12. Rozen WM, Tran TMN, Ashton MW, et al. Refining the course of the thoracolumbar nerves: a new understanding of the innervation of the anterior abdominal wall. Clin Anat. 2008;21:325–33.

13. Flack SH, Martin LD, Walker BJ, et al. Ultrasound-guided rectus sheath block or wound infiltration in children: a randomized study of analgesia and bupivacaine absorption. Paediatr Anaesth. 2014;24:968–73.

14. Dutton TJ, McGrath JS, Daugherty MO. Use of rectus sheath catheters for pain relief in patients undergoing major pelvic urological surgery. BJU Int. 2014;113:246–53.

Analgesia for Laparoscopic/Open Cholecystectomy

12

Arunangshu Chakraborty

Case Scenario

A 41 year old lady is scheduled for an elective laparoscopic cholecystectomy. She has no other comorbidities. She is not on any chronic medicines apart from oral contraceptives.

1. **Describe the surgical incisions of laparoscopic cholecystectomy.**

Laparoscopic cholecystectomy does not generally require any incision. 3–4 ports are entered in the abdominal cavity by piercing the abdominal wall using a trocar.

Sometimes, due to surgical difficulty and or anatomical challenges, a laparoscopic surgery may need to be converted to an open surgery. The typical incision for an open cholecystectomy is a subcostal incision of length 10–15 cm. The incision may need to be extended at times.

Of the laparoscopic ports, the biggest one, i.e. the 10 mm port is made just above the umbilicus. Generally this port is closed in layers.

2. **Describe the somatic innervations of the port sites of laparoscopic cholecystectomy.**

The anterior abdominal wall above umbilicus is innervated by thoracic spinal nerves T7 to 10, which enter the abdominal wall as a continuation of the intercostal nerves in the plane between the transversus abdominis muscle (TAM) and the internal oblique muscle (IOM).

3. **What are the choices for perioperative analgesia in this patient?**

The PROSPECT working group recommends basic analgesic techniques:

- Paracetamol + non steroidal antiinflammatory drugs (NSAID) or cyclooxygenase-2(COX-2) specific inhibitor + surgical site local anaesthetic infiltration. Paracetamol and NSAID should be started before or during operation with dexamethasone (GRADE A).
- Opioid should be reserved for rescue analgesia only (GRADE B).
- Gabapentanoids, intraperitoneal local anaesthetic, and transversus abdominis plane (TAP) blocks are not recommended (GRADE D) unless basic analgesia is not possible.
- Surgically, it has been recommended for low-pressure pneumoperitoneum, postprocedure saline lavage, and aspiration of pneumoperitoneum (GRADE A). Single-port incision techniques are not recommended to reduce pain (GRADE A).

4. **What regional anaesthesia techniques can be used in this patient?**

The most widely practised and highly recommended regional anaesthesia technique for laparoscopic cholecystectomy is local anaesthetic (LA) infiltration by the operating surgeon.

A. Chakraborty (✉)
Sultan Qaboos Comprehensive Cancer Care and Research Centre, Muscat, Oman

Other choices of regional anaesthesia include:

  (a) Oblique subcostal TAP (OSTAP) block,

  (b) Block of the lateral branches of the intercostal nerves in the middle axillary line (**BRILMA**)

  (c) TAP block

  (d) Rectus sheath block

  (e) Intraperitonial LA instillation through laparoscopic port

  (f) Thoracic Paravertebral block (TPVB)

  (g) Erector spinae block and

  (h) Thoracic epidural analgesia

  (i) Quadratus lumborum block

5. **The surgery could not be completed laparoscopically and had to be converted to an open cholecystectomy. How will you manage analgesia now?**

Open cholecystectomy causes significantly more pain compared to laparoscopic cholecystectomy. The pain management strategies need to be boosted accordingly in a scenario like this and a dynamic approach needs to be taken on a case to case basis based on the analgesic modalities already deployed.

If the patient has already received a block such as a fascial plane block or TPVB or thoracic epidural, she would not require another block. If the patient did not receive any block preoperatively, the following can be considered-

  (a) OSTAP block

  (b) Erector spinae plane block (ESPB)

  (c) BRILMA

  (d) TPVB

  (e) Thoracic epidural.

A strong opioid may need to be added to the analgesic regime.

6. **What is your plan of perioperative analgesia for an elective open cholecystectomy in this patient?**

Elective open cholecystectomy is conducted under general anaesthesia. A multimodal opioid sparing analgesia regime is favoured that includes at least one element of regional analgesia. Systemic paracetamol, NSAIDs, dexamethasone and weak opioids are included unless contraindicated otherwise.

The choice of regional anaesthesia are-

  (a) LA infiltration along the incision line by the surgeon

  (b) Continuous wound infiltration of LA

  (c) OSTAP block

  (d) TPVB

  (e) BRILMA

  (f) Thoracic epidural

  (g) ESPB

If the patient requires a strong opioid in spite of the above-mentioned approach, a patient controlled analgesia (PCA) pump with morphine or fentanyl may be added.

7. **In an ERAS regimen, what are the objectives for the analgesia regime?**

The objectives for the analgesic regime within the ERAS protocol are-

  (a) Early ambulation

  (b) Early respiratory physiotherapy

  (c) Opioid sparing

  (d) To minimise complications

Suggested Reading

1. Barazanchi AWH, MacFater WS, Rahiri JL, Tutone S, Hill AG, Joshi GP, PROSPECT collaboration. Evidence-based management of pain after laparoscopic cholecystectomy: a PROSPECT review update. Br J Anaesth. 2018;121(4):787–803. https://doi.org/10.1016/j.bja.2018.06.023. Epub 2018 Aug 7.

2. Shin HJ, Oh AY, Baik JS, Kim JH, Han SH, Hwang JW. Ultrasound-guided oblique subcostal transversus abdominis plane block for analgesia after laparoscopic cholecystectomy: a randomized, controlled, observer-blinded study. Minerva Anestesiol. 2014;80(2):185–93. Epub 2013 Oct 31.

3. Saravanan R, Venkatraman R, Karthika U. Comparison of ultrasound-guided modified BRILMA block with subcostal transversus abdominis plane block for postoperative analgesia in laparoscopic cholecystectomy – a randomized controlled trial. Local Reg Anesth. 2021;14:109–16. https://doi.org/10.2147/LRA.S316320. PMID: 34239324; PMCID: PMC8259940.

4. Wang W, Wang L, Gao Y. A meta-analysis of randomized controlled trials concerning the efficacy of transversus abdominis plane block for pain control after laparoscopic cholecystectomy. Front Surg. 2021;8:700318. https://doi.org/10.3389/

fsurg.2021.700318. PMID: 34422893; PMCID: PMC8371254.

5. Jeong HW, Kim CS, Choi KT, Jeong SM, Kim DH, Lee JH. Preoperative versus postoperative rectus sheath block for acute postoperative pain relief after laparoscopic cholecystectomy: a randomized controlled study. J Clin Med. 2019;8(7):1018. Published 2019 Jul 11. https://doi.org/10.3390/jcm8071018.

6. Das NT, Deshpande C. Effects of intraperitoneal local anaesthetics bupivacaine and ropivacaine versus placebo on postoperative pain after laparoscopic cholecystectomy: a randomised double blind study. J Clin Diagn Res. 2017;11(7):UC08–12. https://doi.org/10.7860/JCDR/2017/26162.10188.

7. Ibrahim M. Erector spinae plane block in laparoscopic cholecystectomy, is there a difference? a randomized controlled trial. Anesth Essays Res. 2020;14(1):119–26. https://doi.org/10.4103/aer.

AER_144_19. Epub 2020 Feb 3. PMID: 32843804; PMCID: PMC7428093.

8. Ökmen K, Metin Ökmen B, Topal S. Ultrasound-guided posterior quadratus lumborum block for postoperative pain after laparoscopic cholecystectomy: a randomized controlled double blind study. J Clin Anesth. 2018;49:112–7. https://doi.org/10.1016/j.jclinane.2018.06.027. Epub 2018 Jun 18.

9. Paladini G, Di Carlo S, Musella G, et al. Continuous wound infiltration of local anesthetics in postoperative pain management: safety, efficacy and current perspectives [published correction appears in J Pain Res. 2020 Mar 30;13:659]. J Pain Res. 2020;13:285–94. Published 2020 Jan 31. https://doi.org/10.2147/JPR.S211234.

10. Lillemoe HA, Aloia TA. Enhanced recovery after surgery: hepatobiliary. Surg Clin North Am. 2018;98(6):1251–64. https://doi.org/10.1016/j.suc.2018.07.011.

Analgesia for Lap/Open Nephrectomy

13

Arunangshu Chakraborty

Case Scenario

A 38-year-old male patient has presented for a nephrectomy due to RCC. What would be your plan of analgesia for this patient?

1. **Describe the cutaneous innervation of the anterolateral abdominal wall.**

The cutaneous supply is derived from the anterior rami of the lower six thoracic nerves and the first lumbar nerve. The thoracic nerves are the continuation of the lower five intercostal and subcostal nerves. Iliohypogastric and ilioinguinal nerves represent the first lumbar nerve (Fig. 13.1).

2. **Describe the nerve supply of the kidney.**

The sympathetic nerve supply of the kidney is derived from the preganglionic fibres originating from T8-L1 segments and converging at the celiac plexus and aortic renal ganglia. Postganglionic fibres originate from the celiac and aorticorenal ganglia. Some sympathetic fibres may reach via the splanchnic nerves. Parasympathetic supply is from the vagus nerve.

3. **What is the mechanism of pain following laparoscopic nephrectomy?**

Postoperative pain after laparoscopic nephrectomy has both somatic and visceral components. Gas distension of the abdominal wall, abdominal port placement and dissection in the abdominal cavity, low abdominal incisions (to retrieve the kidney) and diaphragmatic irritation from residual pneumoperitoneum would cause somatic and visceral pain from both hemiabdomen arising from the umbilical area (T9–T11), the epigastric area (T6–T9) as well as the lower part of the abdomen (T10–T12).

4. **What are the key considerations in this patient?**
   1. Comorbidities [(diabetes mellitus (DM), hypertension (HTN), atrial fibrillation (AF)]
   2. Major surgery with a high risk of perioperative bleeding
   3. Postoperative decline in renal function
   4. Risk of venous thromboembolism and stroke postoperatively

5. **What are this patient's analgesic options for intraoperative and postoperative pain management?**

Multimodal opioid-sparing analgesia is recommended for this patient.

A. Chakraborty (✉)
Sultan Qaboos Comprehensive Cancer Care and
Research Centre, Muscat, Oman

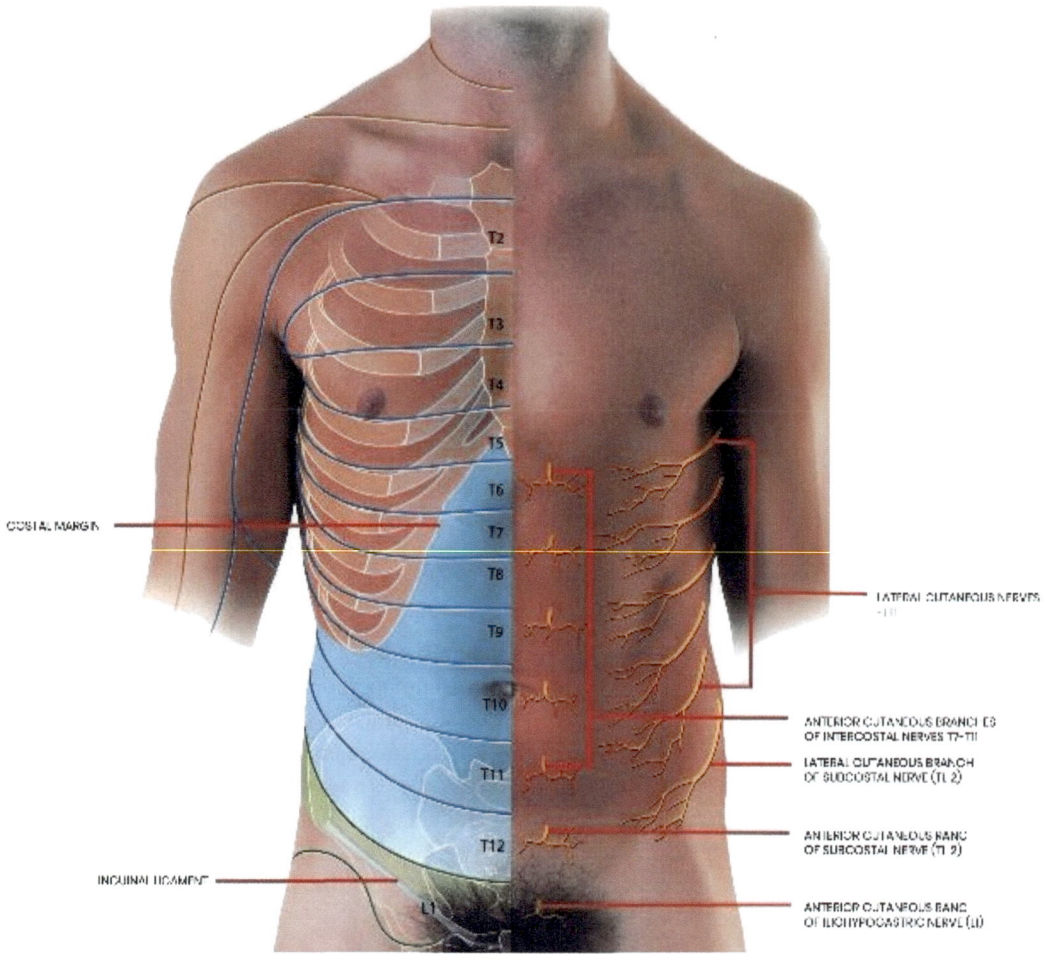

COSTAL MARGIN

T2
T3
T4
T5
T6
T7
T8
T9
T10
T11
T12
L1

LATERAL CUTANEOUS NERVES

ANTERIOR CUTANEOUS BRANCHES
OF INTERCOSTAL NERVES T7-T11

LATERAL CUTANEOUS BRANCH
OF SUBCOSTAL NERVE (T12)

ANTERIOR CUTANEOUS BRANC
OF SUBCOSTAL NERVE (T12)

INGUINAL LIGAMENT

ANTERIOR CUTANEOUS BRANC
OF ILIOHYPOGASTRIC NERVE (L1)

Fig. 13.1 Cutaneous innervation of the anterolateral abdominal wall

The options are:

- Paracetamol
- Strong opioids- fentanyl, oxycodone (caution with opioids and renal function and in the elderly)
- Dexamethasone 4-8 mg intravenous single dose
- Low-dose Ketamine
- Other adjuncts- Alpha-2 agonists (clonidine, dexmedetomidine)
- Single shot spinal with or without local anaesthetic (LA)-Bupivacaine and hydrophilic opioids- morphine, diamorphine

- Port site infiltration with LA at the end of surgery by the surgical team with either standard bupivacaine or liposomal bupivacaine.
- Unilateral paravertebral block
- Fascial Plane Blocks (FPB) either at the beginning or after the end of surgery- such as subcostal TAP block, external oblique fascia plane block, erector spinae block, serratus plane block, quadratus lumborum block
- Other techniques, such as low thoracic epidural with LA and the opioid mix could be used, but it has gone out of favour in the enhanced recovery after surgery (ERAS) Protocols.

Postoperative pain relief:

- In addition to paracetamol and weak opioids—codeine, dihydrocodeine, tramadol.
- Patients who may need strong opioids either orally or via IV-PCA for the first 24 h.

6. **Would you prefer to use NSAIDs and cox-2 inhibitors?**

It is preferable not to use them as patients undergoing radical nephrectomy are left with significantly reduced renal reserve and are at a higher risk of developing moderately severe chronic kidney disease. Moreover, NSAIDs should be used with caution in elderly patients with other significant comorbidities (in this patient, hypertension, diabetes mellitus and warfarin).

7. **Would you prefer a thoracic epidural, considered the gold standard in open surgeries?**

Despite being considered the gold standard in open nephrectomies, it is not recommended in minimally invasive surgeries. Epidural has gone out of favour as the need for analgesia is substantially lesser than open surgery due to its side effects, such as hypotension and risks of epidural hematoma. This patient has a higher risk of postoperative stroke; hence, anticoagulants would need to be started at the earliest opportunity in the postoperative period, and the presence of an epidural catheter may complicate the situation.

8. **What about the use of intrathecal opioids?**

The use of single doses of intrathecal hydrophilic opioids like morphine or diamorphine has recently gained popularity as it provides good analgesia for 18-24 h, reduces IV opioid consumption, and at doses below 300mcg, the risk of respiratory depression is negligible.

9. **What fascial plane blocks can be used in laparoscopic or robotic nephrectomy?**

The options are Transversus Abdominis Plane (TAP) block, Quadratus Lumborum block (QLB) and Erector Spinae Plane (ESP) block.

10. **What approaches would you use for the TAP block?**

No single approach will suffice since the ports are in both the upper and lower abdomen. Bilateral subcostal and anterior/lateral approaches will cover all the quadrants. Exercise caution not to exceed the maximum allowable weight-based local anaesthetic dosage.

11. **What approaches would you prefer for the QLB block?**

No studies confirm the superiority of one approach over the other among QLB 1(lateral), QLB2 (posterior), or QLB 3 (anterior/transmuscular) blocks, although transmuscular approaches have often been used for laparoscopic nephrectomy.

12. **What is the proposed mechanism of action for postoperative analgesia in the case of anterior QLB?**

The spread of injectate with the QLB approaches is cephalad from the lumbar point of administration between the quadratus lumborum and psoas major muscles, predominantly via a pathway posterior to the arcuate ligaments and into the thoracic paravertebral space to reach the somatic nerves and the thoracic sympathetic trunk in the intercostal and paravertebral spaces.

13. **What is the evidence regarding the use of ESP blocks in laparoscopic nephrectomy:**

There are no published studies of the use of ESP blocks in laparoscopic nephrectomy, but considering its success in various abdominal surgeries, including open nephrectomy, it can be a viable alternative.

Level of an ESP block:

ESP block is conventionally used for thoracic surgeries and is performed in the high thoracic region (approximately T4 level). ESP block is performed in the low thoracic region (approximately T10 level) for upper abdominal surgeries.

14. **What will be your plan for analgesia in a case of open subcostal nephrectomy:**
    1. Low thoracic Epidural, with postoperative LA+ opioid mix infusion or patient-controlled epidural.
    2. Paravertebral catheter (Low Thoracic T7-T10)
    3. Subcostal TAP, QLB or ESP catheters
    4. Liposomal Bupivacaine wound infiltration
    5. Wound infusion catheters
    6. IV PCA with opioids

15. **What would be the timing of prophylaxis with low molecular weight heparin and catheter insertion/removal in a patient with an epidural catheter (Table 13.1)**

16. **What would be your choice of fascial plane techniques for the rooftop incision which crosses the midline in a case of open nephrectomy**

Regarding fascial plane blocks, the following options could be explored:

- Bilateral subcostal TAP block
- Bilateral ESP block
- Bilateral anterior QL block

Questions
1. Dosage adjustment of local anaesthetic in patients with impaired renal function
2. What is the influence of renal dysfunction on the choice & dosage of opioids?
3. Describe a typical dose of local anaesthetic infusion rate for Ropivacaine or Bupivacaine?
4. What are the risks and complications associated with a QL block?
5. Regional anaesthesia and potential benefits in cancer surgery

Table 13.1 Guidelines for the management of low molecular weight heparin

	Hold medication	Restart medication
Prophylactic once daily dose	12 h before needle placement	12 h after needle/catheter placement 4 h after catheter removal
Prophylactic twice daily dose	12 h before needle placement	Indwelling catheters should be removed before initiation of LMWH The first dose of LMWH should be no earlier than 12 after needle/catheter placement and in the presence of adequate hemostasis

Suggested Reading

1. Gee WF, Ansell JF. Pelvic and perineal pain of urologic origin. In: Bonica JJ, editor. The management of pain. 2nd ed. Philadelphia: Lea & Febiger; 1990. p. 1368–78.
2. Mathuram Thiyagarajan U, Bagul A, Nicholson ML. Pain management in laparoscopic donor nephrectomy: a review. Pain Res Treat. 2012;2012:201852. https://doi.org/10.1155/2012/201852. Epub 2012 Oct 23. PMID: 23150820; PMCID: PMC3488408.
3. Lau W, Blute M, Weaver A, Torres V, Zincke H. NoMatched comparison of radical nephrectomy vs nephron-sparing surgery in patients with unilateral renal cell carcinoma and a normal contralateral kidney title. Mayo Clin Proc. 2000;75:1236–42.
4. Koning MV, Klimek M, Rijs K, Stolker RJ, Heesen MA. Intrathecal hydrophilic opioids for abdominal surgery: a meta-analysis, meta-regression and trial sequential analysis. BJA. 2020;125:358–72.
5. Elsharkawy H, El-Boghdadly K, Barrington M. Quadratus Lumborum Block: anatomical concepts, mechanisms, and techniques. Anesthesiology. 2019;130:322–35. https://doi.org/10.1097/ALN.0000000000002524.
6. Horlocker TT, Vandermeulen E, Kopp SL, Gogarten W, Leffert LR, Benzon HT. Regional anesthesia in the patient receiving antithrombotic or thrombolytic therapy: American Society of Regional Anesthesia and Pain Medicine Evidence-Based Guidelines (Fourth Edition). Reg Anesth Pain Med. 2018;43(3):263–309. https://doi.org/10.1097/AAP.0000000000000763.

Anaesthesia for Caesarean Delivery

14

Matthew Sinnott

Case scenario

A 38-year primigravida presents for emergency cesarean section. Her vitals are stable, and she has no comorbidities. What would be your plan for anaesthesia in this patient?

1. What are the anaesthetic options for Caesarean delivery (CD)?

The anaesthetic choices can be broadly divided into general (GA) or neuraxial regional anaesthetic techniques. Commonly used RA options include single-shot spinal, epidural, or combined spinal-epidural (CSE) anaesthesia.

2. What are the advantages of RA over GA for CD?

GA carries significant risks in the obstetric population. The anatomical and physiological changes of pregnancy are associated with an increased risk of a difficult airway and aspiration risk. The risk of accidental awareness under GA is also significantly higher in the obstetric population. A RA technique allows these potential adverse events to be avoided and minimises fetal drug transfer.

In addition to avoiding the risks of GA, RA techniques confer additional benefits. Neuraxial opioid administration improves postoperative analgesia, reducing the requirement for further systemic opioids. RA is associated with reduced post-operative nausea and vomiting and venous thromboembolism risk.

Allowing patients to remain awake and aware throughout their delivery and in the presence of their partner improves maternal satisfaction and neonatal bonding [1].

3. Please discuss the relative advantages and disadvantages of the neuraxial techniques commonly used for CD

A single-shot spinal injection provides a fast onset of reliable anaesthesia. The low local anaesthetic (LA) dose requirement means the risk of systemic toxicity is negligible. However, the duration of anaesthesia is limited and cannot be supplemented intra-operatively, which may increase the risk of the patient experiencing pain in prolonged procedures. It is also associated with significant sympatholysis, and the clinician must be alert to the risk of hypotension (and resultant impaired uteroplacental perfusion) and manage this proactively.

Epidural anaesthesia can be titrated to achieve an adequate block and is associated with less haemodynamic instability. This is valuable in high-risk patients, for example, those with cardiac disease. However, the resultant block is often less

M. Sinnott (✉)
Anaesthetic Department, Ashford and St Peter's Hospital NHS Foundation Trust, Chertsey, Surrey, UK
e-mail: matthewsinnott@doctors.org.uk

reliable than that achieved with intrathecal dosing. Epidural catheters sited in labour are also at risk of migration with resulting intravascular or intrathecal drug administration, and the high volumes of LA required pose a risk of toxicity and high/total spinal.

A CSE may combine the benefits of both procedures, as a low intrathecal dose may be extended with subsequent epidural drug administration. However, this must be balanced against the increased technical difficulty of this procedure and the time taken to perform it. Concerns exist, too, regarding the safety of using an 'untested' epidural catheter and exposing a patient to the risks of two procedures rather than one [1, 2].

4. When is neuraxial anaesthesia for CD contra-indicated?

Absolute contra-indications for neuraxial anaesthesia include:

- Maternal refusal
- Overlying infection and systemic sepsis
- Significant coagulopathy or recent anti-coagulant therapy
- Significant uncorrected hypovolaemia
- LA allergy
- Raised intracranial pressure

However, risks must be balanced against the alternative of GA, particularly in the presence of factors such as a predicted difficult airway or unfasted state. This requires an individualized, shared decision-making approach involving the patient and a senior clinician.

5. At what platelet count is it considered safe to perform neuraxial anaesthesia?

Neuraxial anaesthesia is usually considered safe at>70–75 x 10^9/L platelet count. The etiology of thrombocytopenia, clinical signs and symptoms of bleeding, and rate of drop must also be considered. Evidence supporting the role of a concurrent coagulation screen is limited, although a normal INR may provide additional reassurance. Again, it is

essential to balance the alternative of *not* performing neuraxial anaesthetic, especially in patients with a higher predicted risk from GA [2, 3].

6. What are the risks associated with neuraxial anaesthesia?

The risks of neuraxial anaesthesia are:

- Failure, resulting in inadequate analgesia or anaesthesia. The risk of inadequate analgesia from a labour epidural is approximately 1 in 10. The risk of intra-operative pain after epidural top-up is 1 in 20 and 1 in 50 for spinal anaesthesia.
- Hypotension, nausea, motor weakness and itch (transient)
- Post-dural puncture headache: 1 in 100
- Transient, minor neurological dysfunction (patch of numbness or weakness in the leg or foot): 1 in 1000
- Long-lasting minor neurological dysfunction: 1:13,000
- Spinal/ epidural abscess, meningitis and haematoma: 1:50,000 or rarer
- Accidental unconsciousness: 1:100,000
- Permanent severe neurological dysfunction (including paralysis): 1:250,000 [4]

7. What are the surface landmarks available for siting a neuraxial anaesthetic?

Tuffier's line is drawn between iliac crests and intersects the L4 vertebral body. While the conus medullaris is traditionally considered to end at L1/L2, in a significant proportion of the population, it may extend down to L3. For this reason, most anaesthetists advocate avoiding spinal insertion any higher than the L3/4 interspace.

8. What is the role of US when performing neuraxial anaesthesia? What are its potential benefits and drawbacks?

The accuracy of vertebral level prediction based on anatomical landmarks is variable, even by experienced anaesthetists. Pre-procedural US can accurately assess the intervertebral level, depth to epidural space, and optimal needle trajectory. This has been shown to improve first-pass success rate and reduce complications. It is especially useful in patients in whom difficulty is predicted, for example, the obese or those with scoliosis. Concerns about increased procedure performance time have yet to be proven in the meta-analysis [5].

9. What dose of intrathecal LA is commonly used?

0.5% bupivacaine is most frequently used, presented as a hyperbaric formulation (in combination with glucose 8%). The glucose increases the drug's baricity relative to the CSF, so it can be manipulated with patient positioning. Practice varies among anaesthetists, but the usual dose ranges are 10–15 mg bupivacaine. The ED95 of hyperbaric bupivacaine in combination with opioids (10 mcg fentanyl and 200 mcg morphine) is 11.2 [1].

10. What factors affect the spread of LA in intrathecal space?

Drug factors include the dose of LA, baricity, and any prior epidural drug administration. Patient factors include increased CSF pressure from high BMI and/or the gravid uterus and spinal canal abnormalities. Technique factors include the insertion level, barbotage use, and patient positioning following injection [6].

11. What adjuncts are commonly used with LA in spinal anaesthesia for CD?

The most used adjuncts are opioids. Diamorphine is used at a dose of 300 micrograms or morphine 100 micrograms. To improve the speed of onset, intrathecal fentanyl (15–20 micrograms) is often combined with morphine. Higher doses do not confer additional analgesic benefits but increase the risk of side effects, including sedation, itching, and respiratory depression.

12. What options are available for the conversion of a labour epidural for surgical anaesthesia?

2% lidocaine is associated with the fastest onset of anaesthesia. The high concentration and volume necessitate the addition of adrenaline at a concentration of 1:200,000 to minimise systemic absorption and increase the safe dose. Speed of onset can be further enhanced with 50–100 micrograms of fentanyl and/or 2 ml preservative-free 8.4% sodium bicarbonate. However, the preparation time and potential for drug errors may offset benefits.

0.5% bupivacaine is associated with increased duration of anaesthesia, although the time for block onset is slower. 075% ropivacaine may allow some motor sparing and is associated with a reduced need for intra-operative supplementation [7].

13. What is the 'test dose' role when 'topping up' an epidural?

An epidural 'test dose' is designed to detect a misplaced epidural catheter via administering a small dose of local anaesthetic before the total dose is given. An intrathecal catheter would produce a very dense block in a short time frame. Adding adrenaline 1:200,000 will increase maternal heart rate if the catheter is intravascular. However, the test dose does not guarantee safety and may delay establishing adequate analgesia/anaesthesia.

14. What factors are associated with failed conversion of epidural analgesia for surgical anaesthesia?

Factors which have been proven to increase the risk of failure to 'top up' an epidural catheter include increased number of clinician interventions to maintain adequate labour analgesia, increasing pain in the 2 hours before CD, urgency of CD, and the presence of a non-specialist obstetric anaesthetist [7].

15. How do we test for adequacy of neuraxial block before starting surgery?

In general, it is accepted that a block to cold to T4 and a light touch to T5 are required before starting surgery. The motor block should be assessed and ensured that the patient cannot straight leg raise. The caudal spread should be evaluated by testing the sacral dermatomes.

16. How would you proceed if a spinal anaesthetic failed to achieve adequate distribution on testing before starting surgery?

Adequate time should be given to allow the block to reach the required level, and adjusting the table so the patient is head-down can help spread hyperbaric LA solutions. The dose of LA to use if repeating the spinal is challenging and depends on the block distribution of the first spinal. A 'regular dose' risks a high block, while under-dosing risks another inadequate block. A safe approach is to site a CSE and use a low volume of intra-thecal LA. The epidural catheter can then supplement this if the block remains low. However, the time required to perform this must be factored in for emergencies. General anaesthesia is an option but carries the risks discussed above.

17. What are the options available in the event of a failed epidural top-up for CD? What are their benefits and risks?

This is a challenging situation, and each case must be assessed individually. Continuing to use the existing epidural catheter may be unsuccessful, risk LA toxicity, and introduce delays. Removing the epidural catheter and inserting a spinal is again complicated by the above uncertainty over optimal intrathecal dosing. Many anaesthetists use a 20% dose reduction of intrathecal LA as a CSE. Again, the clinical urgency may mean this is impossible, with GA as an alternative.

18. How do you manage a patient complaining of pain intra-operatively during CD?

Actions depend on the procedure stage and whether an epidural catheter is present. The surgery should be paused to allow a full assessment, including what the patient feels and the block's level. The block can be supplemented with fast-acting LA if an epidural catheter is present. If not, analgesic options include Entonox, IV paracetamol and IV opioids. Fast-onset opioids, such as fentanyl or alfentanil, are typically used. The surgical team can infiltrate LA If the procedure is close to finishing. If the baby has not yet been delivered, opioids are often avoided due to concerns of fetal drug transfer, and the neonatal team should be informed if they are administered. A general anaesthetic may be required, mainly if pain occurs early in the procedure, and should always be offered to the patient. Documenting what has happened and thoroughly debriefing the patient afterwards is vital.

19. What regional anaesthesia options are available for patients who undergo CD under GA?

Transversus abdominis plane (TAP) and quadratus lumborum (QL) blocks can provide analgesia when neuraxial block is not possible. Both offer similar analgesic benefits in the absence of intra-thecal morphine, although the benefit is not seen when intrathecal morphine administration has been possible. The choice of block is influenced by practitioner experience and practicalities, including patient positioning—TAP blocks can be easily performed in the supine position. In contrast, QL blocks usually require the patient to be rolled into the lateral position. The QL block may also cause leg weakness if LA spreads to the lumbar plexus. GA is often performed in emergencies, and complete informed consent is challenging. This should be considered and regional blocks only performed if felt to be in the patient's best interests, with a complete discussion and explanation as soon as possible after the procedure [8].

20. What are the PROSPECT pain management recommendations for elective CD?

These are as follows:

- Implementation of strategies to minimise opioid consumption after elective CD
- Intrathecal morphine 50–100 mcg or diamorphine 300 mcg, or in the presence of epidural catheter, epidural morphine 2–3 mg or diamorphine 2–3 mg
- Paracetamol and non-steroidal anti-inflammatory post-delivery and regularly post-operatively
- Single IV dexamethasone dose post-delivery
- Consideration of single injection of LA infiltration, continuous wound LA infusion +/− fascial plane blocks if intrathecal morphine is not used
- Surgical technique to include Joel-Cohen incision, non-closure of peritoneum and abdominal binders
- Consider TENS as an analgesic adjunct [9]

References

1. Armstrong SL, Walters M, Cheesman K, O'Sullivan G. Neuraxial anaesthesia for caesarean delivery. In: Oxford textbook of obstetric anaesthesia. Oxford: OUP; 2016.

2. Sinnott M, Fernando R. Obstetric anaesthesia. In: Lee's synopsis of anaesthesia. Elsevier.

3. Bauer ME, et al. The society for obstetric anesthesia and perinatology interdisciplinary consensus statement of neuraxial procedures in obstetric patients with thrombocytopenia. Anesth Analg. 2021;132(6):1531–44.

4. Obstetric Anaesthetists' Association. Epidural information card. March 2021 Edition. Available from: https://www.labourpains.com/Epidural-Information-Card. Accessed 22 Mar 22.

5. Young B, Onwochei D, Desai N. Conventional landmark palpation vs preprocedural ultrasound for neuraxial analgesia and anaesthesia in obstetrics–a systematic review and meta-analysis with trial sequential analyses. Anaesthesia. 2020;76(6):818–31.

6. Newman B. Complete spinal block following spinal anaesthesia. Anaesthesia tutotial of the week 180 2010

7. Desai N, Carvalho B. Conversion of labour epidural analgesia to surgical anaesthesia for emergency intrapartum Caesarean section. BJA Educ. 2020;1:26–31.

8. El-Boghdadly K, Desai N, Halpern S, Blake L, Odor PM, Bampoe S, Carvalho B, Sultan P. Quadratus lumborum block vs transversus abdominis plane block for caesarean delivery: a systematic review and network meta-analysis. Anaesthesia. 2021;76:393–403.

9. Roofthooft E, Joshi GP, Van de Velde M, on behalf of the PROSPECT Working Group of the European Society of Regional Anaesthesia and Pain Therapy and supported by the Obstetric Anaesthetists' Association. PROSPECT guideline for elective caesarean section: updated systematic review and procedure-specific postoperative pain management recommendations. Anaesthesia. 2021;76:665–80.

Labour Analgesia

15

Matthew Sinnott

Case Scenario You have been asked to assess a 24-year-old primiparous patient. She has no significant past medical history and is in spontaneous labour after an uncomplicated pregnancy. She is 5 cm dilated, contracting 3 in 10, and enquiring about pain relief options.

1. Please describe the pathways by which labour pain is transmitted

The first stage of labour is produced via uterine contractions and cervical dilation. It is conveyed via sympathetic fibres, which enter the spinal cord at T10–L1. It is poorly localised and visceral in character. The second stage of labour is secondary to vaginal and perineal stretch and actual tissue damage and is conveyed via the pudendal nerve (S2–S4).

2. What analgesic options are available for labour?

These can be broadly divided into pharmacological and non-pharmacological therapies. Within pharmacological treatment, there are both neuraxial and non-neuraxial options.

3. Please list non-pharmacological options for labour analgesia

Non-pharmacological options include temperature modulation, hydrotherapy, massage, acupuncture, aromatherapy, hypnosis, and transcutaneous electrical nerve stimulation (TENS). The analgesic benefit is variable, but all have the advantage of avoiding drugs and their associated placental passage.

4. Please describe standard non-neuraxial pharmacological therapies used for labour

Commonly used non-neuraxial pharmacological therapies include inhalational agents, simple systemic analgesics, and opioid-based therapy. All have variable efficacy, and none are complete analgesics. Nitrous oxide in a 50:50 mixture with oxygen (Entonox) provides moderate analgesia and the parturient controls administration. However, it often produces nausea, sedation and dizziness and is not always tolerated. It is also necessary to time inhalation before contractions begin. Systemic opioids may be administered IM or IV. Commonly used IM opioids include pethidine (1 mg/kg IM) and diamorphine (5–7.5 mg IM). These may produce more sedation than analgesia, however, and cross the placenta, which can cause increased sleepiness and delays in

M. Sinnott (✉)
Anaesthetic Department, Ashford and St Peter's Hospitals NHS Foundation Trust, Chertsey, Surrey, UK
e-mail: matthewsinnott@doctors.org.uk

© The Author(s), under exclusive license to Springer Nature Switzerland AG 2026
S. Phillips et al. (eds.), *Regional Anaesthesia*, https://doi.org/10.1007/978-3-032-05165-3_15

establishing breastfeeding in the neonate. IV opioids are usually administered via patient-controlled analgesia (PCA).

5. Please discuss remifentanil PCA in labour in further detail

Remifentanil delivered via PCA is helpful in situations where central neuraxial techniques are impossible or undesirable. This includes maternal coagulopathy or anticoagulant therapy, local infection overlying the insertion site, failure to site central neuraxial techniques, or maternal refusal or preference for an alternative. A typical regimen would be 40 microgram boluses with a lockout time of 2 min. It is important to explain to the parturient that this is an off-label drug use and that the drug crosses the placenta (where it undergoes rapid fetal metabolism). While the analgesia is inferior to that provided by central neuraxial techniques, it is superior to other opioids and associated with high maternal satisfaction rates and favourable delivery and neonatal outcomes. There is no difference in fetal Apgar scores compared with central neuraxial techniques, and it is associated with better neonatal outcomes when compared to IM pethidine. Risks include maternal respiratory depression and rare reports of maternal respiratory and cardiac arrest, mandating 1:1 midwifery care, supplemental oxygen to keep oxygen saturations >/= 94%, and capnography is recommended.

6. Please compare the neuraxial techniques available for labour analgesia

Neuraxial techniques include epidural analgesia, combined spinal-epidural (CSE), and the dural-puncture epidural (DPE). Epidural catheters are the most used, have a long safety record and produce minimal cardiovascular effects. A CSE produces a faster onset of analgesia, which is particularly useful in the latter stages of labour or in patients with previous failed or inadequate epidural analgesia. The intrathecal dosing may produce a more reliable sacral spread of analgesia, and CSF backflow confirms midline epidural placement. However, intrathecal opioids are associated with fetal bradycardia in a dose-dependent manner and cause maternal pruritis. There are increased maternal CVS effects secondary to the intrathecal LA. 'Topping up' the epidural for surgical anaesthesia shortly after insertion requires extra vigilance to exclude intrathecal placement, as the intrathecal dosing of the CSE may disguise this.

The DPE involves the same technique as a CSE, except that no drugs are delivered intrathecally. The hole in the dura may allow the translocation of epidural medication. However, there is limited evidence to support its use and concerns exist over puncturing the dura for no direct benefit.

7. What layers does the Tuohy needle pass through to the epidural space?

The layers passed through are as follows:

- Skin
- Subcutaneous tissue
- Supraspinous ligament
- Interspinous ligament
- Ligamentum flavum
- Epidural space

8. What drugs and at what dose are typically administered epidurally for labour analgesia

Usually, a low-concentration LA is used in combination with an opioid. Commonly used regimens include bupivacaine 0.0625–0.125% or ropivacaine 0.1–0.2%, in combination with either fentanyl 2 mcg/ml or sufentanil 0.2–0.5 mcg/ml. The addition of an opioid allows LA dose reduction of up to 50%, reducing motor block and preserving the mother's ability to push. Low concentration LA (</=0.1% bupivacaine) is accordingly not associated with any increase in instrumental delivery rates or duration of the second stage.

9. What drugs are usually used for the intrathecal component of a CSE?

2–3 ml of a pre-prepared low-dose mix is commonly used, or 1.25–2.5 mg bupivacaine with 10–15 micrgrams of fentanyl prepared separately. Higher doses of opioid (>20 micrograms fentanyl) are associated with increased fetal heart rate abnormalities and itch, whereas higher LA doses will increase the risk of maternal CVS instability.

10. **Aside from providing optimal analgesia, what other benefits do epidurals confer in labour?**

Epidurals provide a safety net in patients at high risk of operative delivery, e.g., patients with obesity or multiple pregnancies, as a well-functioning labour epidural can be rapidly converted to provide surgical anaesthesia. They may also improve function in patients with medical co-morbidities, e.g., blood pressure control in pre-eclampsia, and reduce cardiovascular stress in patients with cardiac disease.

11. **What different ways exist for delivering epidural drugs during labour?**

Epidural drugs can be administered via intermittent clinician boluses as required by the patient. However, this creates a high clinician workload, and pain relief is often interrupted by the regression of analgesia. This results in inconsistent analgesia and poses potential toxicity and sterility concerns as the administration set is repeatedly uncapped.

Continuous epidural infusions (CEI) of 10–15 ml/h of a low dose mix confer advantages over intermittent clinician boluses, although they can result in high LA doses and increased motor block. Programmed intermittent epidural boluses (PIEB) deliver doses of up to 15 ml per hour in divided doses. They may provide a more uniform spread of LA in the epidural space compared to continuous infusions. They result in better pain scores and reduce LA consumption compared with CEI.

Patient-controlled epidural analgesia (PCEA) results in high maternal satisfaction rates. PCEA can be administered in isolation, commonly with 5 ml boluses and a 10-min lockout, 10 ml boluses with a 20-minute lockout, or combined with CEI or PIEB.

12. **Why does breakthrough pain occur during epidural analgesia?**

Breakthrough pain may be due to the natural progression of labour (pain increases), or catheter migration (out of the epidural space, laterally, or intravascularly), displacement, or incorrect initial placement. It is associated with the Currently used lower LA concentrations and may be seen in a correctly sited catheter if there is inadequate dosing or spread within the epidural space[1].

13. **How would you manage an inadequate labour epidural?**

It is essential to assess the parturient for progression and stage of labour. Objectively map the distribution of the block, for example, with ethyl chloride spray. Assess the dosing of LA administered so far. Ensure the catheter has not become dislodged or migrated intravascularly or subdurally. A subdural catheter typically presents with a patchy and unexpectedly high block. If the catheter appears correctly positioned but the distribution is inadequate, higher volumes of low-dose mix may promote spread within the epidural space. Patient positioning may influence spread, and placing the patient 'bad side down' in the case of the unilateral block, or sitting fully upright if sacral sparing is often practised. However, the evidence supporting this is limited. A unilateral block may also be helped by withdrawing the epidural catheter 1–2 cm before giving a bolus. If the distribution is adequate but density insufficient, then higher concentrations of LA e.g. 0.25% bupivacaine with or without adjuncts such as fentanyl or clonidine can be attempted.

If the epidural remains inadequate despite repeated troubleshooting attempts, then an honest discussion should be held about re-siting the catheter. Aside from improving analgesia, repeated interventions have been associated with increased failure rates if there is a need to convert to anaesthesia for operative delivery. On rare occasions, patients may have a resistance to LA, e.g. in Ehler's Danlos syndrome. Ask about previous failed local anaesthesia history, such as during dental treatment.

14. **How should a patient be monitored while epidural analgesia is provided?**

When establishing epidural analgesia, NICE (National Institute for Health and Care Excellence, UK), recommends BP readings every 5 min for 15 min and continuous CTG, cardiotocography) for at least 30 min. Sensory level should be assessed every hour. Straight leg raise should be used to determine the motor block every hour, and the inability to do so should prompt early assessment by an anaesthetist to exclude an acute space-occupying lesion. (i.e a haematoma within the spinal canal), which can cause permanent and devastating neurological injury if not rapidly identified and treated.

15. **How would you manage a parturient with an unwitnessed disconnection of her epidural?**

In general, the epidural should be removed and re-sited due to the risk of introducing infection. However, clinical judgment is required for a patient whose initial insertion was very challenging, and the risk of operative delivery is high. If the uncapped end of the epidural catheter has been protected from soiling, it may be appropriate to trim the catheter with sterile scissors and apply a fresh filter. However, this needs shared decision-making with the mother, balancing the minor but potentially catastrophic risk of epidural infection versus the possible complications from unsuccessful regional and subsequent general anaesthesia during an operative delivery. Chlorhexidine solution should not be used to clean the epidural catheter as this may spread to the epidural space via capillary action and result in neurotoxicity.

16. **A woman develops a fever whilst in labour and has a working epidural, how do you manage this?**

The patient should be reviewed, and the cause of the fever should be sought. Infectious and non-infectious intrapartum fever are associated with adverse maternal and neonatal outcomes, and early management, including broad-spectrum antibiotics, antipyretics, and informing neonatal teams, is indicated.

Provided treatment has been initiated, short-term epidural presence is not associated with increased risk of epidural infection. However, the patient should be carefully followed up to exclude the development of epidural abscess or meningitis.

17. **Can you briefly outline epidural related fever and also what you would do if a woman has a temperature before siting an epidural?**

Epidural-related fever is a non-infectious phenomenon observed in a quarter of patients receiving epidural analgesia. It is thought to be due to immune or thermoregulatory changes caused by LA in parturients.

Intra-partum fever is not a contra-indication to epidural insertion, but the cause of fever should be sought and treatment initiated with an observed reduction in temperature prior to siting the epidural. These women should be carefully followed up to exclude the development of epidural infection. Haemodynamic instability secondary to sepsis, or local infection overlying the insertion site would however preclude safe epidural insertion, and alternative methods of analgesia should be offered.

18. **Please describe the pudendal nerve block. When is it indicated?**

Pudendal nerve blocks are performed for instrumental vaginal deliveries in the absence of a central neuraxial technique, for example, if the mother has refused or there is limited time available due to fetal compromise.

The pudendal nerve arises from S2–S4 and is the main nerve supplying sensation to the external genitalia and skin of the perineum. It runs behind the sacrospinous ligament and is located 1 cm anteromedial and posterior-medial to the ischial spines. The ischial spines are palpated approximately 1 finger's length into the vagina at the 4 o'clock and 8 o'clock positions, and a needle is then inserted either antero- or posterio-medially to a depth of 1 cm. Approximately 7 ml of 1% lidocaine can be injected on each side, and a further 6 ml infiltrated in the perineum. The pudendal blood vessels lie nearby the nerves so it is important to aspirate to rule out intravascular injection.

Questions

1. **Consent and risk of central neuraxial block in obstetrics**
2. **Role of ultrasound and the implications of coagulopathy.**

Suggested Reading

1. Shatil B, Smiley R. Neuraxial analgesia for labour. BJA Educ. 2020;20(3):96–102.
2. McClune G, Hill D. Non-pharmacological methods of pain relief and systemic analgesia in labour. In: Oxford textbook of obstetric anaesthesia. Oxford: OUP; 2016.
3. Ronel I, Weiniger CF. Non-regional analgesia for labour: remifentanil in obstetrics. BJA Educ. 2019;19(11):357–61.
4. Wang T-T, Sun S, Huang S-Q. Effects of epidural analgesia with low concentrations of local anaesthetics on obstetric outcomes: a systematic review and meta-analysis of randomized controlled trials. Anesth Analg. 2017;124(5):1571–80.
5. Wong CA. Epidural and spinal analgesia: anaesthesia for labour and vaginal delivery. In: Chestnut's obstetric anaesthesia: principles and practice. 6th ed. Elsevier; 2020. p. 490–5.
6. Van der Vyer M, Halpern S, Joseph G. Patient-controlled epidural analgesia versus continuous infusion for labor analgesia: a meta-analysis. BJA. 89(3):459–65.
7. Nanji JA, Carvalho B. Pain management during labor and vaginal birth. Best Pract Res Clin Obstet Gynaecol. 2020;67:100–12.
8. George R, Allen TK, Habib AS. Intermittent epidural bolus compared with continuous epidural infusions for labor analgesia: a systematic review and meta-analysis. Anaesth Analg. 2013;116(1):133–44.
9. Desai N, Carvalho B. Conversion of labour epidural analgesia to surgical anaesthesia for emergency intrapartum Caesarean section. BJA Educ. 2020;1:26–31.
10. National Institute for Health and Care Excellence. Clinical guideline [CG190]: Intrapartum care for healthy women and babies, 2014 (revised 2017). London: NICE, 2017. https://www.nice.org.uk/guidance/cg190. Accessed 7 May 22.
11. Yentis SM, Lucas DN, Brigante L, Collis R, Cowley P, Denning S, Fawcett WJ, Gibson A. Safety guidelines: neurological monitoring associated with obstetric neuraxial block 2020. Anaesthesia. 2020;75(7):913–9.
12. Patel S, Sultan P. Intrapartum fever. In: Quick hits in obstetric anaesthesia. Springer; 2022. p. 353–7.
13. Royal College of Obstetricians and Gynaecologists. eLearning and Simulation for Instrumental Delivery. https://elearning.rcog.org.uk/tutorials/technical-skills/elearning-and-simulation-instrumental-delivery-easi. Accessed 9 May 22.

Arunangshu Chakraborty

Case Scenario

A 74-year-old male weighing 54 Kg and with a BMI of 17.8 Kg/m^2 is scheduled for an emergency inguinal hernia repair for acute strangulation of an inguinal hernia. He is diabetic (type II), hypertensive and suffering from COPD and ischemic heart disease. Chronic medications include oral aspirin, clopidogrel, amlodipine, hydrochlorothiazide and inhaled salmeterol+fluticasone. He usually takes a glass of wine before dinner twice a week, used to be a chain smoker but has reduced to 10 cigarettes a day for the last 3 months. He used to walk in the local park daily and was independent in his daily activities. On admission, his BP was 90/60, his pulse rate was 112/min, and his temperature was 101.2 degrees F.

1. **Describe the sensory innervation of the areas involved in an open inguinal hernia surgery**

The cutaneous nerve supply is derived from the descending branches of the thoracolumbar spinal nerves, such as the ilioinguinal nerve (IIN) and iliohypogastric nerve (IHN) (T12, L1). The genital branch of the genitofemoral nerve (GFN) (L1–2) travels in the inguinal canal alongside or within the spermatic cord. It provides motor supply to the cremasteric muscle and sensory innervation to the anterior part of the scrotal skin.

2. **What is the nerve supply of the testes? Why is it pertinent for inguinal hernia surgery?**

The testis is innervated either by
1. Nerve fibres that arise from the tenth and eleventh thoracic spinal segments via the renal and aortic plexuses and accompany the testicular vessels or
2. Fibres that arise from the pelvic plexus and accompany the vas deferens. Some afferent and efferent nerves have been shown to cross over to the contralateral pelvic plexus.

Sometimes, due to the descent of the hernial sac into the scrotum (inguinoscrotal hernia) or a coexisting hydrocele, exploration of the scrotum may be necessary for inguinal hernia surgery. In such cases, adequate analgesia to the testes and the scrotal skin is required.

3. **What are the key clinical considerations in this patient?**
1. Emergency surgery, fasting status
2. Strangulated hernia, possible sepsis and shock- as indicated by low blood pressure and tachycardia
3. Comorbidities (Diabetes, hypertension, ischaemic heart disease, COPD), smoker
4. Drug history: Aspirin, clopidogrel- low platelet aggregation activity and anticipated increased risk of bleeding- relative contraindication for neuraxial anaesthesia

A. Chakraborty (✉)
Sultan Qaboos Comprehensive Cancer Care and Research Center, Muscat, Oman

© The Author(s), under exclusive license to Springer Nature Switzerland AG 2026
S. Phillips et al. (eds.), *Regional Anaesthesia*, https://doi.org/10.1007/978-3-032-05165-3_16

5. High risk of postoperative pulmonary complications following administration of a general anaesthetic given COPD and advanced age
6. Postoperative analgesia
7. Risk of venous thromboembolism and stroke postoperatively

4. **What are the choices of regional anaesthesia for inguinal hernia surgery?**

The choices are-
(a) Surgical site infiltration by the surgeon before incision
(b) Wound infiltration by the surgeon after the surgery
(c) Field block with 30–40 ml local anaesthetic (LA)
(d) IIN-IHN block along with spermatic cord or Genitofemoral nerve (GFN) block
(e) Neuraxial anaesthesia such as spinal anaesthesia, epidural anaesthesia, combined spinal-epidural anaesthesia, caudal anaesthesia
(f) Paravertebral block at T10-L2 levels.
(g) Quadratus lumborum block
(h) Anterior TAP block
(i) Fascia Transversalis block

5. **Would you prefer to use a caudal epidural?**

Caudal (aka sacral) epidural is a well-established modality for perineal and pelvic surgeries in children. As the dermatomal blockade required is up to T10 in adult patients, a very high volume is needed for the caudal route if surgical anaesthesia or effective postoperative analgesia is to be produced. For this reason, caudal epidural is not preferred in adults for inguinal hernia repair surgery. In addition, the risk of motor block and urinary retention at larger volumes and higher concentrations precludes their use, especially if the procedure is planned as a day case.

6. **How is the field block performed for inguinal hernia surgery?**

The field block can be performed using a landmark-based technique or with ultrasound guidance. A total volume of 30mls of 0.25–0.375% Levobupivacaine with or without adrenaline can be used. In children, the dose is 2 mg/kg of 0.25% levobupivacaine, which can be diluted to a larger volume.

The basic principles are-
(a) A skin wheal is made 1.5 cm medial and cephalad to the anterior superior iliac spine (ASIS). A 22 G short bevel needle, fixed to a syringe containing the LA mixture, is directed perpendicular to the skin through the skin wheal. Following the first pop/click as the needle penetrates the external oblique aponeurosis, 5–8 mls of LA is injected to block the iliohypogastric nerve. The needle is advanced deeper until a second click/pop or loss of resistance is felt as the internal oblique is penetrated. A further 5–8 mls of LA is needed to block the ilioinguinal nerve. As the needle is withdrawn, a fanwise subcutaneous infiltration of 5mls of LA above the aponeurosis will block the lower intercostal and subcostal nerves.
(b) A second skin wheal is raised 1–1.5 cm above the mid inguinal point (location of the deep inguinal ring), and 5 ml of LA is injected to block the genital branch of the genitofemoral nerve.
(c) A third skin wheal is made over the pubic tubercle (PT), and 5 ml LA is injected fanwise to block the contralateral innervation.
(d) The surgeon may employ an additional intra-operative injection of 5–10 ml LA in the neck of the hernia sac to supplement the block.

7. **What fascial plane blocks can be used in this case?**

The options are

(a) IIN-IHN block with GFN block
(b) Anterior TAP block
(c) Fascia transversalis block
(d) Quadratus lumborum block.

8. Which is superior, postoperative subfascial or subcutaneous wound infiltration?

Postoperative subfascial LA infiltration was compared with subcutaneous LA infiltration, using a single dose of 10 ml 1% lidocaine through a catheter in the wound. Subfascial infiltration was superior to subcutaneous infiltration for reducing pain scores at rest at 30 min, on mobilisation at 30 and 60 min, and on coughing at 15 and 30 min. The need for supplementary analgesia was similar in the two groups.

9. What will be your choice of anaesthesia regime for this patient?

Considering the advanced age and comorbid conditions such as COPD and heavy smoking, it would be sensible to employ an anaesthetic strategy that will preferably avoid tracheal intubation and mechanical ventilation. A detailed consent should be discussed, including the risks and benefits of the proposed plan and alternatives in case of failure or intraoperative conversion.

After volume resuscitation, once the patient becomes haemodynamically stable, a carefully administered low dose (2 ml) spinal anaesthesia with a 25-27G pencil point needle, ultrasound-guided II&IH nerve block, and GFN block.

For postoperative analgesia, multimodal opioid-sparing analgesia with paracetamol, COX-II inhibitor, and weak opioids will be the choice of drugs for this patient.

10. What are the complications of inguinal block?
1. Intraperitoneal injection and bowel injury
2. Intravascular injection
3. Inadvertent femoral nerve block and quadriceps motor weakness

11. How can a femoral nerve block happen after an inguinal block?

Injection of LA can spread under the fascia iliaca as the iliacus muscle lies in close relation to the ASIS, causing an inadvertent fascia iliaca/femoral nerve block.

12. What is the evidence-based analgesic options for intraoperative and postoperative pain management in this patient?

The PROSPECT collaboration suggests the plan of anaesthesia as follows:

1. Preoperative/intraoperative: Regional anaesthesia (field block ± wound infiltration) or general anaesthesia in combination with regional anaesthetic techniques
2. Postoperative 0–6 h including post anaesthesia care unit (PACU): In addition to above, conventional NSAIDs or COX-2-selective inhibitors (weak opioids should be used when conventional NSAIDs/COX-2-selective inhibitors are contraindicated), combined with paracetamol. Weak opioids should be added when VAS score > 30 but <50*. Strong opioid is to be added when VAS score ≥ 50*
3. Postoperative >6 h: Wound infusion of long-acting local anaesthetic, when possible. Standard medication to be continued: conventional NSAIDs or COX-2-selective inhibitors (use weak opioids when conventional NSAIDs/COX-2-selective inhibitors are contraindicated), combined with paracetamol. Add weak opioid when VAS score > 30 but <50*. Add strong opioid when VAS score ≥ 50*

*Pain ratings on a 1–100-mm visual analogue scale (VAS): score 30 or less, low-intensity pain; over 30 but less than 50, moderate-intensity pain; 50 or more, high-intensity pain. PACU, postanaesthesia care unit; NSAID, non-steroidal anti-inflammatory drug; COX, cyclo-oxygenase.

13. What are the risk factors for chronic pain after inguinal hernia surgery?

Risk factors for chronic postoperative inguinal pain (CPIP) with solid evidence include female gender, young age, high intensity of preoperative pain, high early postoperative pain intensity, history of chronic pain other than CPIP, operation for a recurrent hernia, and open repair technique.

14. **What are the benefits of regional anaesthesia over general anaesthesia in hernia surgery (adults, children, pre-term infants)?**

Regional anaesthesia has various benefits over general anaesthesia (GA) in hernia surgery.

1. In infants: A recently concluded meta-analysis reported that there is moderate-quality evidence to suggest that in infants- [7]

   (a) The administration of spinal in preference to general anaesthesia without pre- or intraoperative sedative administration may reduce the risk of postoperative apnoea by up to 47% in preterm infants undergoing inguinal herniorrhaphy at a postmature age.

   (b) For every four infants treated with spinal anaesthesia, one infant may be prevented from having an episode of postoperative apnoea (NNTB = 4).

   (c) In infants without preoperative apnoea, there is low-quality evidence that spinal rather than general anaesthesia may reduce the risk of preoperative apnoea by up to 66%.

   (d) Although the effect of newer, rapidly acting, quickly metabolised general anaesthetic agents on safety about the risk of postoperative apnoea and neurotoxic exposure has not so far been established in randomised trials, there is potential for harm from postoperative apnoea and direct brain toxicity from general anaesthetic agents superimposed upon pre-existing altered brain development in infants born at very to extreme preterm gestation.

2. In children: Regional anaesthesia is thought to improve the postoperative experience of both children and their parents or caregivers and facilitate the efficient use of hospital facilities. The use of regional anaesthesia in children is expected to continue growing in popularity. Regional anaesthetic techniques, especially ultrasound-guided fascial plane blocks, are safe and should provide the correct balance between risks and benefits for the children.

3. In adults: A recently published systematic review reported that pain scores at 4 and 12 h were higher in the GA group compared to the spinal anaesthesia group. Also, patient satisfaction was more significant in the SA group in both open and laparoscopic inguinal hernia surgeries.

15. **How would you perform a caudal block in children?**

Caudal block in children can be performed using landmark-based techniques and ultrasound guidance.

Position: Left/ right lateral decubitus, with the hips and knees flexed,

Technique:

Landmark: Important landmarks to palpate and identify are-

(a) the posterior superior iliac spines
(b) the line between both spines (Tuffier's line) representing the base of an equilateral triangle, the tip of which indicates the position of the sacral hiatus
(c) the sacral cornua
(d) The sacral hiatus
(e) The sacrococcygeal ligament

The sacrococcygeal ligament can be palpated between the two sacral cornua, where the needle should penetrate the skin at an approximate 45° angle. Once the ligament has been pierced, a flatter angle is assumed before the needle can be advanced to the final position.

It should be noted that Tuffier's line does not seem to be an adequate reference point in neonates placed in a lateral flexed position, as it will shift to a significantly more caudal position in this scenario. Before the local anaesthetic can be applied, cautious aspiration or passive drainage must rule out an accidental intravascular or spinal needle location.

Ultrasound Technique

With a sterile preparation, a high-frequency ultrasound probe is placed transversely on the L5 spine and scanned caudally until it reaches the sacral hiatus. Placing the probe longitudinally in a position slightly paramedian to the lumbar spine, with the cephalad end of the probe on the L5 spine and the caudal end just above the sacral hiatus, the dural sac and the epidural space is identified. The block needle can enter the plane, and a small volume of air or saline can be injected to confirm the needle's position. In the correct position, the caudal epidural space is seen to be swelling up and depressing the dural sac down. A catheter can be passed using a Tuohy needle.

It has been found that the best single indicator of successful caudal epidural injection was visualising by ultrasound in real time the turbulence generated by the local anaesthetic/saline within the caudal space. Since then, more evidence supporting the benefit of ultrasound guidance in neuraxial blocks has been gathered. A recent Cochrane Review has found that using ultrasound improves the success rate of blocks and increases their duration, especially in young children.

16. **What volume of LA will you use for a paediatric caudal block to produce different segmental level blocks (lumbosacral, thoracolumbar, mid-thoracic)?**

Armitage provided the description of dosage for paediatric caudal block in 1979. According to his formula, 0.5 ml/kg may be expected to reach sacral, 1.0 ml/kg lumbar, and 1.25 ml/kg mid-thoracic dermatomes.

Suggested Reading

1. Joshi GP, Rawal N, Kehlet H. on behalf of the PROSPECT collaboration, evidence-based management of postoperative pain in adults undergoing open inguinal hernia surgery. Br J Surg. 2012;99(2):168–85. https://doi.org/10.1002/bjs.7660.

2. Klein SM, Pietrobon R, Nielsen KC, Steele SM, Warner DS, Moylan JA, Eubanks WS, Greengrass RA. Paravertebral somatic nerve block compared with peripheral nerve blocks for outpatient inguinal herniorrhaphy. Reg Anesth Pain Med. 2002;27(5):476–80. https://doi.org/10.1053/rapm.2002.35147.

3. Ahmed A, Fawzy M, Nasr MAR, Hussam AM, Fouad E, Aboeldahb H, Saad D, Osman S, Fahmy RS, Farid M, Waheb MM. Ultrasound-guided quadratus lumborum block for postoperative pain control in patients undergoing unilateral inguinal hernia repair, a comparative study between two approaches. BMC Anesthesiol. 2019;19(1):184. https://doi.org/10.1186/s12871-019-0862-z. PMID: 31623572; PMCID: PMC6798412.

4. López-González JM, López-Álvarez S, Jiménez Gómez BM, Areán González I, Illodo Miramontes G, Padín Barreiro L. Ultrasound-guided transversalis fascia plane block versus anterior transversus abdominis plane block in outpatient inguinal hernia repair. Rev. Esp Anestesiol Reanim. 2016;63(9):498–504. https://doi.org/10.1016/j.redar.2016.02.005. Epub 2016 Apr 8.

5. Frassanito L, Zanfini BA, Pitoni S, Germini P, Del Vicario M, Draisci G. Ultrasound-guided genitofemoral nerve block for inguinal hernia repair in the male adult: a randomised controlled pilot study. Minerva Anestesiol. 2018;84(2):189–95. https://doi.org/10.23736/S0375-9393.17.11948-6. Epub 2017 Jul 5.

6. Yndgaard S, Holst P, Bjerre-Jepsen K, Thomsen CB, Struckmann J, Mogensen T. Subcutaneously *versus* subfascially administered lidocaine in pain treatment after inguinal herniotomy. Anesth Analg. 1994;79:324–7.

7. Jones LJ, Craven PD, Lakkundi A, Foster JP, Badawi N. Regional (spinal, epidural, caudal) versus general anaesthesia in preterm infants undergoing inguinal herniorrhaphy in early infancy. Cochrane Database Syst Rev. 2015;2015(6):CD003669. Published 2015 Jun 9. https://doi.org/10.1002/14651858.CD003669.pub2.

8. Li L, Pang Y, Wang Y, et al. Comparison of spinal and general anesthesia in inguinal hernia repair in adults: a systematic review and meta-analysis. BMC Anesthesiol. 2020;20:64. https://doi.org/10.1186/s12871-020-00980-5.

9. Wiegele M, Marhofer P, Lönnqvist PA. Caudal epidural blocks in paediatric patients: a review and practical considerations. Br J Anaesth. 2019;122(4):509–17. https://doi.org/10.1016/j.bja.2018.11.030.

Analgesia for Total Hip Arthroplasty

Namita Sharma and Chetan Mehra

Clinical Scenario

A 75 year old male with advanced osteo-arthritis of the left hip joint is scheduled for a total hip arthroplasty. He is a hypertensive and diabetic on medications. His exercise tolerance is severely restricted because of painful knee and hip joints. He has been prescribed enalapril, metoprolol, aspirin and oral hypoglycemic agents. His renal profile is marginally deranged, while the rest of the blood investigations are within acceptable limits. Cardiac evaluation reveals an ejection fraction of 35% with a negative dobutamine stress echocardiography. His spine appears lordotic at the lumbar level.

1. Describe the innervation of the hip joint.

- The anterior portion of the joint capsule is supplied by direct branches of the femoral nerve (L1–L4) that run along the iliopsoas muscle.
- Anteromedial portion is supplied by a branch of the obturator nerve (L1–L4).
- Posterior portion is supplied by branches of the sciatic nerve.

- Posteromedial portion of the hip capsule is supplied by ramus from the nerve of the quadratus femoris muscle (L5–S2).
- Posterolateral portion is supplied by rami of the superior gluteal nerve (L4–S1).

The relevant cutaneous innervation for hip surgery include:

- The lateral femoral cutaneous nerve (L1 to L3)
- The lateral cutaneous branch of the iliohypogastric nerve (L1)
- The subcostal nerve (T12) for incisions that extend cranially

2. Indications for total hip arthroplasty.

As formulated by the EUROHIP(European collaborative database of cost and practice patterns of THR) the indications for THR include:

- Pain
  - Severity
  - At rest
  - At night
  - With activity
- Function
  - Walking distance
  - Need for cane
  - Need for analgesics
  - Difficulty in climbing stairs
  - Difficulty in putting on shoes or socks

N. Sharma (✉)
Ashford and St Peter's Hospital, Chertsey, UK
e-mail: namita.sharma@nhs.net

C. Mehra
Department of Anaesthesia, Indraprastha Apollo Hospital, New Delhi, Delhi, India

© The Author(s), under exclusive license to Springer Nature Switzerland AG 2026
S. Phillips et al. (eds.), *Regional Anaesthesia*, https://doi.org/10.1007/978-3-032-05165-3_17

- Physical Examination
  - Range of motion
- Radiograph findings

Amount of joint space preserved on x-ray.

3. Approaches to Total Hip Arthroplasty

Surgical approaches to total hip arthroplasty include:

- Posterior Approach (Southern or Moore approach): Most employed approach worldwide. Performed with the patient in the lateral decubitus position.
- Direct Lateral Approach (Hardinge or Transgluteal approach): Can be performed in lateral decubitus or supine position.
- Direct Anterior Approach—first described by Smith-Petersen for reducing congenital hip dislocations. Performed in supine position.

4. What are the anaesthesia considerations in a patient undergoing Total Hip Arthroplasty?

Pre-operative
These are usually elderly patients with multiple underlying medical issues. Preoperative assessment and optimization is essential given the multiple issues such as hypertension, diabetes mellitus, ischaemic heart disease, autonomic dysfunction, neuropathy, parkinsonism and chronic kidney disease. These patients are usually on multiple medications for their medical conditions, including blood thinners, antidepressants, oral opioids.

Clinical assessment of the cardiorespiratory reserve in these patients is often difficult due to their limited mobility. An ECG and 2D ECHO can only provide an assessment of the patients in the resting state. A pharmacological stress test may be necessitated to further assess the dynamic function of the cardiovascular system.

Prolonged analgesic usage, which may include NSAIDS may compromise their renal parameters. Pre-operative use of opioids, antidepressants and anti-convulsants necessitate dose adjustments in the perioperative period.

Parkinsonism is an age related issue which may have effects on positioning and lie supine/lateral for a long time.

These patients may have multiple joint involvement especially if they are also suffering from rheumatoid arthritis. They may have cervical spine and temporomandibular joint involvement which can make airway management difficult. Patients suffering from ankylosing spondylitis may have restrictive lung disease making ventilation difficult. Patients with ankylosing spondylitis may also prove to be a challenge for central neuraxial anaesthesia.

A review of the patient's regular medications is an absolute necessity. They might be on various medications like anti-hypertensives, oral hypoglycaemic's and oral anti-coagulants many of which may require modification.

Intra-operative
Irrespective of the anaesthetic technique, certain issues are common to all the patients undergoing total hip arthroplasty. These include:

- Haemorrhage
- Hypotension
- Deep vein thrombosis
- Pulmonary embolism
- Bone Cement Implantation Syndrome (BCIS)
- Over sedation as a result of the sedative drugs used intra-operatively leading to airway compromise

Postoperative
The major concern in the postoperative phase is patient mobilization and adequate analgesia. Multiple options are available for pain management. Regional anaesthesia technique is the cornerstone of multimodal analgesia (MMA) regime for the post-operative analgesia following total hip arthroplasty. These include epidural analgesia, fascia iliaca block, lumbar plexus block, PENG block, intrathecal/intravenous morphine or fentanyl PCA, etc. Non-opioid analgesics such as cox-2 inhibitors, paracetamol are used as a component of multimodal analgesia because of their synergistic action on pain pathways.

5. What are the choices of anaesthetic techniques for total hip arthroplasty?

The surgery can be performed under:

- General Anaesthesia (GA) Central neuraxial anaesthesia: spinal, epidural, combined spinal and epidural anaesthesia
- GA with peripheral nerve blocks
- Peripheral nerve blocks

There are certain advantages to using regional anaesthesia over general anaesthesia. These include reduced blood loss, lower incidence of blood transfusion, lower incidence of deep vein thrombosis and pulmonary embolism, better post-op pain scores and reduced cost and disadvantages of GA like stress responses to intubation can be avoided.

General anaesthesia on the other hand may be preferable for patients with fixed cardiac output states, infection at site of needle insertion for neuraxial blocks, bleeding diathesis/coagulopathy who cannot lie down for prolonged periods or who refuse for regional anaesthesia.

6. What are the options for analgesia in patients undergoing total hip arthroplasty?

Recommendation for analgesia in total hip arthroplasty is given by the PROSPECT guidelines (procedure specific postoperative pain management). These include:

Pre and Intra-operative Interventions:
- Pre-operative exercise and education are recommended (Grade A)
- The basic analgesic regimen should include a combination of paracetamol and a non-steroidal anti-inflammatory drug or a cyclo-oxygenase-2-selective inhibitor administered preoperatively or intraoperatively and continued postoperatively (Grade A)
- Spinal or general anaesthesia is recommended (Grade A)

- A single intraoperative dose of intravenous dexamethasone 8–10 mg is recommended for its analgesic and anti-emetic effects (Grade A)
- A single-shot fascia iliaca block or local infiltration analgesia (Grade D)
- If the patient has received spinal anaesthesia for the surgery, intrathecal morphine 0.1 mg (Grade D) could be considered.

Post-operative Interventions:
- Paracetamol (Grade A)
- NSAIDS or COX 2 selective inhibitors (Grade A)
- Opioids should be reserved as rescue analgesics in the postoperative period (Grade D)

Regional Analgesia Options Include:
1. Epidural analgesia
2. Lumbar plexus block
3. Lumbar rector spinae plane block
4. Quadratus lumborum block
5. Fascia iliaca block
6. PENG block
7. Femoral nerve block
8. Lateral femoral cutaneous nerve block, Ilioinguinal, ilio-hypogastric, selective T12 nerve, cluneal nerve blocks (for skin incision only)
9. Local infiltration analgesia (LIA)

7. Describe in detail the fascia iliaca compartment block.

Fascia iliaca compartment is a potential space lying between the fascia iliaca and the iliacus and psoas muscle posteriorly. Femoral, obturator and the lateral cutaneous nerve of the thigh run through this space. Deposition of local anaesthetic in this space has the potential to block all three nerves.

Block Technique: With the advent of ultrasound, the landmark approach has fallen out of favour. Ultrasound allows for a suprainguinal approach to fascia iliaca block which provides a more reliable block of the obturator and lateral cutaneous nerve of the thigh.

Landmark Guided Technique The anatomical landmarks required for the block are the anterior superior iliac spine, pubic tubercle, and inguinal ligament. The inguinal ligament is divided into thirds. The needle insertion point is 1 cm below the lateral third and medial two-thirds of the inguinal ligament. A short blunt bevelled needle is inserted perpendicular to the skin. It is advanced further till two distinct "pops" are felt as the needle punctures first the fascia lata followed by fascia iliaca. This is followed by injection of 25–30 ml of the local anaesthetic after negative aspiration of blood.

Ultrasound Guided Technique A high frequency (6-14 MHz) probe is used. The operator may choose a supra-inguinal or infra-inguinal approach. For the infra-inguinal approach the probe is placed at the inguinal crease and the femoral artery is identified along with the femoral nerve as a hyperechoic structure lateral to the artery. The iliacus muscle along with the overlying fascia iliaca will be seen further laterally. With an in-plane technique the needle is placed just below the fascia iliaca and local anaesthesia is injected and its spread visualized. An optimally performed block will lift the fascia iliaca off the iliacus muscle.

For the supra-inguinal approach a high frequency probe is placed over the ASIS in the sagittal plane. The probe is then moved medially till the characteristic "bowtie sign" is seen, formed by the internal oblique muscle cranially, sartorius caudally and the iliacus muscle inferiorly with the fascia iliaca overlying it inferiorly. The deep circumflex femoral artery serves as a landmark to identify the plane between the internal oblique muscle and the iliacus muscle. The needle is introduced by an in-plane approach caudo-cranially. The goal is to pierce the fascia iliaca and then using hydro dissection the fascia is separated from the iliacus muscle. At this point the local anaesthetic can then be injected. FICBs

decreases the consumption of opioids perioperatively.

8. **What are the alternative regional anaesthesia techniques to FICB for post-op analgesia?**

The alternative regional anaesthesia techniques include:

- Epidural Anaesthesia
- Lumbar plexus block
- Anterior quadratus lumborum (QLB) block
- Femoral Nerve Block
- Femoral 3-in-1 Block
- PENG Block (Pericapsular Nerve Group Block)

9. **Are you aware of any motor sparing block for THR surgery?**

PENG block.

First described in 2018 as a novel technique to reduce post-op pain and opioid consumption following hip surgery. Performed under ultrasound guidance, the goal of the block is to deposit the local anaesthetic in the myofascial plane between psoas tendon anteriorly and the pubic rami posteriorly.

The anterior capsule of the hip joint has abundant nociceptors, whereas the posterior capsule of the hip has abundant proprioceptors. For analgesia, anterior capsule should be our target.

The anterior capsule of the hip joint is supplied by the articular branches of the femoral, obturator and accessory obturator nerve. These articular branches are the target for the PENG block. Since the PENG block targets the sensory, articular branches of the femoral nerve, it avoids the motor weakness of quadriceps caused by the femoral nerve block. This helps in early ambulation and recovery.

10. **Describe the PENG block?**

The block is performed with the patient in supine position with the operator standing on the side of the affected limb. A low frequency curvilinear probe is used. The probe is initially placed transversely over the ASIS and then rotated counter-clockwise by 45 degrees. The femoral artery along with the iliopectineal eminence, iliopsoas tendon and the pectineus muscle can be identified over the pubic ramus. The needle is introduced in a lateral to medial direction via an in-plane approach targeting the plane between the iliopsoas tendon and the pubic rami. After negative aspiration the local anaesthetic is deposited. The psoas tendon can be seen lifting up from the linear hyperechoic pubic ramus. The ramus serves as an end point for safe needle insertion.

20–30 ml of 0.25% Bupivacaine, 0.25% levobupivacaine, 0.375% of ropivacaine is usually adequate for this block. The lateral cutaneous nerve of the thigh can be separately targeted in patients for whom the posterior or direct lateral approach to hip surgery is used.

11. What is the mechanism of action of the erector spinae plane block?

In the Lumbar ESP block, the local anaesthetic is deposited between the erector spinae muscle and transverse process of the lumbar vertebrae. The local anaesthetic spreads into the paravertebral space and diffuses to block the ventral rami and dorsal rami and blocks both dorsal and ventral rami of the lumbar spinal nerves.

12. The Fascia iliaca catheter gets displaced on the first post-operative day and the patient is unable to mobilise due to the pain. What would your plan be for analgesia?

We should continue on multimodal anaesthesia such as NSAIDS/COX-2 inhibitors and oral opiods. However, the interventional strategy can be:

- Reinsertion of the catheter into fascia iliaca with ultrasound guidance
- Targeting both femoral Nerve and lateral femoral cutaneous nerve under ultrasound guidance

13. While performing hydrodissection for suprainguinal fascia iliaca plane block, you notice the circumflex femoral artery being pushed down. What should you do next

This shows the needle placement is superficial to the fascia iliaca. The needle needs to be redirected in the correct plane between fascia iliaca and iliacus muscle. The pulsating deep circumflex femoral artery can be further identified using the doppler mode. The local anaesthetic should be seen spreading under this artery.

14. The patient scheduled for total hip arthroplasty surgery is on oral morphine, gabapentinoids, SSRIs. How will you modify his postoperative analgesia schedule

The elderly patients are often prescribed polypharmacy for their medical conditions. Anti-convulsants, anti-depressants and oral opioids should be continued in the peri-operative period. A caution should be observed in case of the use of opioids used peri-operatively by any other route. A neurology opinion can be sought for dose adjustments of mood-altering medications.

15. Patient has received a PENG block. He complains of buckling of knee and weakness in knee extension. What can be the reason for this and how will you modify your treatment plan?

The PENG block classically blocks the articular branches of the femoral nerve. However, the femoral nerve can inadvertently be blocked by the superficial deposition of the local anaesthetic, rather than under the psoas tendon. This leads to quadriceps weakness. In such cases, the patient is reassured and advised not to mobilise for next 12–24 h till the effect of the block is weaned off.

Questions

- What are the complications associated with peripheral nerve blocks for total hip arthroplasty?
- Can total hip arthroplasty be performed solely under peripheral regional anaesthesia? What will be your plan of anaesthesia?
- Can you mention few advantages of suprainguinal fascia iliaca plane block over infrainguinal fascia iliaca block.
- What are different drug combinations used for LIA? What is the evidence of LIA in comparison to peripheral and central neuraxial anaesthesia?
- An elderly patient is taking acitrom (warfarin) following aortic valve surgery, and needs a THR. Discuss the anaesthetic management.
- What is the current role of sacral plexus block for post-operative analgesia following THR?

Suggested Reading

1. Dreinhöfer KE, Dieppe P, Stürmer T, Gröber-Grätz D, Flören M, Günther K, et al. Indications for total hip replacement: comparison of assessments of orthopaedic surgeons and referring physicians. Ann Rheum Dis. 2006 Oct;65(10):1346–50.

2. Moretti VM, Post ZD. Surgical approaches for total hip arthroplasty. Indian J Orthop. 2017 Aug;51(4):368.

3. Anger M, Valovska T, Beloeil H, Lirk P, Joshi GP, Van de Velde M, et al. PROSPECT guideline for total hip arthroplasty: a systematic review and procedure-specific postoperative pain management recommendations. Anaesthesia. 2021;76(8):1082–97.

4. Bohacek I. Applications and critical evaluation of fascia iliaca compartment block and quadratus lumborum block for orthopedic procedures. Acta Clin Croat. 2019;58(Suppl. 1):108–13.

5. Kumar K, Pandey RK, et al. Comparison of conventional infrainguinal versus modified proximal suprainguinal approach of fascia Iliaca Compartment Block for postoperative analgesia in total hip arthroplasty. A prospective randomized study. Acta Anaesthesiol Belg. 2015;66(3):95–100.

6. Desmet M, Vermeylen K, Van Herreweghe I, et al. A longitudinal supra-inguinal fascia Iliaca compartment Block reduces morphine consumption after total hip arthroplasty. Reg Anesth Pain Med. 2017;42(3):327–33.

7. Kukreja P, Avila A, Northern T, et al. A retrospective case series of Pericapsular Nerve Group (PENG) block for primary versus revision total hip arthroplasty analgesia. Cureus. 12(5):e8200.

8. Lei X, Leng JC, Elsharkawy H, et al. Replacement of Fascia Iliaca Catheters with continuous Erector Spinae Plane Blocks within a clinical pathway facilitates early ambulation after total hip arthroplasty. Pain Med. 2020;21(10):2423–9.

9. Andersen L, Kehlet H. Analgesic efficacy of local infiltration analgesia in hip and knee arthroplasty: a systemic review. Br J Anaesth. 113(3):360–74.

Analgesia for Total Knee Replacement and Cruciate Ligament Surgery

18

Namita Sharma and Chetan Mehra

Clinical Scenario

A 73-year-old man presents for an elective total knee arthroplasty. He weighs 104 kg and is 170 cm tall, with a BMI of 36. He has hypertension, gout and a 20-pack-year history of smoking. His home medications include naproxen, which he stopped a week ago, allopurinol and atenolol.

1. **What are the key clinical considerations in this patient?**

Anaesthetic

Obesity: In the United Kingdom, a BMI of 30–39.9 kgm^2 is classified as obese, and a BMI of 40 kgm2 and above is classified as severely obese. Obesity can pose technical difficulties and delay cannulation, regional anaesthesia placement, central neuraxial blockade placement, and potential difficulties in bag-mask ventilation and endotracheal intubation. With a more significant proportion of body fat, the pharmacokinetics of drugs may be affected.

Smoking: Increased airway reactivity, mucous production and coughing during the procedure (if awake) and a possibility of undiagnosed COPD and/or IHD.

Hypertension: Increased lability of the patient's blood pressure intraoperatively can be expected.

Surgical

Obesity: Potentially more difficult to position this patient and conduct surgery in the affected joint.

Smoking: Delayed wound healing and increased chance of infection.

Patient

Obesity: Functional residual capacity and expiratory residual volume are reduced in obese patients. These patients can desaturate quickly and often have obstructive sleep apnea. There is an increased incidence of IHD, HTN, and CCF in the obese, with increased gastric acidity and fluid volume increasing the risk of aspiration.

Hypertension: Increased myocardial oxygen demand due to high systemic vascular resistance and high left ventricular end-diastolic pressure in these patients can make them prone to subendocardial ischaemia,

N. Sharma (✉)
Ashford and St Peter's Hospital, Chertsey, UK
e-mail: namita.sharma@nhs.net

C. Mehra
Department of Anaesthesia, Indraprastha Apollo Hospital, New Delhi, Delhi, India

S. Phillips et al. (eds.), *Regional Anaesthesia*, https://doi.org/10.1007/978-3-032-05165-3_18

Table 18.1 The sensory innervation of Knee

Compartment	Nerves	Considerations	Joint supply	Cutaneous supply
Anterior	Femoral nerve	Crosses behind the inguinal ligament and lateral to the femoral artery and provides branches to innervate each muscular component of the quadriceps muscle (Vastus medialis, intermedius and lateralis branches)	The vastus medialis to the medial collateral ligament. The vastus lateralis branches end at the quadriceps tendon without innervating the knee capsule.	The vastus medialis to the superomedial aspect. The vastus intermedius to the anterosuperior aspect of the knee
	Common fibular nerve	Provides articular (genicular) branches to the knee, lateral superior, lateral inferior, recurrent.	The inferolateral capsule of the knee joint Proximal tibio fibular joint	The lateral aspect of the knee
	Saphenous nerve	Cutaneous branch of the femoral nerve Runs in the adductor canal	Infrapatellar branch Descending branch Antero inferior capsule of the knee joint	The medial and inferior aspects of the knee
Posterior	Tibial nerve	The branch of the sciatic nerve provides the posterior articular nerve	Articular (genicular) branches to knee: Medial superior, medial inferior; middle, and capsular branches	The medial portion of the capsule, retinaculum, collateral ligaments of the knee joint, and proximal and distal tibiofibular joint.
	Obturator nerve	Originates two main branches: Anterior and posterior	Posterior branch to the joint capsule, cruciate ligaments and synovial membrane	Anterior branch to the medial aspect and mid-thigh

Table 18.2 Plexuses supplying knee joint

Plexuses	Contributors to the plexus	Sensory innervation
Peri patellar	Femoral nerve; medial, lateral and intermediate femoral cutaneous nerves; saphenous nerve; infrapatellar branch of the retinacular nerves; medial and lateral nerve to vastus intermedius	Skin anterior, superior, medial and lateral to the patella; retinacula; collateral ligaments and capsule of the knee joint
Subsartorial	Saphenous nerve; infrapatellar branch of the obturator nerve; anterior division of the medial femoral cutaneous nerve; nerve to vastus medius	Cutaneous to the medial side of the knee, retinaculum, collateral ligaments and capsule of the knee joint
Popliteal	Tibial, sciatic and obturator nerve	Retinaculum, anterior and posterior cruciate ligaments, collateral ligaments and capsule of the knee joint

2. **Describe the sensory innervation of the knee (Tables 18.1 and 18.2)**

3. **What are the choices of regional anaesthesia for total knee replacement? (Table 18.3)**

4. **What are the choices of regional anaesthesia for cruciate ligament surgery (Table 18.4)**

Current evidence suggests that LAI and ACB for cruciate ligament surgery provide similar analgesic efficacy, but neither analgesic technique impacts early or late functional outcomes.

Recent systematic reviews comparing regional analgesic techniques concluded that LAI provides effective post-operative pain relief and can be recommended, unlike ACB and FNB, which resulted in conflicting results when compared to placebo.

Table 18.3 Regional anesthesia options for total knee replacement

Analgesic procedure	Advantages	Disadvantages	Contraindications
Intrathecal analgesia	Relatively easy technique Bilateral analgesic effect for bilateral TKA	Effect on sympathetic innervation (urinary retention and hypotension) Respiratory depression related to intrathecal use Pruritis Unnecessary bilateral block Risk of infection and nerve damage Delays mobilisation	Elevated intracranial pressure Infection on the injection site Risk of hypotension (hypovolaemia) Thrombocytopaenia or coagulopathy Patient inability to get into position Allergy to LA Bleeding diatheses
Femoral nerve block	Easy access with or without ultrasound guidance Excellent analgesia Good predictable course of the catheter with ultrasound guidance	Delays mobilisation High risk of falls	Infection on the injection site If there is no US/S guidance, anatomical anomalies affecting landmark identification Pre-existing neuropathies affecting the distribution of the block
Sciatic nerve block (posterior)	Analgesia to the posterior aspect of the knee Adjuvant effects on anterior compartment blocks	Relatively deep block Requires semi-prone/prone position Delays mobilisation	Infection on the injection site If there is no US/S guidance, anatomical anomalies affecting landmark identification Pre-existing neuropathies affecting the distribution of the block
Adductor canal block (ACB)	Allows early mobilisation and recovery times Continuous techniques provide the highest analgesic effect Higher opioid sparing than LAI Easy ultrasound-guided access	Tunnelling is required in some cases	Infection on the injection site If there is no US/S guidance, anatomical anomalies affecting landmark identification Pre-existing neuropathies affecting the distribution of the block
iPACK	Adjuvant analgesic effect with ACB Analgesia on the posterior aspect of the knee Minimal impact on mobilisation	Limited to single-shot technique Short analgesic effect Risk of foot drop	Infection on the injection site If there is no US/S guidance, anatomical anomalies affecting landmark identification Pre-existing neuropathies affecting the distribution of the block
Local Anaesthetic infiltration (LAI)	Easy intraoperative mobilisation Adjuvant analgesic effect	Increased risk of toxicity Short analgesic effect Risk of infections with intraarticular catheter	
Genicular nerve block	Low risk of toxicity	Requires fluoroscopy and trained staff US/S guidance, still in investigation Scarce clinical evidence	Infection on the injection site Bleeding diatheses
Cryoanalgesia	No risk of toxicity (no LA use)	Unpredictable analgesic duration Risk of permanent motor and sensory block Scarce clinical evidence	Raynauds syndrome Cryoglobulinaemia Bleeding diatheses Infection on the injection site

Adapted from Pulsed radiofrequency of the composite nerve supply to the knee joint as a new technique for relieving osteoarthritic pain: a preliminary report. Pain Physician.2014;17(6):493–506.

Table 18.4 Regional anesthesia options for cruciate ligament surgery

Analgesic procedure	Advantages	Disadvantages	Contraindications
Femoral nerve block	Easy access with or without ultrasound guidance Excellent analgesia Good predictable course of the catheter with ultrasound guidance	Delays mobilisation High risk of falls	Infection on the injection site If there is no US/S guidance, anatomical anomalies affecting landmark identification Pre-existing neuropathies affecting the distribution of the block
Intrathecal analgesia	Relatively easy technique Bilateral analgesic effect for bilateral TKA	Effect on sympathetic innervation (urinary retention and hypotension) Respiratory depression related to intrathecal use Pruritis Unnecessary bilateral block Risk of infection and nerve damage Delays mobilisation	Elevated intracranial pressure Infection on the injection site Risk of hypotension (hypovolaemia) Thrombocytopaenia or coagulopathy Patient inability to get into position Allergy to LA Bleeding diatheses
Adductor canal block (ACB)	Allows early mobilisation and recovery times Continuous techniques provide the highest analgesic effect Higher opioid sparing than LAI Easy ultrasound-guided access	Tunnelling is required in some cases	Infection on the injection site If there is no US/S guidance, anatomical anomalies affecting landmark identification Pre-existing neuropathies affecting the distribution of the block
Local Anaesthetic infiltration (LAI)	Easy intraoperative mobilisation Adjuvant analgesic effect	Increased risk of toxicity Short analgesic effect Risk of infections with intraarticular catheter	

Adapted from Pulsed radiofrequency of the composite nerve supply to the knee joint as a new technique for relieving osteoarthritic pain: a preliminary report. Pain Physician.2014;17(6):493–506.

5. **Would you prefer central neuraxial block-ade (CNB) or general anaesthesia in joint arthroplasty?**

I prefer to use CNB.

Perlas et al. reported that both 30-day mortality and length of stay were reduced with CNB.

A meta-analysis also found that GA may increase early postoperative cognitive dysfunction in joint arthroplasty.

Multiple studies have found that SA reduces significant complications after total joint arthroplasty. (Table 18.5).

Regarding opioid usage in CNB, I would avoid adding them in favour of local anaesthetic only. Ideally, this would be done with short-acting agents and regional anaesthetic techniques such as adductor canal blocks with LAI. Intrathecal morphine increases pruritis and decreases patient satisfaction while showing inferior opioid-sparing effects when compared to LAI.

6. **What would your analgesia regime of choice be for this patient?**

Table 18.5 Comparison of spinal anaesthesia and general anaesthesia for outpatient total joint arthroplasty

Perioperative factor	Evidence favours SA	Evidence favours GA	Comments
Perioperative mortality Pulmonary complications Acute renal failure Infections	+		Consensus based on existing evidence
Deep vein thrombosis Pulmonary embolism	+/−		SA may confer small benefits but may provide no difference in modern practice.
Surgical bleeding Transfusion	+/−		There is limited evidence that SA reduces bleeding, but anti-fibrinolytics may eliminate these differences.
Major adverse cardiac events	−	−	No difference based on existing evidence
PONV	+/−		SA may confer small benefits but may be no difference with modern total intravenous anaesthesia techniques and fluid replacement.
Urinary retention		+	Lower odds with GA
Early physical therapy participation		+	GA may be advantageous, especially compared with bupivacaine.
Postoperative pain	−	−	Early pain may be higher with GA, but after 6 h, SA results in more pain10. Multimodal analgesia may minimise differences.

+ likely benefit; +/− possible benefit; − no difference

This would follow the PROSPECT published guidance:

- Spinal anaesthesia using short-acting local anaesthetic only without intrathecal opioids. Intrathecal opioids could be considered when adductor canal block and LAI is not possible.
- NSAIDS and COX 2 inhibitors are recommended pre-, intra and post-operatively and reduce postoperative opioid requirements along with Paracetamol.
- A single preoperative or intra-operative dose of dexamethasone ($\geq$10 mg, iv) is recommended.
- A single-shot ACB is recommended and preferably combined with LIA. Continuous ACB is not recommended because of inconsistent benefits.
- I would not conduct a femoral or sciatic nerve block (SNB) due to the resulting quadriceps weakness. LAI is as effective as SNB for postoperative analgesia and opioid requirements.
- Continuous LIA or continuous intra-articular local anaesthetic infusion are not recommended because of inconsistent benefits and concerns of potential infection.
- Post-operative NSAIDs and paracetamol are recommended.
- Opioids would be reserved as rescue medications

7. **What components can feature in an ERAS pathway for TKR?**

Pre operative

- *Preoperative patient education* has been shown to reduce pre-operative anxiety across several systematic reviews, but how and when it should be delivered has not been studied adequately. Despite this, it is still a strong recommendation within ERAS.

- *Smoking and alcohol cessation programmes*—strongly recommended
- *Anaemia correction*- strongly recommended
- *Preoperative physiotherapy*—not recommended; prehabilitation (nutrition therapy and psychological preparation for exercise regimes) has shown improvements in recovery for general surgical patients, but there are no procedure-specific studies in knee replacement
- *Preoperative carbohydrate treatment*—in knee replacement, it may well increase patient well-being but has not been shown to accelerate the achievement of discharge criteria or reduce complications, so it is not currently recommended as essential for an ERAS programme

Intraoperative

- *General anaesthesia versus neuraxial blockade*—Modern general anaesthesia and neuraxial techniques may both be used as multimodal anaesthetic techniques.
- *Spinal opioids*—where spinal anaesthesia is used, spinal opioids should not form part of the ERAS pathway
- *Local infiltration of anaesthetic (LIA) and nerve blockade* –
- *Avoid surgical drains and use of tourniquet*—strongly recommended
- *Perioperative fluid management*—judicious intravenous fluids intraoperatively and oral intake encouraged postoperatively.
- *Urinary catheters*—are not recommended or used less than 24 h

Postoperative

- *Prevention of post-operative nausea and vomiting (PONV)*—*it is strongly recommended to screen patients for PONV and to use* multimodal strategies to prevent PONV.
- *Tranexamic acid*—prevention of perioperative blood loss and, therefore, allogenic blood transfusion is strongly recommended

- *Paracetamol and NSAIDs*—use of these, barring contraindications, is strongly recommended
- *Gabapentanoids*
- *Supplemental opioid analgesia*- ERAS programmes seek to minimise opioid analgesia. Oxycodone may be used as a multimodal approach
- *Maintaining normothermia*—normal body temperature should be maintained peri and postoperatively through pre warming and the active warming of patients intraoperatively
- *Antimicrobial prophylaxis*—patients should receive systemic antimicrobial prophylaxis by local policy and availability
- *Antithrombotic prophylaxis treatment*— *Patients should be mobilised as soon as possible after surgery and receive antithrombotic* prophylaxis treatment as per local policy.
- *Post-operative nutritional care*—*an early return to regular diet should be encouraged*
- *Early mobilisation*—patients should be mobilised as early as they are able
- *Criteria-based discharge*—team-based discharge criteria should be met to facilitate discharge back to patients' home
- *Continuous audit and improvement*

Suggested Reading

1. Stebler K, Martin R, Kirkham KR, Lambert J, Sede A, Albrecht E. Adductor canal block versus local infiltration analgesia for postoperative pain after anterior cruciate ligament reconstruction: a single centre randomised controlled triple-blinded trial. Br J Anaesth. 2019;123(2):e343–a349.
2. Sehmbi H, Brull R, Shah UJ, et al. Evidence basis for regional anaesthesia in ambulatory arthroscopic knee surgery and anterior cruciate ligament reconstruction: Part II: adductor canal nerve block-a systematic review and meta-analysis. Anesth Analg. 2019;128:223e38.
3. Yung EM, Brull R, Albrecht E, Joshi GP, Abdallah FW. Evidence basis for regional anaesthesia in ambulatory anterior cruciate ligament reconstruction: Part III: local instillation analgesia-a systematic review and meta-analysis. Anesth Analg. 2019;128:426e37.
4. Vorobeichik L, Brull R, Joshi GP, Abdallah FW. Evidence basis for regional anaesthesia in ambulatory anterior cruciate ligament reconstruc-

tion: Part I-femoral nerve block. Anesth Analg. 2019;128:58e65.

5. Perlas A, Chan VWS, Beattie S. Anaesthesia technique and mortality after total hip or knee arthroplasty: a retrospective, propensity score-matched cohort study. Anaesthesiology. 2016;125:724–31.

6. Zywiel MG, Prabhu A, Perruccio AV, et al. The influence of anaesthesia and pain management on cognitive dysfunction after joint arthroplasty: a systematic review. Clin Orthop Relat Res. 2014;472:1453–66.

7. Memtsoudis SG, Sun X, Chiu Y-L, et al. Perioperative comparative effectiveness of anaesthetic technique in orthopaedic patients. Anaesthesiology. 2013;118:1046–58.

8. Johnson RL, Kopp SL, Burkle CM, et al. Neuraxial vs general anaesthesia for total hip and total knee arthroplasty: a systematic review of comparative-effectiveness research. Br J Anaesth. 2016;116:163–76.

9. Sansonnens J, Taffé P, Burnand B, et al. Higher occurrence of nausea and vomiting after total hip arthroplasty using general versus spinal anaesthesia: an observational study. BMC Anesthesiol. 2016;16:44.

10. Harsten A, Kehlet H, Ljung P, et al. Total intravenous general anaesthesia vs. spinal anaesthesia for total hip arthroplasty. Acta Anaesthesiol Scand. 2015;59:542–3.

11. Schwenk ES, Johnson RL. Spinal versus general anaesthesia for outpatient joint arthroplasty: can the evidence keep up with the patients? Reg Anesth Pain Med. 2020;45:11.

12. Lavand'homme PM, Kehlet H, Rawal N, Joshi GP. Pain management after total knee arthroplasty. procedure specific postoperative pain management recommendations. Eur J Anaesthesiol. 2022;39(9):743–57.

13. Soffin EM, YaDeau JT. Enhanced recovery after surgery for primary hip and knee arthroplasty: a review of the evidence. Br J Anaes. 2016;117(suppl 3).

14. Wainwright TW, Gill M, Mcdonald DA, Middleton G, et al. Consensus statement for perioperative care in total hip replacement and total knee replacement surgery: Enhanced Recovery After Surgery (ERAS®) Society recommendations. Acta Orthopaedica. 2019;91(1):3–19.

Analgesia for Lower Limb Amputation

19

Namita Sharma and Chetan Mehra

Case Scenario

A 62-year-old man presented to the ER in a state of stupor and was managed for diabetic ketoacidosis. He also has a chronic, non-healing, infected ulcer in his right foot, extending above ankle level. He is scheduled for a right-sided below-knee amputation. He is a chronic smoker and has a history of 40 pack years.

1. **What are the indications for lower extremity amputation (LEA)**
- Major trauma
- Gangrene of various etiologies
- Malignant tumor
- Infections
  - Chronic osteomyelitis
  - Surgical site infection
  - Necrotizing fasciitis
- Others
  - Madura foot
  - Lymphedema
  - Severe burns

2. **What are the anaesthesia considerations for patients who are undergoing amputation?**

N. Sharma (✉)
Ashford and St Peter's Hospital, Chertsey, UK
e-mail: namita.sharma@nhs.net

C. Mehra
Department of Anaesthesia, Indraprastha Apollo Hospital, New Delhi, Delhi, India

There is usually a paucity of time for preoperative optimisation of such patients. However, it is prudent to rectify the reversible patient factors prior to surgery. Broadly, we can divide them into preoperative, intraoperative, and postoperative.

Pre-operative:

Anaesthesia implications for this patient include:

- Chronic smoking
- Elderly age group
- Uncontrolled diabetes with limited exercise tolerance

Intra-operative

Choice of anaesthesia depends on the severity of the patient's co-morbidities.

Although general anaesthesia offers a better control over hemodynamic parameters, with minimal interference with perioperative anticoagulation, it may lead to respiratory compromise with use of perioperative opioids, muscle relaxants and invasive ventilation.

Central neuraxial anaesthesia eliminates the risks associated with opioids and invasive ventilation. It may however, lead to precipitous hypotension inpatients with autonomic dysfunction and interfere with use of perioperative anticoagulants.

A combined spinal epidural gives the advantage of using a low dose sub arachnoid block which does not cause significant haemodynamic changes. The epidural catheter can then be used

S. Phillips et al. (eds.), *Regional Anaesthesia*, https://doi.org/10.1007/978-3-032-05165-3_19

to prolong the duration of anaesthesia or provide postoperative analgesia.

Peripheral regional anaesthesia provides excellent working conditions with minimal interference with patient's hemodynamics.

Post-operative

These patients may require HDU or ICU care in the postoperative period.

A multimodal approach to pain management is ideal for such patients, where the use of epidural or peripheral regional analgesia techniques allows a significant reduction in the use of NSAIDs and opioids.

3. **Enumerate the advantages of regional block for amputation.**

Advantages offered by regional anaesthesia over general anaesthesia include:

- Improved stump flow
- Superior postoperative analgesia
- Avoidance of basal atelectasis caused by mechanical ventilation
- Decrease in incidence of cognitive dysfunction. This assists in better compliance with medical therapy and functional recovery and decreases the length of hospital stay.
- Using a pre-emptive peripheral nerve block has been reported to significantly lower the incidence of septic shock and re-exploration of the stump, possibly because of increased blood flow and reduced inflammatory response.
- Reduction in the incidence of peri-operative blood transfusion.

General anaesthesia also carries a considerable safety profile, as comparative evidence regarding outcomes of RA for LEA is limited to observational studies with conflicting results.

Post-operative pulmonary complications are a leading cause of morbidity and mortality.

The various options include:

- Spinal anaesthesia
- Combined spinal epidural anaesthesia
- Sciatic nerve block at the popliteal level combined with saphenous nerve block (adductor canal block/saphenous nerve block at the level of tibial tuberosity)
- Lumbar Plexus block along with sciatic nerve block
- 3-in-1 femoral nerve block along with sciatic nerve block

A sciatic nerve block at an appropriate level combined with a lumbar plexus block or a 3-in-1 block can anaesthetize the whole lower limb. A continuous catheter technique can also be used for postoperative analgesia.

If chosen, central neuraxial or general anaesthesia should be complemented by peripheral regional anaesthesia techniques.

4. **Enumerate sensory innervation of the lower limb**

The nerve supply of the lower limbs is derived from the lumbar and sacral plexus. (Figs. 19.1, 19.2, 19.3, 19.4, 19.5, 19.6, 19.7, and 19.8).

The lumbar plexus is derived from the anterior rami of L1 to L4 along with a contribution from the T12 thoracic nerve.

The components of lumbar plexus include:

- Femoral nerve (L2, L3, L4): Innervates the skin over the anterior thigh and medial leg.
- Obturator nerve (L2, L3, L4): Innervates the skin over the medial thigh.
- Lateral cutaneous nerve of thigh (L2—L3): Innervates the skin over the anterior and lateral thigh down to the level of knee.
- Iliohypogastric nerve (T12—L1)
- Ilioinguinal nerve (L1)
- Genitofemoral nerve (L1—L2)

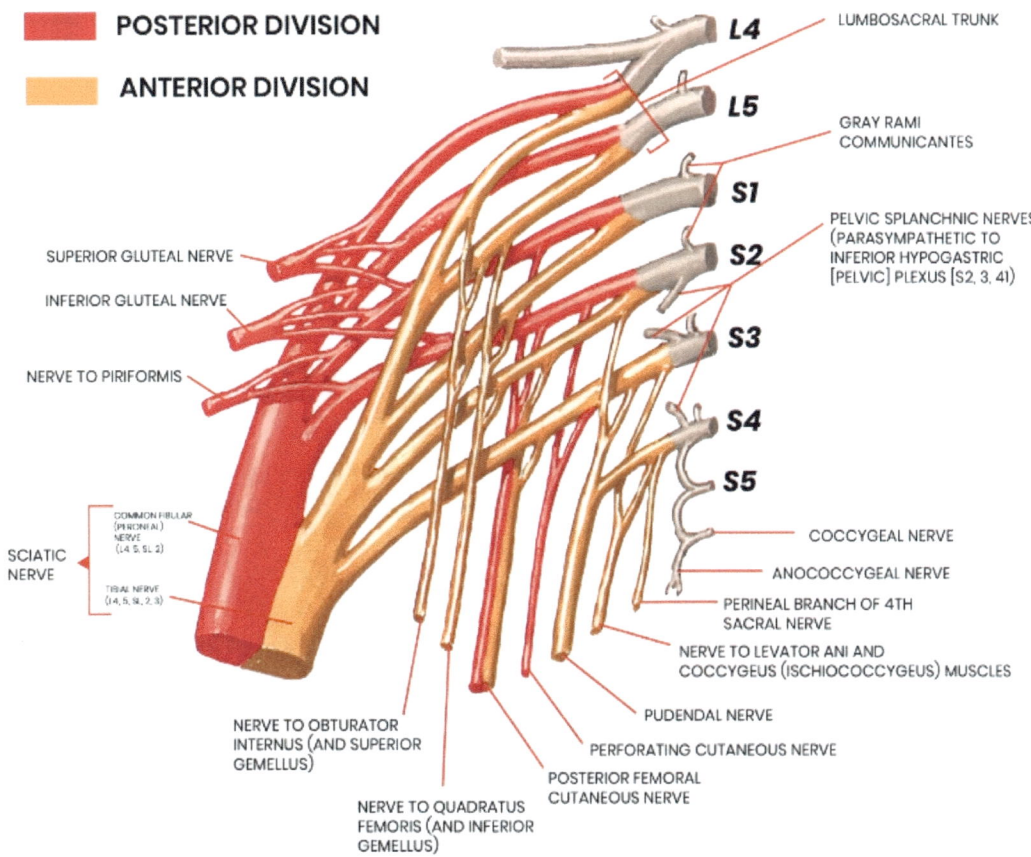

POSTERIOR DIVISION

ANTERIOR DIVISION

Fig. 19.1 Schema of the sacral plexus showing the posterior and anterior divisions

The sacral plexus is derived from the anterior rami of S1, S2, S3 and S4 spinal nerves.

The components of sacral plexus include:

- Sciatic nerve (L4, L5, S1, S2, S3): It has two components: the common peroneal and tibial nerve.
  - The tibial component supplies the skin on the posterolateral leg, lateral foot and lateral sole.
  - The common peroneal component supplies the skin of the lateral leg and dorsum of foot.
- Posterior femoral cutaneous nerve (S1, S2, S3): Innervates the skin over posterior thigh and leg. It also innervates the perineum.
- Pudendal nerve (S2, S3, S4)
- Superior gluteal nerve (L4, L5, S1)
- Inferior gluteal nerve (L5, S1, S3)

5. **What are the approaches to ultrasound guided sciatic nerve block**
- Sacral plexus block (Parasacral approach) (Fig. 19.9):
  - Targets the components of sacral plexus while exiting the greater sciatic foramen.
  - Pyriformis muscle and posterior border of ischium act as ultrasound landmarks for locating sciatic nerve.
  - The superior gluteal artery lies in close vicinity of the nerve. It should be used with caution in patients with deranged coagulation profile.
  - A curvilinear probe is used for imaging the sciatic nerve at this level.

Fig. 19.2 Lumbar
plexus

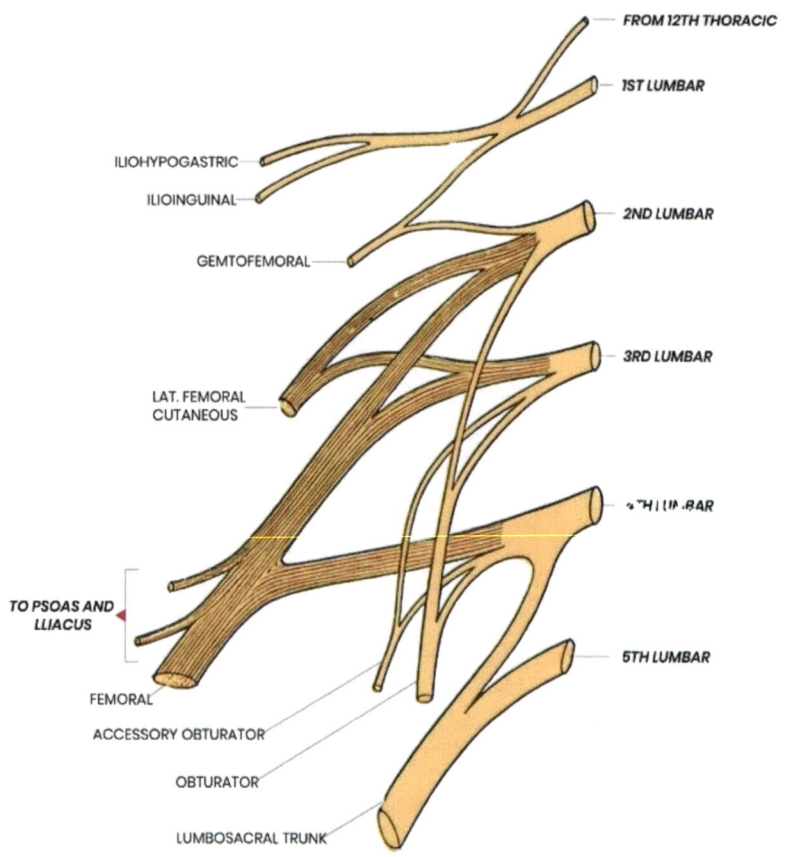

- Anterior approach (Fig. 19.10):
  - It is useful when the patient can't be placed in a lateral position due to pain or the presence of an external fixator.
  - It is technically difficult as the scan is performed on the anteromedial thigh.
  - It is not ideal for catheter insertion as the nerve lies quite deep.
  - A curvilinear probe is used for imaging the sciatic nerve at this level.
- Transgluteal approach:
  - Sciatic nerve is identified deep to gluteus maximus.
  - The probe is placed between the ischial tuberosity and the greater trochanter on the buttock.
  - Imaging requires a curvilinear probe given the depth at which the sciatic nerve is usually imaged at this level.

- Subgluteal approach (Fig. 19.11):
  - The ultrasound probe is placed just inferior to the transverse gluteal crease.
  - The nerve is quite superficial at this level and can be imaged with a linear probe.
  - Ideal approach for a continuous catheter technique.
- Sciatic nerve block at popliteal level (Fig. 19.12):
  - The sciatic nerve at the level of popliteal fossa can be approached posteriorly or from the lateral side of the leg.
  - The sciatic nerve is usually divided into its respective tibial and common peroneal nerve components. These lie in the common paraneural sheath covering of the sciatic nerve. A subparaneural spread of local anaesthetic is desirable.

Fig. 19.3 Cutaneous innervation of lower limb

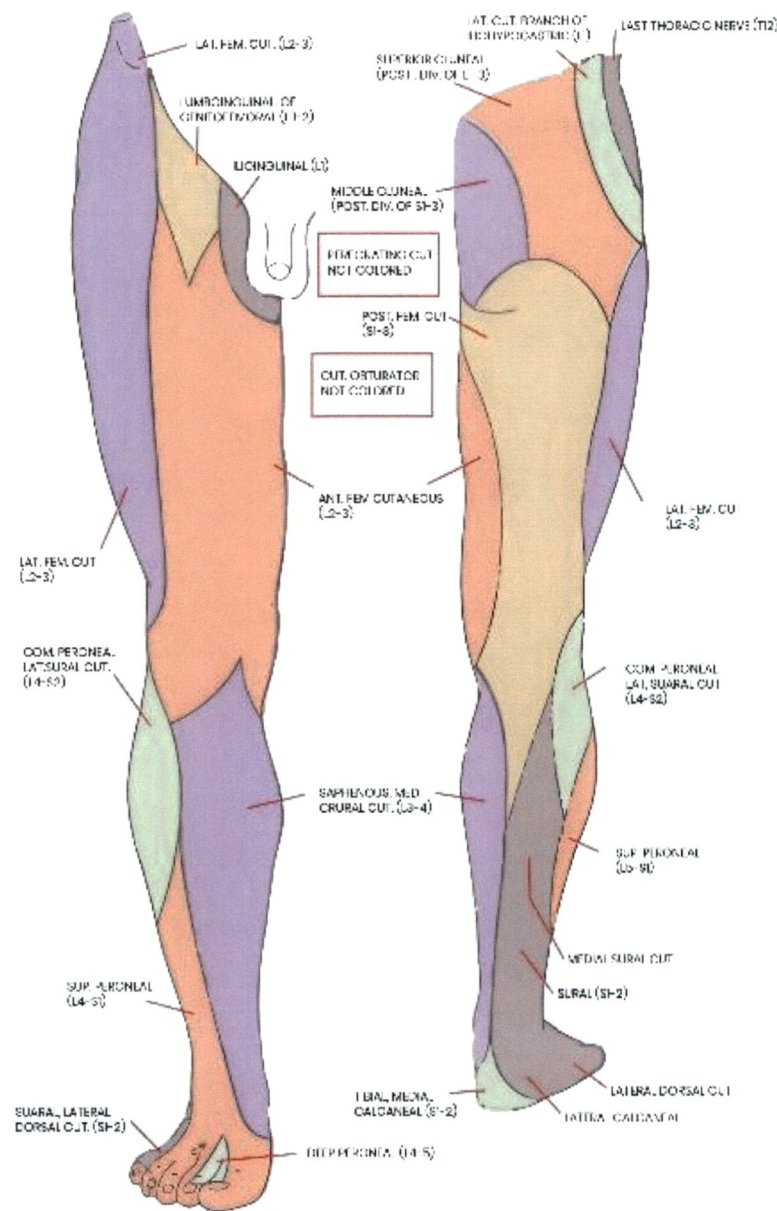

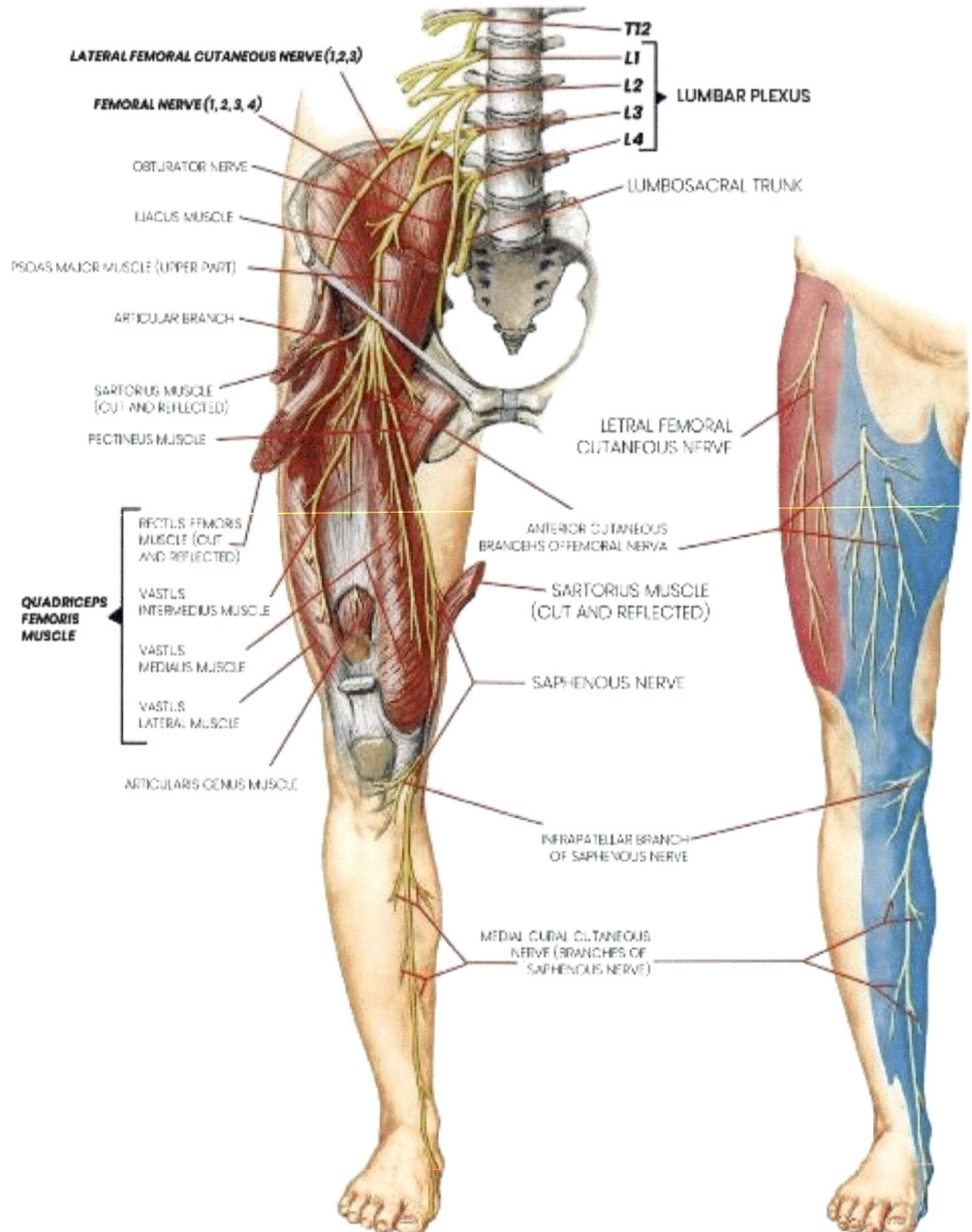

Fig. 19.4 Lumbar plexus and innervation of the anterior thigh

Fig. 19.5 *Innervation of the lower leg and foot—peroneal nerve branches and distribution*

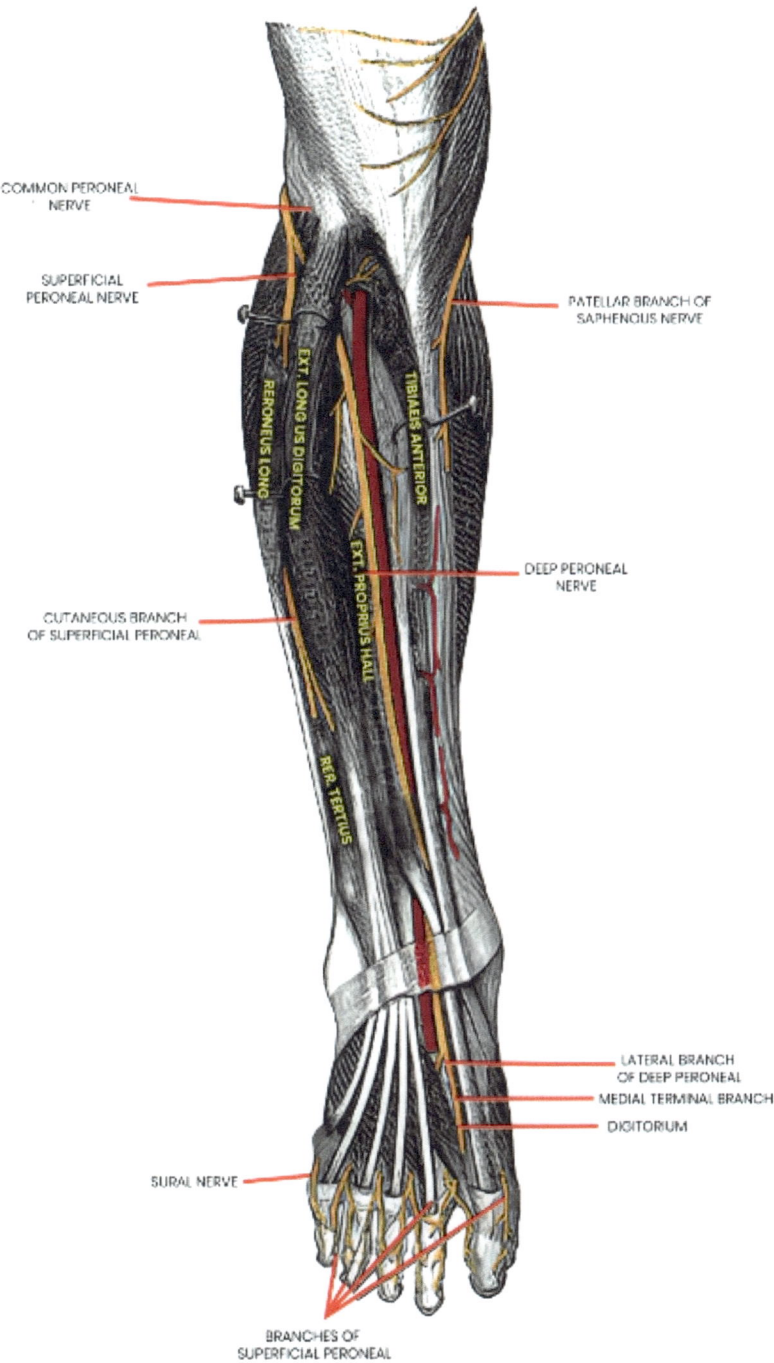

COMMON PERONEAL NERVE

SUPERFICIAL PERONEAL NERVE

PATELLAR BRANCH OF SAPHENOUS NERVE

EXT. LONG US DIGITORUM

PERONEUS LONG

TIBIALIS ANTERIOR

EXT. PROPRIUS HALL

DEEP PERONEAL NERVE

CUTANEOUS BRANCH OF SUPERFICIAL PERONEAL

PER. TERTIUS

LATERAL BRANCH OF DEEP PERONEAL

MEDIAL TERMINAL BRANCH

DIGITORUM

SURAL NERVE

BRANCHES OF SUPERFICIAL PERONEAL

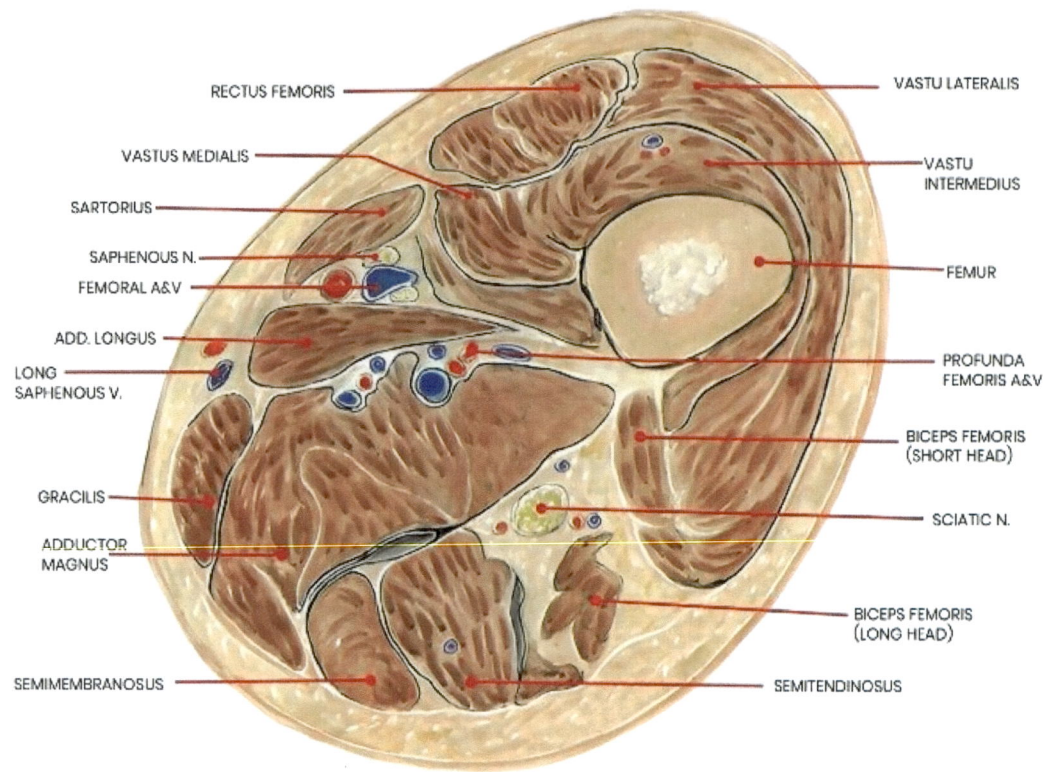

RECTUS FEMORIS

VASTU LATERALIS

VASTUS MEDIALIS

VASTU INTERMEDIUS

SARTORIUS

SAPHENOUS N.

FEMORAL A&V

FEMUR

ADD. LONGUS

LONG SAPHENOUS V.

PROFUNDA FEMORIS A&V

BICEPS FEMORIS (SHORT HEAD)

GRACILIS

SCIATIC N.

ADDUCTOR MAGNUS

BICEPS FEMORIS (LONG HEAD)

SEMIMEMBRANOSUS

SEMITENDINOSUS

Fig. 19.6 Cross-sectional anatomy of the mid-thigh

- The sciatic nerve can be targeted at a superficial depth, making this a preferred approach for surgeries below the level of knee.
- It can be used for perineural catheter placement.

6. What are possible peripheral nerve block combinations for amputations

The peripheral regional blockade will depend on the site of amputation. The common sites of amputation include below-knee amputation (BKA), above-knee amputation (AKA), hindquarter amputation, upper limb amputation, or pre-quarter amputation.

BKA
- Sciatic nerve catheter at the popliteal level, although any of the proximal approaches can be used
- Sub-sartorial/adductor canal catheter (preserves quadriceps strength). The femoral nerve block can also be used instead (Fig. 19.13)

AKA
- Proximal approaches of sciatic nerve block (subgluteal, parasacral, anterior), and
- Femoral nerve or fascia iliaca catheter or lumbar plexus catheter (Fig. 19.14)
- Lateral cutaneous of thigh and obturator nerve blocks to be supplemented in case of sole

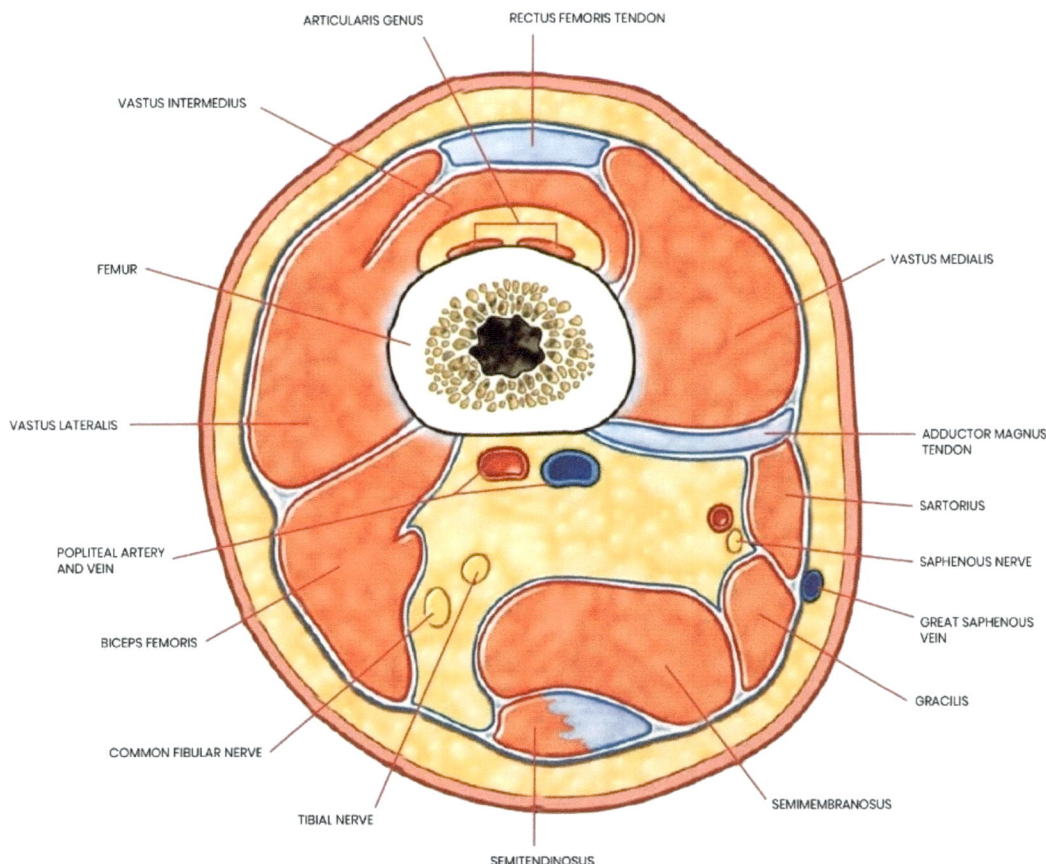

Fig. 19.7 Cross-sectional anatomy of the distal thigh

regional anaesthesia technique (Figs. 19.15, 19.16 and 19.17)

Hindquarter Amputation
The following can be used as a supplement for the purpose of perioperative analgesia

- Lumbar plexus catheter (Figs. 19.18 and 19.19)
- Lumbar erector spinae plane catheter

Upper Limb Amputations
Brachial plexus catheters at appropriate level depending upon level of amputation and patient related factors such as respiratory issues.

The intercostobrachial nerve has to be targeted separately, as it arises from the second intercostal nerve.

Forequarter Amputation
- Interscalene approach of brachial plexus block
- Cervical erecter spinae plane block
- Cervical plexus block can supplemented as required

Anesthesia for mid-foot amputation using peripheral nerve blocks.
The nerve supply of foot is derived from the distal branches of the sciatic and the femoral nerves.

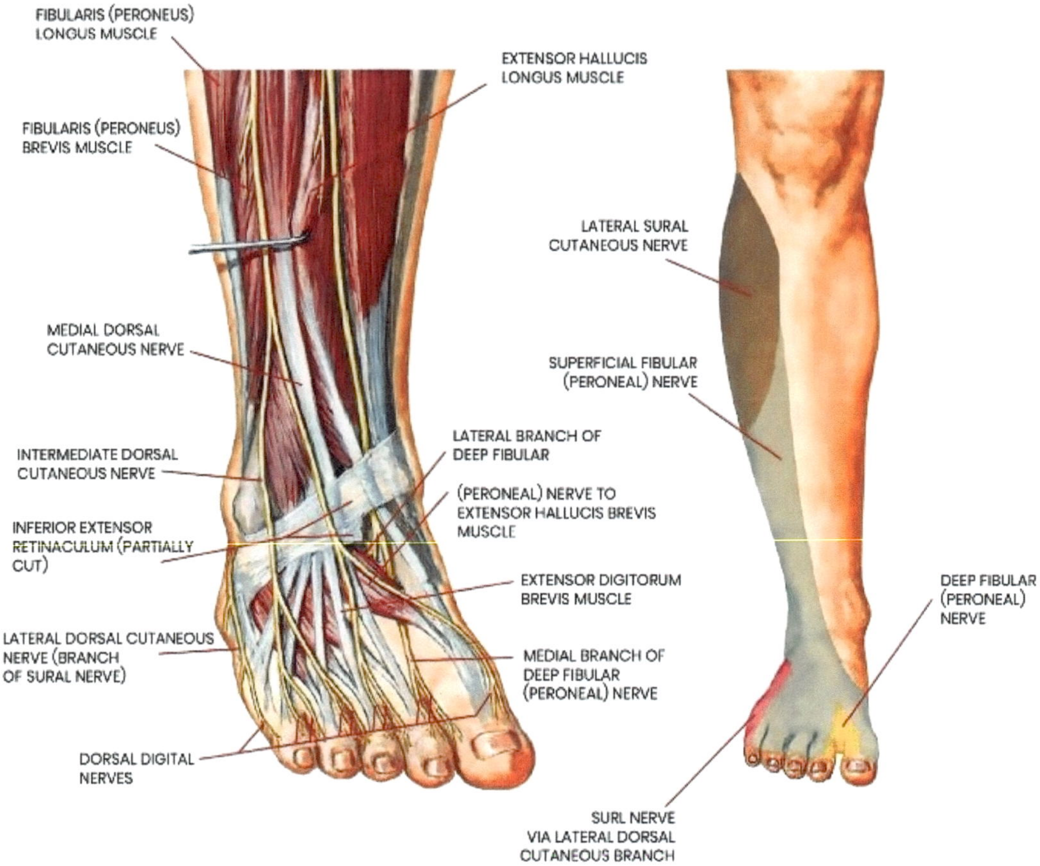

FIBULARIS (PERONEUS) LONGUS MUSCLE

FIBULARIS (PERONEUS) BREVIS MUSCLE

EXTENSOR HALLUCIS LONGUS MUSCLE

LATERAL SURAL CUTANEOUS NERVE

MEDIAL DORSAL CUTANEOUS NERVE

SUPERFICIAL FIBULAR (PERONEAL) NERVE

INTERMEDIATE DORSAL CUTANEOUS NERVE

LATERAL BRANCH OF DEEP FIBULAR

(PERONEAL) NERVE TO EXTENSOR HALLUCIS BREVIS MUSCLE

INFERIOR EXTENSOR RETINACULUM (PARTIALLY CUT)

EXTENSOR DIGITORUM BREVIS MUSCLE

DEEP FIBULAR (PERONEAL) NERVE

LATERAL DORSAL CUTANEOUS NERVE (BRANCH OF SURAL NERVE)

MEDIAL BRANCH OF DEEP FIBULAR (PERONEAL) NERVE

DORSAL DIGITAL NERVES

SURL NERVE VIA LATERAL DORSAL CUTANEOUS BRANCH

Fig. 19.8 Innervation of the dorsal foot and lower leg

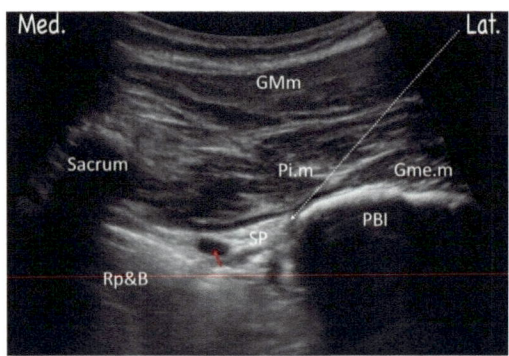

Fig. 19.9 Ultrasound image showing the anatomy for a sacral plexus block from medial (Med.) to lateral (Lat.) view, including gluteus maximus muscle (GMm), piriformis muscle (Pi.m), gluteus medius muscle (Gme.m), posterior border of ilium (PBI), sacrum, sacral plexus (SP), and retroperitoneal space and bowel (Rp&B). The red arrow is the inferior gluteal artery, the dotted white line indicates the needle path targeting the sacral plexus for local anesthetic injection

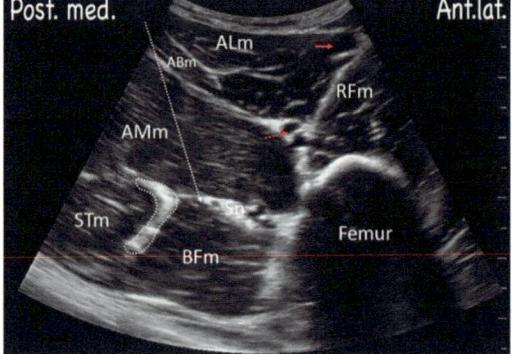

Fig. 19.10 Ultrasound image showing the anatomy for an anterior approach to the sciatic nerve block from posteromedial (Post. med.) to anterolateral (Ant. lat.) view, including adductor longus muscle (ALm), adductor brevis muscle (ABm), adductor magnus muscle (AMm), rectus femoris muscle (RFm), biceps femoris muscle (BFm), semitendinosus muscle (STm), and sciatic nerve (Sn). The dotted white line indicates the needle path, the solid red arrow marks the femoral artery, and the dotted arrow points to the location of the sciatic nerve

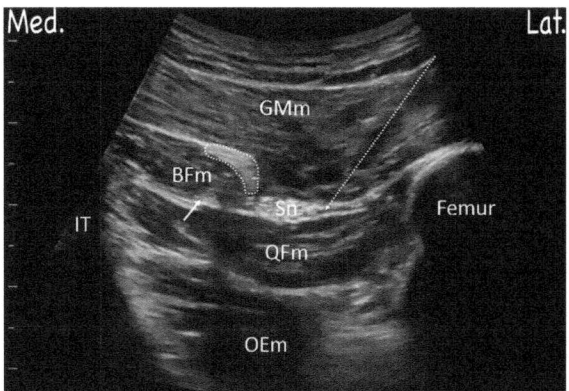

Fig. 19.11 Ultrasound image showing the anatomy for an infragluteal approach to the sciatic nerve block from medial (Med.) to lateral (Lat.) view, including gluteus maximus muscle (GMm), biceps femoris muscle (BFm), quadratus femoris muscle (QFm), obturator externus mus-

cle (OEm), sciatic nerve (Sn), femur, and ischial tuberosity (IT). The dotted white line indicates the needle path for the block, and the white arrow points to the biceps femoris muscle

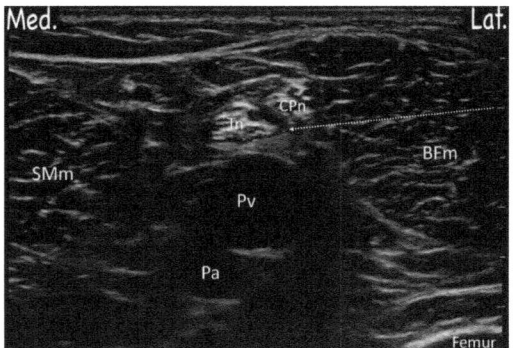

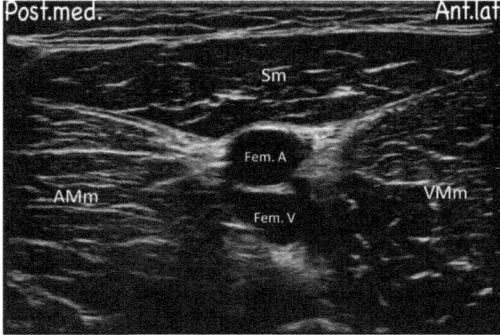

Fig. 19.12 Ultrasound image showing the anatomy for a sciatic nerve block at the popliteal fossa from medial (Med.) to lateral (Lat.) view, including semimembranosus muscle (SMm), biceps femoris muscle (BFm), tibial nerve (Tn), common peroneal nerve (CPn), popliteal vein (Pv), popliteal artery (Pa), and femur. Dotted line is needle trajectorty

Fig. 19.13 Ultrasound image showing the anatomy for an adductor canal block from posteromedial (Post. med.) to anterolateral (Ant. lat.) view, including sartorius muscle (Sm), adductor magnus muscle (AMm), vastus medialis muscle (VMm), femoral artery (Fem. A), and femoral vein (Fem. V). The double asterisk (**) indicates the saphenous nerve location within the adductor canal

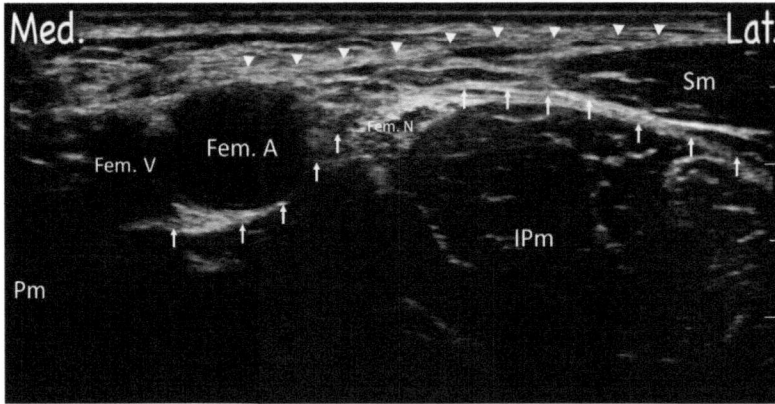

Fig. 19.14 Ultrasound image showing the anatomy for an infrainguinal fascia iliaca block from medial (Med.) to lateral (Lat.) view, including pectineus muscle (Pm), ilio-psoas muscle (IPm), sartorius muscle (Sm), femoral artery (Fem. A), femoral vein (Fem. V), and femoral nerve (Fem. N)

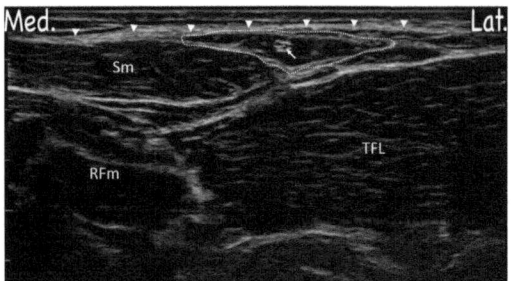

Fig. 19.15 Ultrasound image showing the anatomy for a lateral femoral cutaneous nerve block from medial (Med.) to lateral (Lat.) view, including sartorius muscle (Sm), rectus femoris muscle (RFm), tensor fasciae latae muscle (TFL), and the fascial plane. The white arrowheads indicate the fascia iliaca, the dotted outline shows the potential space for the injection, and the small white arrow points to the lateral femoral cutaneous nerve within the interfascial plane

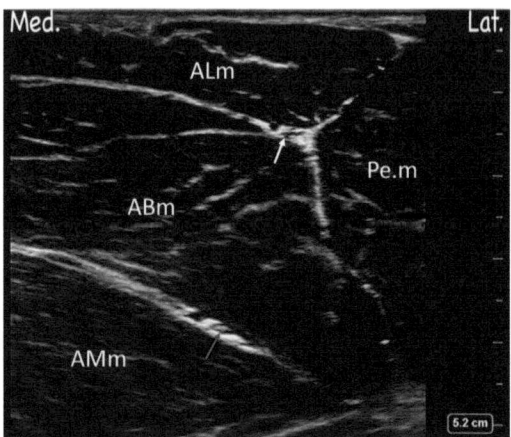

Fig. 19.16 Ultrasound image showing the anatomy for the division of the obturator nerve from medial (Med.) to lateral (Lat.) view, including adductor longus muscle (ALm), adductor brevis muscle (ABm), adductor magnus muscle (AMm), and pectineus muscle (Pe.m). The white arrow indicates the anterior division of the obturator nerve, while the red arrow points to the posterior division of the obturator nerve as it courses between the adductor muscles

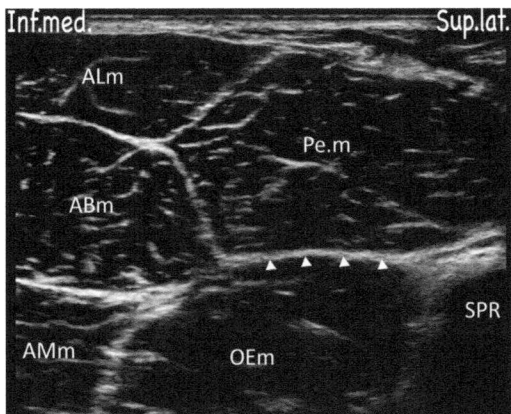

Fig. 19.17 Ultrasound image showing the anatomy of the subpectineal plane for the obturator nerve block from inferomedial (Inf. med.) to superolateral (Sup. lat.) view, including adductor longus muscle (ALm), adductor brevis muscle (ABm), adductor magnus muscle (AMm), obturator externus muscle (OEm), pectineus muscle (Pe.m), and superior pubic ramus (SPR). The white arrowheads indicate the subpectineal plane

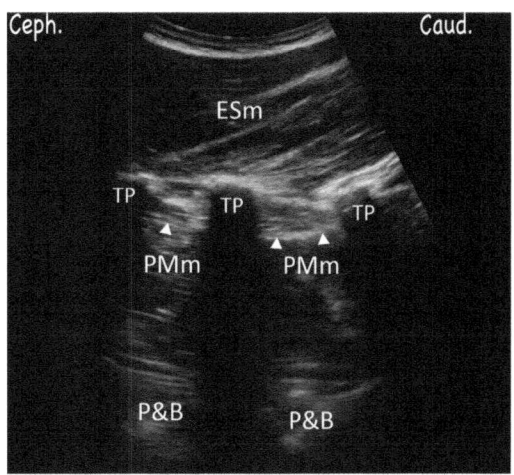

Fig. 19.19 Ultrasound image showing the anatomy for a lumbar plexus block using the Trident sign from cephalad (Ceph.) to caudal (Caud.) view, including erector spinae muscle (ESm), psoas major muscle (PMm), transverse processes (TP), and peritoneum and bowel (P&B). The white arrowheads indicate the location of the psoas major muscle between the transverse processes, forming the characteristic Trident sign configuration for the lumbar plexus block

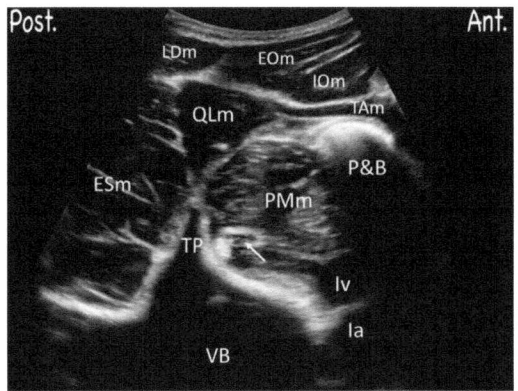

Fig. 19.18 Ultrasound image showing the anatomy for a lumbar plexus block using the Shamrock sign from posterior (Post.) to anterior (Ant.) view, including latissimus dorsi muscle (LDm), external oblique muscle (EOm), internal oblique muscle (IOm), transversus abdominis muscle (TAm), quadratus lumborum muscle (QLm), erector spinae muscle (ESm), psoas major muscle (PMm), transverse process (TP), vertebral body (VB), iliac vein (Iv), iliac artery (Ia), and peritoneum and bowel (P&B). The white arrow points to the psoas major muscle, while the dotted interface represents the Shamrock sign configuration for the lumbar plexus block

- Sural nerve (branch of the common peroneal and tibial nerve): supplies the lateral aspect of foot.
- Posterior tibial nerve: supplies the deep ventral structures, muscles and sole of foot.
- Superficial peroneal nerve: supplies the dorsum of foot.
- Deep peroneal nerve: supplies the deeper dorsal structures and the web space between the first and second toe.
- Saphenous nerve: supplies the medial aspect of the foot.

The peripheral regional anaesthesia techniques include:

- Popliteal sciatic nerve block (supplemented with saphenous nerve block)
- Ankle block

Ankle block can be performed using a landmark-guided, peripheral nerve stimulator-guided, or ultrasound-guided approach. Complications associated with this block are minimal. Most of them are associated with the ankle tourniquet or the injection itself. Some patients may develop transient paraesthesias. The incidence of LAST is extremely rare, given the low volume of local anaesthetic used for the block.

7. Enumerate concerns of RA for infected foot amputation

Local anaesthetics act by blocking the sodium channels after crossing the neuronal membrane. In the case of local infections, the pH of the surrounding tissue is acidaemic, thus rendering more of the local anaesthetic molecules in the ionised state. The ionised portion of the local anaesthetic does not cross the neuronal membrane, making it less effective.

The fraction of ionisation depends upon the pKa of the local anaesthetic. A local anaesthetic agent with a pKa close to the tissue pH will have lower ionization and be more effective. This explains why lignocaine with a pKa of 7.8 has a faster onset of action than bupivacaine with a pKa of 8.1. So, to improve the efficacy of the local anaesthetic agent, bicarbonate may be added to the solution, which makes the pH more alkaline. This increases the unionized fraction of local anaesthetic available.

8. Describe the WALANT technique used for limb amputation

WALANT (wide-awake, local anaesthesia, no tourniquet technique) has recently become popular for upper and lower limb surgeries, especially in patients with significant comorbidities.

This technique involves injecting dilute local anaesthetic in and around the operative area. Lignocaine is the commonly used local anaesthetic for the WALANT technique. The local anaesthetic is mixed with normal saline to increase the volume of the solution and infiltrate a larger area.

Carpal tunnel release, tendon transfer, ankle fixations, and toe amputations are some of the surgeries performed under the WALANT technique.

9. Perineural catheters (PNCs) for major lower limb amputation

PNCs are inserted close to the major nerves, such as the tibial and sciatic nerve, for below and above knee amputations. The surgeons place the catheters intra-operatively, under direct vision. The use of PNCs has been associated with lower post-op pain scores and opioid consumption. The evidence of PNCs effect on chronic stump pain, phantom limb pain and mortality is lacking.

10. Discuss about pain following amputation

Pain intensity before amputation has been established to be a reliable risk factor for experiencing post-operative pain of varying intensity.

The types of pain associated with lower limb amputations include:

- Ischaemic limb pain
- Residual limb pain: It typically begins within 1–2 weeks post-amputation and may be severe in 5–10% of patients. The pain will lessen as the wound heals, but it may get prolonged if complications such as infection, wound dehiscence, or osteomyelitis set in.
- Phantom limb pain: It typically begins within 1–7 days. It may be severe in 5–10% of patients and persist for months to years. It may be intermittent or constant, and the nature of pain can vary from aching to shooting, stabbing, burning, or throbbing.
- Phantom limb sensation: onset within 1–7 days. It is seen in up to 90% of patients. It can persist for months to years. Patients experience non-painful sensations, often perceived as the existence of a deformed or twisted limb.
- Other musculoskeletal pain: this may occur because of a change in mechanics due to the amputated limb. Patients may have back, hip or knee pain and occasional gait abnormalities.

11. **Analgesia modalities used for phantom limb pain (PLP)**

The pathophysiology of PLP is multifactorial. It is believed to be mediated via peripheral, spinal cord, and cerebral mechanisms.

It manifests as persistent postoperative pain and phantom sensations, which are resistant to frequently used analgesic and psychotropic drugs.

A multidisciplinary approach starting before amputation should be attempted, which includes patient information, multi-modal analgesia regime and psychological assessment, but these are met with inconsistent results.

Peripheral nerve block techniques have been suggested as the best method for attenuating phantom limb pain. This has been theorized to be due to the inhibition of peripheral nociceptive stimuli and prevention of the establishment of central sensitisation by using LA at the site of nerve trauma.

12. **Enumerate peri-operative multi-modal analgesia for limb amputation**

Preoperative Stage
Patient information and assessment of psychological status.

Insert an epidural or peripheral regional catheter for infusion of LA preoperatively.

Intraoperative Stage
Establish regional anaesthesia (neuraxial or nerve block) before incision. General anaesthesia, if planned, must be complimented with regional anaesthesia.

Intraoperative ketamine infusion.

Add paracetamol and NSAID (based on renal and liver profile).

IV magnesium or clonidine should be considered.

The use of systemic opioids should be carefully assessed.

Postoperative Phase
Continue the above-mentioned dosing schedule for 24 to 72 h, as tolerated.

Follow a multidisciplinary approach by taking relevant inputs from a pain physician and a psychiatrist.

Gabapentinoids, calcitonin and non-pharmacological therapies should be considered for refractory PLP.

Patient communication and education, especially at the time of discharge.

Questions
1. An elderly patient with an infected amputated stump of leg is now scheduled to undergo amputation above the level of the knee. Which evoked motor response can be accepted for a proximal approach of sciatic nerve block, while using a peripheral nerve stimulator?
2. How will you assess the effectiveness of the obturator nerve block?
3. Discuss non-pharmacological methods of treatment of phantom limb pain.
4. What is the evidence of the role of gabapentinoids for treatment of phantom limb pain?
5. Describe a treatment plan for upper limb amputation.
6. Which superficial nerves should be targeted for tourniquet pain?
7. Discuss the anaesthesia plan for midfoot amputation.
8. What are the anaesthesia implications of local anaesthetic agents in case of infected foot amputation while performing ankle block?
9. What are the analgesia options for stump pain?
10. What is the role of pre-emptive stellate ganglion block for prevention of post-amputation pain for upper limb amputation?
11. Discuss the anaesthesia options for ray amputation of foot.

Suggested Reading

1. Melsom H, Danjoux G. Perioperative care for lower limb amputation in vascular disease. Contin. Educ. Anaesth. Crit. Care Pain. 2011;5(11):162–6.

2. Mufarrih SH, Qureshi NQ, Schaefer MS, Sharkey A, Fatima H, Chaudhary O, Krumm S, Baribeau V, Mahmood F, Schermerhorn M, Matyal R. Regional anaesthesia for lower extremity amputation is associated with reduced post-operative complications compared with general anaesthesia. Eur J Vasc Endovasc Surg. 2021 Sep;62(3):476–84.

3. Malik O, Brovman EY, Urman RD. The use of regional or neuraxial anesthesia for below-knee amputations may reduce the need for perioperative blood transfusions. Reg Anesth Pain Med. 2018;43:25e35.

4. Moreira CC, Farber A, Kalish JA, Eslami MH, Didato S, Rybin D, et al. The effect of anesthesia type on major lower extremity amputation in functionally impaired elderly patients. J Vasc Surg. 2016;63:696–701.

5. Khan S, Qianyi R, Liu C, Ng E, Fook-Chong S, Tan M. Effect of anaesthetic technique on mortality following major lower extremity amputation: a propensity score-matched observational study. Anaesthesia. 2013;68:612e20.

6. Niskakangas M, Dahlbacka S, Liisanantti J, Vakkala M, Kaakinen T. Spinal or general anaesthesia for lower-limb amputation in peripheral artery disease e a retrospective cohort study. Acta Anaesthesiol Scand. 2018;62:226e33.

7. Awad IT, Duggan EM. Posterior lumbar plexus block: anatomy, approaches, and techniques. Reg. Anesth. Pain Med. 2005;30:143–9.

8. Shevlin S, Johnston D, Turbitt. The sciatic nerve block. Br J Anesthesia Educ. 2020;20(9):312–20.

9. Albaqami MS, Alqarni AA. Efficacy of regional anesthesia using ankle block in ankle and foot surgeries: a systematic review. Eur Rev. Med Pharmacol Sci. 2022 Jan;26(2):471–84.

10. Sinnott CJ, Garfield JM, Thalhammer JG, Strichartz GR. Addition of sodium bicarbonate to lidocaine decreases the duration of peripheral nerve block in the rat. Anesthesiology. 2000 Oct;93(4):1045–52.

11. Bajuri MY, Saidfudin NS, Marzli N, Azriq N, Azemi AF. Safety of wide-awake local anesthesia with no tourniquet (WALANT) in for lower limb surgery: a potential alternative in times of emergency. Front. Surg. 2022;9:848422. https://doi.org/10.3389/fsurg.2022.848422.

12. Morey TE, Giannoni J, Duncan E, Scarborough MT, Enneking FK. Nerve sheath catheter analgesia after amputation. Clin Orthop Relat Res. 2002;397:281–9.

13. Borghi B, D'Addabbo M, et al. The use of prolonged peripheral neural blockade after lower extremity amputation: the effect on symptoms associated with phantom limb syndrome. Anesth Analg. 2010;111(5):1308–15.

14. Nikolajsen L, Ilkjaer S, Christensen JH, Krøner K, Jensen TS. Randomised trial of epidural bupivacaine and morphine in prevention of stump and phantom pain in lower-limb amputation. Lancet. 1997;350:1353–7.

15. Naughtin S, Erskine R. Management of postamputation limb pain. R I Med J. 2013;103(4):19–22.

Analgesia for Ankle and Foot Surgery

Namita Sharma

Clinical Scenario

A 54 year old man sustained a stable tri malleolar fracture of his left ankle whilst playing football 5 days previously. He is listed on the trauma list for open reduction and internal fixation of this injury. The swelling around his ankle joint has reduced adequately for surgery to proceed. He has primary polycythaemia rubra vera which is controlled with hydroxyurea and he is a smoker of 10 a day for 30 years.

1. **What are the key clinical considerations in this patient?**

Anaesthetic

Age: Age related changes can occur on all body systems notably the cardiovascular system with atherosclerosis, IHD, hypertension and deep vein thrombosis increasing in frequency.

Hydroxyurea: Effects on bone marrow and cell lines therefore potential increased chance of infection or bleeding.

Smoking: Increased airway reactivity, mucous production and coughing during the procedure (if awake) and a possibility of undiagnosed COPD and/or IHD.

Positioning: Possible lateral positioning of patient which is a consideration for pressure point protection and airway management during general anaesthesia or patient comfort during potential 'awake' surgery with the need for sedation.

Surgical

Polycythaemia: Increased chance of blood clots and therefore meticulous anticoagulation in peri operative period.

Smoking: Delayed wound healing and increased chance of infection.

Tri malleolar fracture: Increased operating time as three fractures to be treated.

2. **What is meant by a tri- malleolar ankle fracture?**

There are three bones which make up the ankle joint (Fig. 20.1):

- Tibia
- Fibula
- Talus

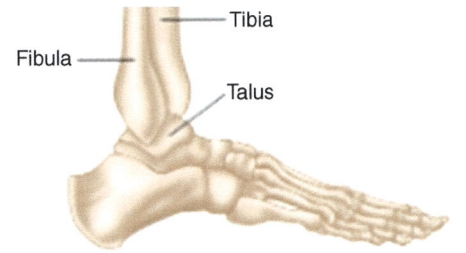

Fig. 20.1 Three bones of ankle joint

N. Sharma (✉)
Ashford and St Peter's Hospital, Chertsey, UK
e-mail: namita.sharma@nhs.net

Two joints are involved in ankle fractures:

- Ankle joint—where the tibia, fibula and talus meet.
- Syndesmosis joint—the joint between the tibia and fibula which is held together by ligaments.
- Ankle fractures can be described as non-displaced; displaced or open fractures.

A trimalleolar fracture involves the lateral malleolus, the medial malleolus, and the distal posterior aspect of the tibia, (the posterior malleolus). A bimalleolar fracture when the both the medial and lateral malleolus are fractured. Since the injuries are on both sides of the ankle the ankle can be quite unstable and often dislocated. They can be treated conservatively or surgically.

A trimalleolar fracture is a bimalleolar injury but with the addition of a fractured posterior malleolus. If the fracture is considered unstable surgical intervention will be required.

3. **Describe the sensory innervation of the foot and ankle (Table 20.1)?**

4. **What are the choices of regional anaesthesia for foot and ankle surgery (Table 20.2)?**

5. **What would be your analgesia regime of choice be in this patient?**

Pre Operatively or Intra Operatively

- Paracetamol, NSAIDs and COX 2 specific inhibitors

Intra operatively

- IV Dexamethasone for PONV prophylaxis and it also enhances the impact of the regional anaesthetic technique
- Adductor canal and popliteal nerve block but a femoral and sciatic nerve would be considered if conducting awake surgery with a thigh tourniquet.
- GA/sedation additional to nerve blocks if deemed necessary but combined adductor canal and popliteal nerve block allows opera-

Table 20.1 Sensory innervation of foot and ankle

Nerves	Considerations	Joint supply	Cutaneous supply
Tibial nerve	Should be blocked first as largest of ankle nerves and therefore longest onset time. Divides into three branches: Medial calcaneal branch; medial and lateral plantar nerves.	Talus Calcaneus Navicular Cunieforms Cuboid Metatarsals Phalanges	Plantar aspect of the foot
Saphenous nerve		Medial malleolus Talus Medial phalanx	Medial aspect of leg and foot
Superficial peroneal nerve			Dorsal aspect of the foot
Deep peroneal nerve		Talus Calcaneus Navicular Cunieforms Cuboid Metatarsals Phalanges	1st webspace of the foot
Sural nerve		Lateral malleolus Talus Calcaneus Cuboid (rarely)	*Lateral malleolus and the fifth phalanx in both plantar and dorsal aspects*

Table 20.2   Various regional blocks for foot and ankle surgery

Analgesic procedure	Advantages	Disadvantages	Contraindications
Intrathecal analgesia	Relatively easy technique Shorter acting agents such as 2 Chloroprocaine and hyperbaric prilocaine allow assessment of neurology quicker Can control thigh tourniquet pain	Effect on sympathetic innervation (urinary retention and hypotension) Respiratory depression related to intrathecal use Pruritis Unnecessary bilateral block Risk of infection and nerve damage Delays mobilisation A dense block could mask compartment syndrome	Elevated intracranial pressure Infection on the injection site Risk of hypotension (hypovolaemia) Thrombocytopaenia or coagulopathy Patient inability to get into position Allergy to LA Bleeding diatheses
Femoral nerve block	Easy access with or without ultrasound guidance Excellent analgesia Good predictable course of catheter with ultrasound guidance Can control thigh tourniquet pain (with sciatic/popliteal block)	Delays mobilisation High risk of falls	Infection on the injection site If no US/S guidance anatomical anomalies affecting landmark identification Pre existing neuropathies affecting the distribution of the block
Adductor canal block (ACB)	Allows early mobilisation and recovery times Continuous techniques provide the highest analgesic effect Easy ultrasound guided access Can control thigh tourniquet pain (with popliteal/sciatic block)	Tunnelling is required in some cases	Infection on the injection site If no US/S guidance anatomical anomalies affecting landmark identification Pre existing neuropathies affecting the distribution of the block
Sciatic nerve block (posterior)	Analgesia to the ankle and foot Provides analgesia for thigh tourniquet	Relatively deep block Requires semi prone/prone position Delays mobilisation A dense block could mask compartment syndrome	Infection on the injection site If no US/S guidance anatomical anomalies affecting landmark identification Pre existing neuropathies affecting the distribution of the block
Popliteal block	Analgesia to the ankle and foot Provides analgesia for a calf tourniquet	Relatively deep block Requires semi prone/prone position Delays mobilisation A dense block could mask compartment syndrome	Infection on the injection site If no US/S guidance anatomical anomalies affecting landmark identification Pre existing neuropathies affecting the distribution of the block
Ankle block	Less impairment of mobility compared to a proximal block Relative easy block to conduct	Does not provide analgesia if a tourniquet is being applied Forefoot and toe surgery only	Infection on the injection site
Local Anaesthetic infiltration (LAI)	Easy intraoperative mobilisation Adjuvant analgesic effect	Increased risk of toxicity Short analgesic effect Risk of infections with intraarticular catheter	

(continued)

Table 20.2 (continued)

Analgesic procedure	Advantages	Disadvantages	Contraindications
Digital nerve blocks	Often landmark guided but can be located with ultrasound Simple to perform Can be performed on all 5 digits 'Rescue block' is needed	Only for distal toe surgery	

tion to be conducted under regional anaesthesia alone.

- Nerve blocks have been found to have a more opiate sparing effect post operatively compared to central neuraxial blockade

Post operatively
- Paracetamol, NSAIDs and COX 2 specific inhibitors continued post operatively
- Opioids for rescue post operative relief
- NSAIDS and COX2 inhibitors should be given for under 2 weeks duration postoperatively to reduce the risk of bone non union to that of patients who do not take NSAIDs post operatively.

6. **Would you conduct regional anaesthesia in patients who are deemed to be at high risk of developing compartment syndrome?**

Acute compartment syndrome has a reported incidence of 3.1 in 100,000 with a range of 1–7.3 in 100,000. It is 10 times more common in men which is accentuated by the fact men suffer the fractures that are associated with ACS more commonly (13:1). Up to 40% of all ACS episodes involve a tibial shaft fracture and approximately 4–5% of all tibial fractures result in ACS.

There is a paucity of high quality data on this topic with most being case reports and case series.

With full informed consent from the patient and a discussion with the surgical team, I would advocate the use of a single shot or peri-neural catheter regional techniques using low dose local anaesthesia such as 0.1–0.25% Ropivicaine or Bupivicaine for single shot and 0.1% for continuous regional anaesthesia. This would be in conjunction with other multimodal strategies in both the adult and paediatric population.

Suggested Reading

1. Moosa F, Allan A, Bedforth N. Regional anaesthesia for foot and ankle surgery. Br J Anaesth Educ. 2022;22(11):424–31.
2. Sort R, Brorson S, et al. Peripheral nerve block anaesthesia and postoperative pain in acute ankle fracture surgery: the AnAnkle randomised trial. Br J Anaesth. 2021;126(4):881–8.
3. Bjorn S, Wong WY, Baas J, et al. The Importance of the Saphenous Nerve Block for Analgesia Following Major Ankle Surgery A Randomized, Controlled, Double-Blind Study. Reg Anaesth Pain Med. 2018;43(5):474–9.
4. Al Farii H, Farahdel L, Frazer A, et al. The effect of NSAIDs on post fracture bone healing: a meta analysis of randomised control trials. OTA Int. 2021;4(2):e092.
5. Klucka J, Stourac P, Stouracova A, Masek M, Repko M. Compartment syndrome and regional anaesthesia: critical review. Biomed Papers. 2017;161:242–51.
6. McQueen M, Gaston P, Court-Brown C. Acute compartment syndrome. Who is at risk? J Bone Joint Surg. 2000;82-B:200–3.
7. Garner M, Taylor S, Gausden E, Lyden J. Compartment syndrome: diagnosis, management and unique concerns in the twenty-first century. Musculoskelet J Hosp Spec Surg. 2014;10:143–52.
8. Mabvuure NT, Malahias M, Hindocha S, Khan W, Juma A. Acute compartment syndrome of the limbs: current concept sand management. Open Orthop. J. 2012;6:535–43.
9. Ganeshan R, Mamoowala N, Ward M, Sochart D. Acute compartment syndrome risk in fracture fixation with regional blocks. BMJ Case Rep. 2015:bcr2015210499.

Analgesia for Perineal Surgery

21

Arunangshu Chakraborty and Amit Dixit

Case Scenario

A 20-year-old male is scheduled for hypospadias surgery. What are the strategies that you will consider for perioperative analgesia?

1. **Describe the Nerve supply of male/female genitalia**

The cutaneous nerve supply of male and female genitalia can be divided into three sections (Fig. 21.1):

1. Nerve supply from descending branches of the thoracolumbar spinal nerves such as ilioinguinal nerve (IIN), iliohypogastric nerve (IHN) (T12, L1), genitofemoral nerve (GFN) (L1–2) which supply the pubic and suprapubic area.
   - IHN innervates the posterolateral gluteal and suprapubic skin.
   - IIN innervates the skin of the proximal medial thigh and the skin over the root of the penis and upper part of the scrotum (anterior third) in males or the skin covering the mons pubis and the adjoining labium majus in females.
   - The genitofemoral nerve, which innervates the skin of the scrotum in males or that of the mons pubis and labium majus in females via its genital branch, plays a critical role in the inguinoscrotal descent of the developing testis. It also innervates the anteromedial skin of the thigh via its femoral branch.

2. Posterior: The posterior cutaneous nerve of the thigh (aka the posterior femoral cutaneous nerve) is a sensory nerve derived from the sacral plexus (S1–3). It arises partly from the dorsal divisions of the S1 and S2 and the ventral divisions of the S2 and S3 sacral spinal nerves. It supplies the skin of the posterior thigh, buttock and posterior aspect of the scrotum or labia.

3. Branches of the pudendal nerve (PN) (S2–4) (Fig. 21.2):
   - Dorsal nerve of the penis/clitoris: innervates the penis/clitoris respectively.
   - Perineal nerve: The perineal nerve is the second and the largest of the three branches of the pudendal nerve. It typically arises in the last portion of the Alcock's canal or just as the pudendal nerve exits it. The perineal nerve bifurcates into deep (muscular) and superficial (cutaneous) perineal nerves.
   - The deep branch supplies the muscles of the urogenital triangle (bulbospongiosus, ischiocavernosus and superficial transverse perineal muscle), the external urethral sphincter and the ante-

A. Chakraborty (✉)
Sultan Qaboos Comprehensive Cancer Care and Research Center, Muscat, Oman

A. Dixit
Department of Anaesthesia, Ruby Hall Hospital, Pune, India

S. Phillips et al. (eds.), *Regional Anaesthesia*, https://doi.org/10.1007/978-3-032-05165-3_21

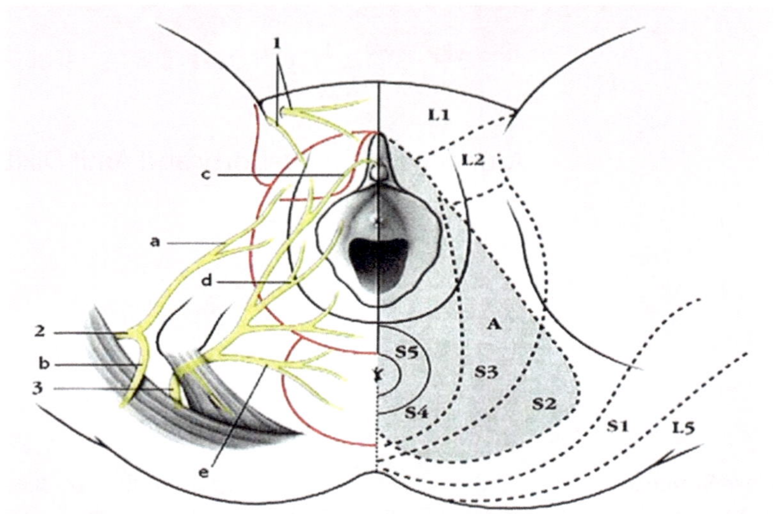

Fig. 21.1 Innervation of the perineum: 1: Ilioinguinal, Iliohypogastric and Genitofemoral nerves; 2: Posterior cutaneous nerve of thigh—a: perineal branch, b: inferior clunial nerve; 3: Pudendal nerve and branches—c: dorsal nerve of clitoris (penis in males), d: perineal nerve, e: inferior rectal nerve; A: Area supplied by the pudendal nerve

Fig. 21.2 Anatomy of pudendal nerve. (Source: Häggström M. Medical gallery of Mikael Häggström 2014. WikiJ Med. 2014:1(2). https:// doi.org/10.15347/ wjm/2014.008. ISSN 2002-4436)

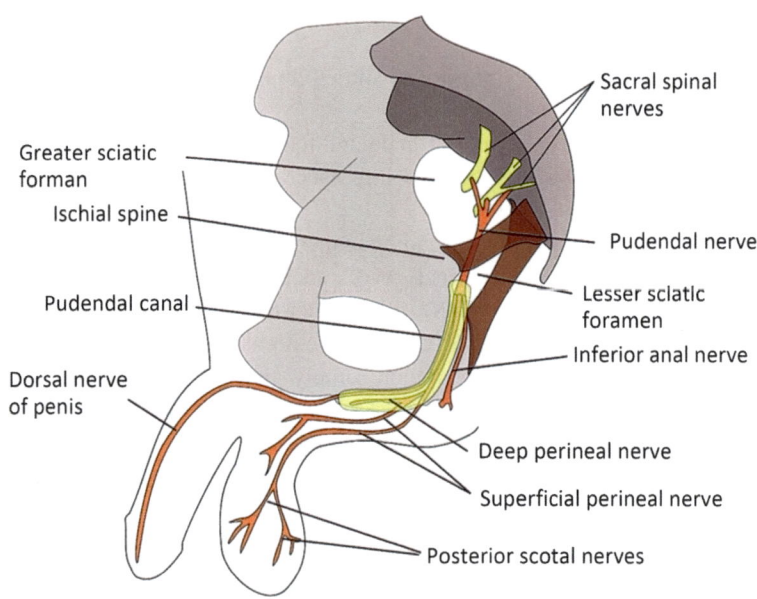

rior parts of the external anal sphincter and levator ani.

- The superficial branch of the perineal nerve provides sensory supply to the posterior scrotal area in males, and the labia minora, vaginal vestibule, lower one-fifth of the vaginal canal and the

posterior aspect of the labia majora in females.

- Inferior rectal nerve (aka inferior anal nerve): It arises directly from the sacral plexus in some individuals. The inferior anal nerve is a mixed nerve that provides sensory supply to the inferior portion of the anal canal (till the pectinate line) and the circumanal skin and motor supply to the external anal sphincter. In addition, the inferior anal nerve may provide sensory innervation to the lower part of the posterior wall of the vagina in females.

Nerve supply of the testes?

The testis is innervated either by

1. Nerve fibres that arise from the tenth and eleventh thoracic spinal segments via the renal and aortic plexuses and accompany the testicular vessels or
2. Fibres that arise from the pelvic plexus and accompany the vas deferens. Some afferent and efferent nerves have been shown to cross over to the contralateral pelvic plexus.

Autonomic innervation of the male/female external genitalia

Ans: The penis/clitoris in male/female respectively derives its autonomic innervation from the pelvic plexus. The nerve supply of the upper vagina is autonomic and derived from the utero-vaginal plexus, which is a subsidiary of the inferior hypogastric plexus.

2. **Discuss the mechanism of pain following gender reassignment surgery**

Ans: Postoperative pain after gender reassignment surgery has both somatic and visceral components. The somatic pain is mediated via the spinal nerves of T12, L1, L2 and S2–4, namely the IHN, IIN, GFN, PN and the posterior cutaneous nerve of the thigh. The visceral component is derived from the innervation of the testes, the 10th and 11th thoracic spinal nerves and the pelvic plexus. Key considerations in a patient undergoing gender reassignment surgery include

(a) Comorbidities and hormone replacement therapy
(b) History of multiple drug abuse
(c) Major surgery with a high risk of perioperative bleeding
(d) Postoperative analgesia
(e) Risk of venous thromboembolism and stroke postoperatively

3. **What are the analgesic options for intraoperative and postoperative pain management in gender reassignment surgery:**

Multimodal opioid-sparing analgesia is recommended for this patient include:
- Paracetamol
- Non-steroidal anti-inflammatory drugs (NSAIDs), including parenteral COX-II inhibitors
- Strong Opioids—Fentanyl, Oxycodone (exercise caution to prevent habit forming). Patient-controlled analgesia (PCA) pumps are provided with caution.
- Dexamethasone 4–8 mg intravenous single dose
- Low-dose Ketamine
- Other adjuncts—Alpha-2 agonists (Clonidine, Dexmedetomidine)
- Single shot spinal Local anaesthetic (Bupivacaine) with or without opioids—Morphine, Diamorphine
- The surgical team infiltrates the local site with local anaesthetics at the beginning and end of the surgery, using either standard bupivacaine or liposomal bupivacaine.
- Fascial Plane Blocks (FPB) are used at the beginning of surgery, such as the IIN and IHN block with additional spermatic cord and penile blocks.
- Caudal epidural—single shot or with continuous catheter

Postoperative pain relief:
- In addition to paracetamol and weak opioids such as Codeine, Dihydrocodeine, Tramadol
- Patients may need potent opioids either orally or via IV-PCA for the first 24 h.
- Continuous caudal analgesia

4. Enumerate the Benefits of using caudal epidural in perineal surgeries:

Caudal (also termed sacral) epidural is a well-established modality for perineal and pelvic surgeries. Caudal epidural is the only modality of regional anaesthesia apart from spinal anaesthesia that can provide complete analgesia for a major perineal surgery such as gender reassignment surgery, as it can cover all three different segments of innervation of the perineum as explained above, with the additional advantage of providing postoperative analgesia.

In a patient who is a reformed opioid abuser, caudal analgesia is preferable as it can allow opioid free perioperative analgesia. Preoperative siting of the caudal epidural catheter would be ideal for this patient. After insertion, the entry site should be wiped dry and covered with a transparent adhesive waterproof dressing. An anaesthetic regime for caudal analgesia can include a bolus dose of 25–30 ml LA (bupivacaine 0.25% or ropivacaine 0.2%) followed by an infusion of 5–8 ml/h, titrated to the degree of analgesia.

5. What are the disadvantages of caudal analgesia in perineal surgeries:

Disadvantages of caudal analgesia include:
  (a) Contraindications in local infections/inflammations/skin disease/excoriations
  (b) The perianal area is a source of faecal infection, and an indwelling catheter inserted through the caudal route bears the risk of infection, leading to meningitis and adhesive arachnoiditis.
  (c) For perineal surgery, the caudal catheter site of entry is close to the area of surgery and thus can get soiled during the operation. Even if it is placed postoperatively, the discharge from the surgical wound can soil/soak it.

6. What is the role of intrathecal opioids

The use of single doses of intrathecal hydrophilic opioids like morphine or diamorphine has recently gained popularity as it provides good analgesia for 18–24 h, reduces IV opioid consumption, and at doses below 300 µg, the risk of respiratory depression is negligible.

7. Discuss the fascial plane blocks that can be used for this patient

Fascial plane blocks that can be used in a case of gender reassignment surgery include the IIN-IHN block and the Sacral Erector Spinae Plane (S-ESP) block.

Mechanism of S-ESP: Although S-ESP blocks mostly the dorsal sacral nerves, the presence of sacral foramina allows some LA to enter the ventral area, which houses the sacral plexus where the pudendal nerve and the posterior cutaneous nerve of the thigh originate from. A recently described modification of the S-ESP, the ultrasound-guided sacral foramen injection (USFI), can reportedly achieve ventral egress of LA and provide perineal analgesia.

In this technique, the injection endpoint is above the opening of the second sacral foramen. Single-shot injection is to be employed on both sides. Catheters can be placed by using a Tuohy needle. An initial bolus of 15–20 ml 0.2% ropivacaine bilaterally is followed by an infusion of 4–5 ml 0.2% ropivacaine in continuous technique.

8. Regional anaesthesia techniques can be contemplated in patients undergoing gender reassignment surgeries:

No single regional anaesthesia technique/block can provide complete analgesia of the perineum, particularly in a major surgery such as this one. A combination of blocks can be helpful to address all the segments of innervation of the perineum, as described above.

1. **Simple perineal infiltration:**

Perineal infiltration is to be performed in two planes:

  (a) the superficial plane represented by the skin and the subcutaneous tissue whose infiltration is performed along the path of the incision;

  (b) The deep plane involving the muscles of the ischiorectal fossa is infiltrated with LA in a fanning manner.

2. **Posterior perineal block:**

This block combines infiltration close to the nerves via the transperineal route and the infiltration of the superficial and deep perianal nerves. It is performed in the patient in a lithotomy position, preferably under general anaesthesia. Extensive disinfection of the perineum and anal canal should be carried out. The essence of the technique lies in introducing a finger in the rectum, which not only allows to guide the needle in the various muscle planes and towards the landmark bone but also, above all, to avoid any penetration of the needle into the rectal lumen. Using a needle 24 G with short bevel of 50 mm and two 20 ml syringes of LA. Three spaces are infiltrated in the following way:

  (a) the presacral space: the intrarectal finger locates the concavity of the sacrum, and 5 ml of LA is injected

  (b) the right and left ischiorectal spaces: the tuberosity ischial bone is identified by a clamp formed by the intrarectal finger and the thumb. The needle is inserted upwards and inwards over 1 cm, and then 7.5 ml of LA is injected on each side

  (c) the peri-sphincter block is performed by injecting 5 ml of LA in the four perianal quadrants (12, 3, 6 and 9 o'clock positions), piercing perpendicular to the sphincter up to 3–4 cm deep.

This block is fraught with the risk of transmission of Hepatitis C infection in this patient and should be avoided.

3. **Pudendal nerve block:**

The pudendal nerve can be blocked using a transperineal approach, a landmark-based approach, or the guidance of a peripheral nerve stimulator (PNS) or ultrasound.

Anatomy

The pudendal nerve arises from the ventral rami of the sacral plexus (S2–4). It is called the nerve of the perineum as it supplies the perineum and muscles within the perineum, penis, external anal sphincter and posterior 2/3 of the scrotum.

PNS-guided technique: The pudendal block is performed with a patient in a lithotomy position, preferably under general anaesthesia or sedation. The point of the puncture is at the intersection of the medial edge of the tuberosity of the ischial bone and a horizontal straight line passing through the upper edge of the anus. After local skin infiltration with LA, a 100 mm short bevel insulated needle connected to PNS is introduced perpendicular to the skin in a horizontal plane and sagittally by walking off the medial edge of the ischial tuberosity. The crossing of the perineal aponeurosis is sometimes noticeable. After decreasing the intensity of the current stimulation between 0.5 and 1 mA, the optimal motor responses sought are:

- a contraction of the sphincter of the anus (lower rectal response) and
- vulvar and bulbocavernosus muscle contraction (perineal response) and
- contraction of the clitoral region (clitoral response) and penile region in males.

These three motor responses may be concurrent often. Refining the search by mobilising the needle slightly up or down is also possible. On a collective of 62 blocks performed in 45 patients, in 52% of cases, the motor response is of the lower rectal and perineal type, in 27% of lower rectal cases, in 11% of perineal cases, in 8% of cases, lower rectum, perineum and clitoris. Lack of motor response was noted in 2% of cases. The average depth is 45.1 ± 11.6 mm (25–80 mm). Ten to 15 ml of LA can be injected on each side, a total of 20–30 ml. Adrenaline should be

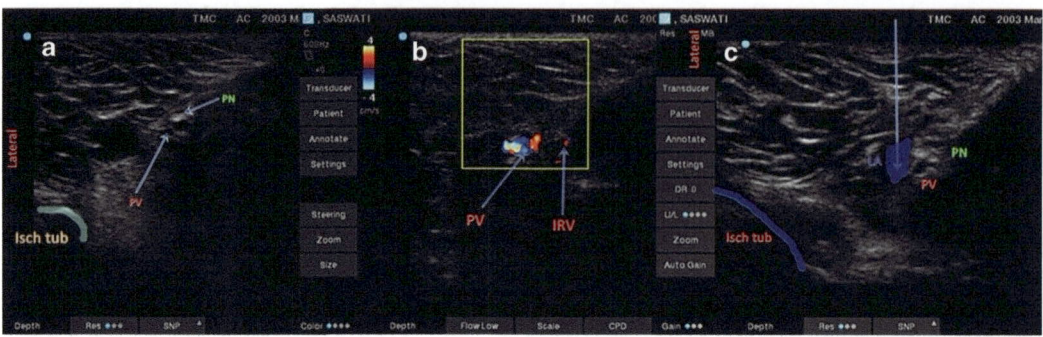

Fig. 21.3 Pudendal nerve block Ultrasound image: (**a**) the initial scanning image, (**b**) Colour Doppler image showing pudendal vessels (PV) and inferior rectal vessels (IRV), (**c**) Pudendal nerve block: the block needle enters out of the plane, LA is deposited around the pudendal nerve (PN). Note that the ischial tuberosity (Isch tub) lies lateral and anus/perineal body medial. The above image is of a pudendal nerve block on the right side

avoided due to the terminal character of the nearby pudendal artery. The block of the perineal branch of the posterior cutaneous nerve of the thigh can be performed either when performing the pudendal block by injection of 5 ml of local anaesthetic in contact with the ischial tuberosity or by subcutaneous infiltration given the ischial tuberosity.

Technique

The ultrasound-guided perineal approach was reported by Parras and Blanco in 2013.

In the lithotomy position, a high-frequency linear probe is placed between the anus and the ischial tuberosity to view the ischiorectal fossa. The hyperechoic curved line laterally indicates the ischial tuberosity, and the hypoechoic area medially represents the anorectal shadow. The ischiorectal fossa lies between the ischial tuberosity laterally and the anorectal shadow medially. The pudendal nerve may be visualised in the fossa as small hyperechoic structures of about 2 mm. Recognition may be impaired because of their small diameter, and colour Doppler is useful for identifying the internal pudendal artery. Once the vascular structure is determined, the needle is advanced out of the plane and injected with a dose of 0.5–1 ml/kg on each side. An out-of-plane approach is used (Fig. 21.3).

Alternatively, an oblique parasagittal probe orientation and in-plane needling can be used with the needle moving from the caudad to the cephalad direction.

The limitations of pudendal nerve block are:

- Need for a bilateral block (hence potential for LA toxicity).
- The spread of LA is not well appreciated due to the fat density that makes it almost as anechoic as that of the LA.
- Potential for artery injury, as visualisation of the pudendal artery is difficult due to its small diameter and sinuous path.
- Success rate of 88%

Questions

1. What is the nerve supply of the perineum?
2. What are the critical considerations in a patient undergoing gender reassignment surgery
3. What are the options for perioperative analgesia in a case of gender reassignment surgery?
4. What is the mechanism of the sacral ESP block?
5. What are the approaches to pudendal nerve block?
6. What are the limitations of the pudendal nerve block?
7. How can the caudal block provide postoperative analgesia in major perineal procedures?

Suggested Reading

1. Cesmebasi A, Yadav A, Gielecki J, et al. Genitofemoral neuralgia: a review. Clin Anat. 2015;28:128–35.
2. Hutson JM, Li R, Southwell BR, et al. Regulation of testicular descent. Pediatr Surg Int. 2015;31:317–25.
3. Rauchenwald M, Steers WD, Desjardins C, et al. Efferent innervation of the rat testis. Biol Reprod. 1995;52:1136–43.
4. Taguchi K, Tsukamoto T, Murakami G. Anatomical studies of the autonomic nervous system in the human pelvis by the whole-mount staining method: left-right communicating nerves between bilateral pelvic plexuses. J Urol. 1999;161:320–5.
5. Bolandard F, Bonnin M, Duband P, Mission JP, Bazin JE. Techniques d'anesthésie locorégionale du périnée: indications en gynécologie, en proctologie et en obstétrique [Perineal regional anaesthesia: indications in gynaecologic and proctologic surgery and in obstetric]. Ann Fr Anesth Reanim. 2006;25(11–12):1127–33. French. https://doi.org/10.1016/j.annfar.2006.06.014. Epub 2006 Oct 4.
6. Chakraborty A, Chakraborty S, Sen S, Bhattacharya T, Khemka R. Modification of the sacral erector spinae plane block using an ultrasound-guided sacral foramen injection: Dermatomal distribution and radiocontrast study. Anaesthesia. 2021;76:1538–9. [PubMed] [Google Scholar].
7. Bolandard F, Bonnin M, Mission JP, Duband P, Bazin JE. A pudendal nerve block with neurostimulation: type and frequency of motor responses. Ann Fr Anesth Reanim. 2004;23:R130.
8. Parras T, Blanco R. Bloqueo pudendo ecoguiado Ultrasond Guided Pudendal Block. Cir Mayor Ambul. 2013;18:31–5.
9. Rofaeel A, Peng P, Louis I, Chan V. Feasibility of real-time ultrasound for pudendal nerve block in patients with chronic perineal pain. Reg Anesth Pain Med. 2008;33:139–45.
10. Gaudet-Ferrand I, De La Arena P, Bringuier S, Raux O, Hertz L, Kalfa N, Sola C, Dadure C. Ultrasound-guided pudendal nerve block in children: a new technique of ultrasound-guided transperineal approach. Pediatr Anesth. 2018;28(1):53–8.

Part II

Complications of Regional Anesthesia

Hisham Harb

Case Scenario

A patient who had a popliteal sciatic block for ankle surgery complains of persistent lower limb paraesthesia and weakness.

1. **What are the Differential diagnoses in this scenario?**

Differential diagnosis of persistent neurological dysfunction following peripheral nerve block (PNB):
- PNB-related Peripheral Nerve Injury (PNI)
- Extrinsic compression
  - Patient positioning
  - Tourniquet
  - Tight cast
- Intrinsic compression
  - Compartment syndrome
  - Perineural haematoma
- Post-surgical inflammatory neuropathy

2. **What is the incidence of nerve injury after regional anaesthesia?**

Postoperative Neurological Symptoms (PONS), usually paraesthesia, can occur in up to 15% of patients. However, it is important to note that this rarely results in permanent injury. The incidence of PONS is 0–2.2% at 3 months, 0–0.8% at 6 months, and 0–0.2% at 1 year. The risk of PNB-related Permanent Neurological Injury (PNI) is difficult to quantify owing to the paucity of accurate data collection on the subject. However, the range reported is between 0.014% and 0.04%.

3. **What is the double crush theory**

The 'double crush' theory suggests that patients with pre-existing neural compromise may be more susceptible to injury at another site when exposed to a secondary insult. This theory is relevant in nerve injury management as it underscores the importance of considering a patient's overall neurological health when assessing the risk of nerve injury.

4. **What are the patient factors that may increase the risk of PNI**

H. Harb (✉)
Frimley Park Hospital, Surrey, UK

- Pre-existing neurological compromise
  - Hereditary peripheral neuropathies
  - Mechanical—spinal stenosis, compression radiculopathy
  - Ischaemic—peripheral vascular disease
  - Toxic—chemotherapy
  - Metabolic—diabetes mellitus
  - Autoimmune—multiple stenosis
- Smoking
- Hypertension
- Anticoagulant therapy

5. **How might the conduct of the PNB be adapted to reduce the risk of PNI**

- Nerve localisation techniques
  - Ultrasound
  - Peripheral nerve stimulation
- Equipment
  - Needle design
    - Smaller gauge
    - Short bevel
    - Echogenic for better ultrasound visualisation
  - Injection pressure monitoring—aim for opening injection pressure <15 psi
- Pharmacological
  - Neurotoxicity of LA—Ropivacaine lowest potential for neurotoxicity
  - Avoidance of vasoconstrictor (vasoconstriction can cause PNI due to ischaemia and also increased time nerve exposure to neurotoxic LA)
- Performance of block
  - Awake patient
  - Planning a trajectory that avoids direct needle contact with the nerve
  - The use of hydrodissection

6. **What current intensity and pulse duration would you be happy with to indicate safe needle-to-nerve placement?**

0.5 mA, 0.1 ms, 2 Hz

7. **What is the pathophysiology of PNI?**

	Seddon's PNI classification		
	Neuropraxia	Axonotmesis	Neurotmesis
Pathology	Myelin sheath damage only	Loss of axonal continuity. Endoneurium intact	Complete transection of nerve
Mechanism	Stretch Compression	Varied	Transaction
Prognosis	Good Recovery in weeks – months	Prolonged recovery May be incomplete	Poor

Sunderland's PNI classification:

> First degree = Seddon's neuropraxia
> Second degree = Seddon's axonotmesis
> Third degree = Lesion in endoneurium.
> Perineurium and epineurium intact
> Fourth degree = Only epineurium remains intact
> Fifth degree = Complete transection of the nerve

8. When would you conduct electrophysiological studies after a suspected nerve injury, and why?

Electrophysiological studies are typically delayed for 2–3 weeks, as this allows sufficient signs of Wallerian (nerve fibre) degeneration to appear. However, in consultation with a neurologist, these studies may be requested earlier, as the presence of EMG changes in this 'early' period may signal pre-existing neurology that is not attributable to an acute PNB-related event.

9. What effects do adjuncts have on nerve injury?

The addition of adrenaline (at concentrations greater than 5 μg/ml) as an adjunct leads to vasoconstriction, which is in addition to the vasoconstriction caused by some local anaesthetics. Therefore, it further reduces neural blood flow, leading to ischaemia and nerve injury.

10. What do you mean by extraneural, perineural and intraneural injection

An injection outside the epineurium is considered extra- or perineural, whereas any injection inside the epineurium is considered intraneural. An intraneural injection can be either extrafascicular (if perineurium is not breached) or intrafascicular (if perineurium is breached). Any damage to the perineurium exposes the protective environment of the fascicles.

11. How can injection pressure monitoring reduce the risk of PNB-related PNI?

To date, no case reports of clinically significant nerve injury have been reported with low opening injection pressures (<15 psi).

Pressure monitoring is highly sensitive to intra-fascicular injections. A low opening injection pressure indicates an injection that is either extraneural (outside the epineurium) or extravascular (inside the epineurium but outside the perineurium).

The distinction between extra or intra-fascicular injection is significant as damaging the perineurium exposes the protective environment of the fascicles. Even small amounts of solution injected intra-fascicularly can lead to axonal degeneration and permanent neural damage.

12. How would you reassure/counsel the patient who presents with nerve injury a week after a peripheral nerve block?

- Establish whether the distribution of neurology is consistent with PNB and whether any features require urgent intervention (see management above)
- Reassure the patient, especially if examination only reveals a mild neurological deficit
- Protect limb—education about caring for a numb bit
- Consider early involvement of chronic pain if allodynia or hyperalgesia is present. This proactive approach can significantly improve patient outcomes.
- Review in 2–4 weeks. If persistent deficit:
  - Refer to neurology
  - MRI
  - Neurophysiology studies

Fortunately, most nerve injuries eventually resolve, with the risk of permanent injury being extremely low. This should provide some reassurance to the patient.

Questions

1. What is the 'double crush' theory?
2. What is triple monitoring and how does it help prevent nerve injury?
3. Which injection is more dangerous for nerve damage: intrafascicular or sub-epineurial?
4. What are the risk factors for cauda equina syndrome after spinal anesthesia?
5. Injury with which type of needle, Blunt or sharp bevelled, will be more disastrous?
6. What is the '**compressed air injection technique**'?
7. What is the level of evidence for using injection pressure monitoring and ultrasound guidance to prevent PNB-related injury?
8. How do you approach a patient who demonstrates a patch of numbness and paraesthesia following an upper limb surgery under a supraclavicular block?

Suggested Reading

1. O'Flaherty D, McCartney CJL, Ng SC. Nerve Injury after peripheral nerve blockade – current understanding and guidelines. BJA Educ. 2018;18(12):384–90.
2. RA-UK guidelines for the management of nerve injury associated with regional anaesthesia. https://www.ra-uk.org/index.php/guidelines-standards.
3. Neal JM, Barrington MJ, Brull R, et al. The second ASRA practice advisory on neurologic complications associated with regional anaesthesia and pain medicine: executive summary 2015. Reg Anesth Pain Med. 2015;40:401–30.
4. Jacob AK, Kopp SL, Hebl JR. Regional anesthesia in the patient with pre-existing neurological disease. NYSORA website.

Simon Bindelle

Case Scenario

A 67-year-old female with a background of type 2 diabetes mellitus patient presents one-week following total hip arthroplasty performed under spinal anaesthesia and sedation. She complains of numbness and weakness affecting her left leg. On examination, there is weakness of knee extension and ankle dorsiflexion, reduced sensation to light touch over the medial malleolus, and loss of patellar reflex.

(L4 nerve root injury pattern)

1. **What is the Incidence of nerve damage following neuraxial block?**
   - The incidence of permanent injury following central neuraxial block has been estimated by the UK's 3rd National Audit Project
   - This gives 'optimistic' and 'pessimistic' figures due to the clinical uncertainty in reported cases:
     - Pessimistic 4.2 per 100,000 (1 in 24,000)
     - Optimistic 2.0 per 100,000 (1 in 54,000)

   - However, risk is individual to patient circumstances. In general, epidural catheterisation poses higher risk than single shot spinal injections, and peri-operative procedures in adults are higher risk than those in obstetrics, chronic pain, and paediatrics

2. **Enumerate possible differential diagnosis:**

There are several causes of perioperative central nerve injury. The clinical picture described above depicts an injury to the L4 nerve root.

Direct trauma
- Due to spinal or epidural needle, catheter, or direct injection of drugs
- Patients may complain of pain or paraesthesia on injection
- Commonly affects a single nerve root

Vertebral canal haematoma (See Chap. 25)

S. Bindelle (✉)
Groupe santé CHC, Liège, Belgium

Infection

Epidural abscess

- Usually results from epidural catheterisation, although spontaneous and haematogenous spread from other sites is possible
- Causative organism, commonly staphylococci
- Risk factors include:
  - Immunosuppression
  - Pre-existing spinal pathology
  - Systemic infection
  - Increased duration of epidural catheterisation
  - Poor asepsis on insertion
- Classical triad (note this is variable and should not be relied upon):
  - Back pain,
  - Fever,
  - Neurologic deficit
- MRI will show the abscess and cord compression, while blood tests will reveal raised inflammatory markers
- Treatment requires broad-spectrum antibiotics. Early surgical decompression is vital to minimise long-term neurological sequelae

Meningitis

- An alternative infective pathology with similar risk factors but which usually follows spinal anaesthesia as there is a dural breach and is typically caused by *Staphylococcus viridans*
- Symptoms include neck stiffness, photophobia, headache, back pain, fever, nausea, lethargy

Chemical injury

- Injected irritants may cause adhesive arachnoiditis, with a widespread inflammatory reaction resulting in interruption of blood supply
- Symptoms are often severe and irreversible, and in extremis raised intracranial pressure may result from obstructed CSF flow
- Chlorhexidine is a critical cause

3. Discuss the treatment plan for nerve damage following neuraxial block.

Prevention

Direct trauma

- May be prevented with pre-procedural ultrasound to estimate the level of needle insertion accurately, given the unreliability of landmark palpation and low-lying conus (below L1/2) in a significant minority of patients
- Any patient-reported pain or paraesthesia on insertion must prompt needle withdrawal and redirection, as lateral deviation may still injure nerve roots

Vertebral canal haematoma

- Time central neuraxial block appropriate according to last dose of anticoagulant or antiplatelet agent
- Screen for platelet count and coagulation status where appropriate (See Chap. 25 for further detail)

Infection

- Expert consensus suggests the following measures:
  - Prior history and examination to identify those at higher risk
  - Strict aseptic technique
  - Bacterial filters for epidural catheters
  - Leave the catheter inserted for the shortest possible time to avoid disconnections
  - Evaluate the insertion site for signs of infection daily

Adhesive arachnoiditis

- Guidelines to minimise the risk of injury secondary to chlorhexidine suggest:
  - Use of 0.5% rather than 2% chlorhexidine solution (same aseptic properties but less neurotoxicity)
  - Carefully checking gloves and equipment for contamination
  - Allow skin to dry completely before proceeding with needle insertion

Investigation and management

- Review urgently
- Vertebral canal haematoma and epidural abscess are space-occupying lesions. Successful management depends on early surgical decompression. Meningitis also carries significant morbidity and even mortality risk
- Urgent imaging of the spine (MRI is the gold standard) is required if any of the following red flags are present on history or examination:
  - Pre-existing risk factors, including coagulopathy, spinal canal deformity and immunosuppression
  - Severe back pain
  - Fever and raised inflammatory markers
  - Bladder or bowel symptoms
  - Motor or sensory deficits are central or radicular (**as per our case scenario**), bilateral or progressive. Return of symptoms after initial resolution is also a red flag.
- If there are no red flags, liaise with a neurologist and consider electrophysiologic studies

4. **How will you assess the outcome in these patients?**

- Outcome is variable and depends on the severity of symptoms at presentation. Bowel and bladder involvement is a late sign and suggests a worse prognosis
- Space-occupying lesions (vertebral canal haematoma and epidural abscess) are time-critical, and any delays to surgery will worsen the prognosis
- There are minimal treatment options for adhesive arachnoiditis

Questions

1. What are common causes of central nerve damage following neuraxial anaesthesia?
2. How can the risk of nerve damage be minimised during a neuraxial block?
3. What steps would you take if a patient exhibits symptoms of nerve damage after a neuraxial block?
4. What diagnostic imaging is most effective in assessing nerve damage in these cases?
5. What are the long-term outcomes after central nerve damage after neuraxial anaesthesia?
6. What role of patient positioning in prevention of nerve injury during the procedure?
7. How would you effectively communicate the risks due to central neuraxial blocks to patients?

Suggested Reading

1. Duncan A, Patel S. Neurological complications in obstetric regional anaesthetic practice. J Obstet Anaesth Crit Care. 2016;6:3–10.
2. Chambers DJ, Howells ACL. Neurological complications in obstetric regional anaesthesia. Anaesth Intensive Care Med. 2016;17(8):372–4.
3. Neal JM, Barrington MJ, Brull R, et al. The second ASRA practice advisory on neurologic complications associated with regional anesthesia and pain medicine Executive Summary 2015. Reg Anesth Pain Med. 2015;40(5):401–30.
4. McCombe K, Bogod D. Learning from the law. A review of 21 years of litigation for nerve injury following central neuraxial blockade in obstetrics. Anaesthesia. 2020;75:541–8.
5. Hewson DW, Bedforth NM, Hardman JG. Spinal cord injury arising in anaesthesia practice. Anaesthesia. 2018;73(Suppl. 1):43–50.
6. Young B, Onwochei D, Desai N. Conventional landmark palpation vs preprocedural ultrasound for neuraxial analgesia and anaesthesia in obstetrics – a systematic review and meta-analysis with trial sequential analyses. Anaesthesia. 2021;76:818–31.
7. American Society of Anesthesiologists Task Force on infectious complications associated with neuraxial techniques. Practice advisory for the prevention, diagnosis, and management of infectious complications associated with neuraxial techniques. Anesthesiology. 2010;112:530–45.
8. Yentis SM, Lucas DN, Brigante L, et al. Safety guideline: neurological monitoring associated with obstetric neuraxial block. A joint guideline by the Association of Anaesthetists and the Obstetric Anaesthetists' Association. Anaesthesia. 2020;2020(75):913–9.

9. Association of Anaesthetists of Great Britain and Ireland. Safety guideline: skin antisepsis for central neuraxial blockade. Anaesthesia. 2014;69:1279–86.

10. O'Neal MA, Chang LY, Salajegheh MK. Postpartum spinal cord, root, plexus and peripheral nerve injuries involving the lower extremities: a practical approach. Anesth Analg. 2015;120(1):141–8.

11. O'Flaherty D, McCartney CJL, Ng SC. Nerve injury after peripheral nerve blockade—current understanding and guidelines. BJA Educ. 2018;18(12):384–90.

12. Cook TM, Counsell D, Wildsmith JAW. Royal College of Anaesthetists Third National Audit Project. Major complications of central neuraxial block: report on the Third National Audit Project of the Royal College of Anaesthetists. Br J Anaesth. 2009;102:179–90.

Local Anaesthetic Systemic Toxicity (LAST)

24

Hisham Harb

Case Scenario

A 60-year-old man underwent a thoracotomy. A paravertebral catheter was inserted. A loading dose of Bupivacaine was administered, followed by an infusion via the catheter. A further bolus dose was given in the post-anaesthetic care unit. Shortly after, he became confused and agitated and then developed a generalised tonic-clonic seizure.

1. **What is the Differential diagnosis in the above clinical scenario?**
   - LAST
   - Seizure
     - Epilepsy
     - Hypoxia

2. **Discuss how you will recognise suspected LA toxicity.**

A patient with LA toxicity may present with
   (a) Sudden alteration in mental status, severe agitation or loss of consciousness, with or without tonic-clonic convulsions
   (b) CVS collapse—may have shockable or non-shockable rhythm
   (c) Note—LAST may occur sometime after the LA administration

3. **Discuss immediate management of LA toxicity.**
   (a) Stop injecting LA
   (b) Call for help
   (c) Airway—secure with tracheal tube if necessary
   (d) Breathing—give 100% Oxygen and establish adequate ventilation
   (e) Circulation—secure IV access and monitor cardiovascular (CVS) status throughout
   (f) Seizure control—benzodiazepines or small incremental doses of propofol or thiopentone

4. **What will you do next after initial stabilisation in this patient?**

   (a) In circulatory arrest
      (i) CPR using usual protocols. Expect prolonged resuscitation
      (ii) Anticipate that arrhythmias may be refractory. Avoid using lidocaine as anti-arrhythmic
      (iii) Consider use of cardiopulmonary bypass if available
      (iv) Give INTRAVENOUS LIPID EMULSION (INTRALIPID)
   (b) Without circulatory arrest
      (i) Supportive treatment for hypotension, bradycardia and arrhythmias
      (ii) Consider INTRAVENOUS LIPID EMULSION

H. Harb (✉)
Frimley Park Hospital, Surrey, UK

© The Author(s), under exclusive license to Springer Nature Switzerland AG 2026
S. Phillips et al. (eds.), *Regional Anaesthesia*, https://doi.org/10.1007/978-3-032-05165-3_24

5. **What is the definitive antidote for LA toxicity?**

INTRAVENOUS LIPID EMULSION 20%
- 1.5 ml/kg over 1 min

Followed by
- 0.25 ml/kg/min infusion

After 5 min, if still unstable:
- Repeat bolus (up to a maximum of three boluses)
- Double infusion rate

Maximum cumulative dose of 12 ml/kg
- Continue for atleast 15 min after hemodynamic stability is restored

6. **What is the risk of LA toxicity as the practice of RA is evolving**

The incidence of LAST is 1.8 per 1000 peripheral nerve blocks. It can present with rapid onset signs and symptoms following accidental intravascular injection or delayed features because of systemic absorption of LA. Presentation patterns are evolving as the practice of ultrasound-guided RA evolves, with delayed presentation of LAST becoming more prevalent.

LAST typically leads to central nervous system (CNS) and CVS effects.

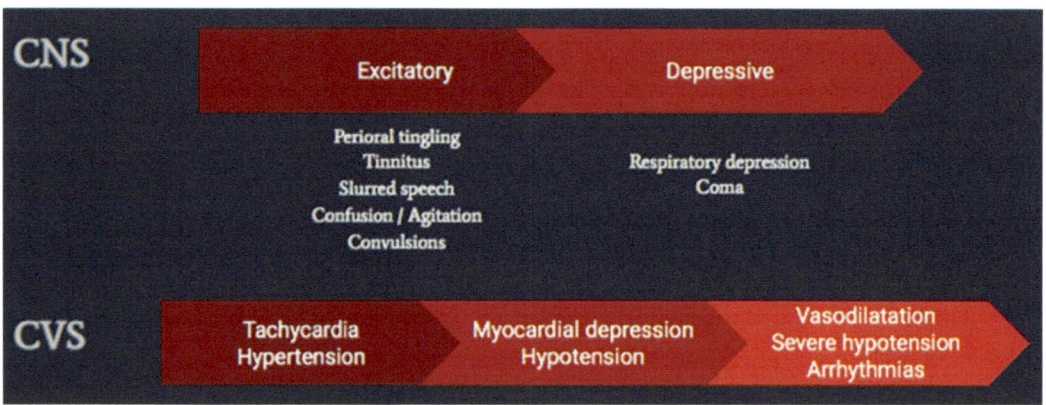

The CVS:CNS ratio refers to the dose required to cause CVS toxicity relative to the dose required to cause CNS toxicity. The ratio for Lidocaine is 7:1, compared to 2:1 for Bupivacaine, meaning that Bupivacaine is much more likely to cause CVS collapse if systemic toxicity occurs. Recovery from LA-induced cardiac arrest may be delayed (>1 h).

7. How might the conduct of the RA technique reduce the risk of LAST?

- Choice of LA
  - CVS:CNS ratio—choose least cardiotoxic e.g. Lidocaine
  - Dose reduction in vulnerable groups
    - Extremes of age
    - Frailty
    - Acidosis
    - Renal/hepatic disease—single dose unaffected, reduced rate of infusion
    - Pre-existing heart disease
- Other techniques
  - Ultrasound-guidance
  - Frequent aspiration
  - Incremental dosing
  - Use of vasoconstrictor

8. What are the relative risks of LAST depending on the block site?

Intercostal > Paravertebral > Caudal > Epidural > Brachial plexus > Femoral/Sciatic > Subcutaneous

There are increasing reports of LAST secondary to fascial plane blocks, where onset of toxicity is delayed.

Questions

1. What are the safe maximum doses of bupivacaine and ropivacaine for administration as a single dose and infusion in infants?
2. What is the recommended test dose in children? What are the clinical signs suggestive of a positive test dose?
3. Why are local anaesthetics less effective in acidic pH such as abscess or inflammation sites?
4. What is the role of Vasopressin in management of LAST?
5. A patient who received supraclavicular brachial plexus block complains of perioral numbness and tingling. The patient is conscious, oriented and haemodynamically stable at this stage. What should be your immediate management?
6. Can calcium channel blockers be used in management of LA toxicity associated arrhythmias?
7. In a case of sciatic nerve block, the patient starts experiencing signs of LAST with Cardiovascular collapse. Lipid emulsion is unavailable in your operation theatre complex. Can you use propofol as a replacement?
8. What is lipid sink theory of lipid emulsion?
9. Where do we insert lipid emulsion administration into the ACLS algorithm?
10. What is the recommended management of local anaesthetic toxicity associated seizures?
11. What is a 'lipid rescue kit'? Where should it be kept?

Suggested Reading

1. MacFarlane AJR, Gitman M, Bornstein KJ, El-Boghdadly K, Weinberg G. Updates in our understanding of local anaesthetic systemic toxicity: a narrative review. Anaesthesia. 2021;76:27–39.
2. Association of Anaesthetists' guidelines for management of severe local anaesthetic systemic toxicity. https://anaesthetists.org/Home/Resources-publications/Guidelines/Management-of-severe-local-anaesthetic-toxicity.

Vascular Puncture and Hemorrhage

25

Simon Bindelle

Case Scenario

After an axillary block is performed to remove a hand tumour surgically, a patient develops a significant axillary swelling accompanied by paresthesias and radial nerve weakness. This case scenario is a typical example of a complication that can arise from a peripheral nerve block, highlighting the importance of understanding and managing vascular punctures and hematomas.

1. **What is the Differential diagnosis**

Differential diagnosis of a swollen arm and nerve
 weakness after axillary block:
   Haematoma
   Abscess
   Venous thromboembolism
   Tourniquet use
   Prior axillary lymph node dissection

2. **Discuss the Management plan for this patient**

History

The following questions should be asked to ascertain the risk. Was there any coagulopathy? Is the patient on anticoagulants? Does the patient have co-morbidities that may increase the risk of nerve injury (diabetes, etc)? Was there a suspicion of a vascular puncture during the block?

Was a positive aspiration (for blood) documented? Was digital pressure applied to the axilla or artery following injection? Did the surgeon use an arm tourniquet (if so, what pressure was used, and what was the duration)? Was the arm positioned during surgery to avoid abduction more significant than 90°?

Examination

Inspection of the arm—Signs of infection (swollen arm, erythema, pain and tenderness to the touch)? What is the differential arm circumference? Is there a subcutaneous fluid collection?

Signs of vascular compromise—Is a distal pulse (a pulse located further away from the heart, such as in the wrist or fingers) present? What is the hand's capillary refill time?

Neurological examination—Is there any neurological deficit in the upper limb? If so, what nerve distribution?

Investigations

Bloods—FBC, coagulation tests, CRP −/+ blood culture

Review of per-operative notes (Anaesthetic and surgical notes)

Imaging of the arm (ultrasound + Doppler/MRI)

Evaluation by a neurologist, nerve conduction studies and electromyography (these investigations are usually performed later and are not part of an urgent management plan for an

S. Bindelle (✉)
Groupe santé CHC, Liège, Belgium

acute recognised hematoma causing nerve compression).

Management

If nerve compression secondary to a hematoma is suspected, urgent investigation and treatment is required. If there were concerns about vascular puncture, immediate digital pressure should have been applied to the skin after the block.

Inform the surgeon

Reversal of any anticoagulation

Elevation of the arm

Active and passive physiotherapy

Consider surgical evacuation of the haematoma if
- The haematoma continues to expand
- The nerve palsy persists or deteriorates
- There is evidence of vascular or lymphatic obstruction

3. **How will you estimate the outcome in this patient**

Haematomas are not a frequently reported complication after peripheral nerve blocks. Large haematomas causing nerve weakness are very uncommon. Contributing factors include coagulopathies and use of anticoagulants, elevated arterial blood pressure, and multiple arterial punctures. Conservative treatment is appropriate in most cases of haematoma after peripheral nerve block. An expanding haematoma within the spinal canal (i.e. an enclosed space) warrants urgent neurosurgical assessment to avoid or reduce the risk of permanent nerve damage. Intravascular injections are the leading causes of local anaesthetic systemic toxicity (see Chap. 26).

4. **Is the transarterial technique for axillary brachial plexus block still recommended?**

No. Since ultrasound guidance is widely used for peripheral nerve blocks, voluntary arterial punctures are avoided, and periarterial techniques are preferred in order to reduce the risk of haematomas. A review of 1062 cases of transarterial axillary blocks was published in 2007. The authors reported a complication rate of 3.2%, including three patients with persistent neuropraxia and an overall success rate of 93%.

5. **Is there a risk of compartment syndrome in the upper arm?**

Compartment syndrome is most common in the lower leg and lower arm. Compartment syndrome in the upper arm is rare but has been reported. The upper arm is divided into three compartments: anterior, posterior, and deltoid. The brachial plexus and axillary artery are located in the anterior compartment.

6. **What are the risk factors for haematoma formation after regional anaesthesia?**

Multiple attempts

Anticoagulant treatment

Coagulopathy

Large needle gauge

Technically difficult procedure

Use of catheter for continuous regional anaesthesia

Increasing age

Female sex

Questions

1. What is the incidence of hematoma after axillary brachial plexus block?
2. What is the most typical complication following the axillary block?
3. What will be your initial management steps if an expanding hematoma is observed following the femoral nerve block?
4. What will be the signs of hematoma following a supraclavicular brachial plexus block?
5. Which approach to the axillary brachial plexus block has the maximum incidence of hematoma?
6. Which nerve blocks have been classified as deep blocks as per the latest ESRA guidelines?

Suggested Reading

1. Bendavid B. The axillary block is complicated by a hematoma and radial nerve injury. Reg Anesth Pain Med. 1999;24(3):264–6.
2. Hudson S, Emamdee R, Htut Y, Pal S. The transarterial brachial plexus block for hand and forearm surgery. Eur J Anaesthesiol. 2007;24(5):470–2.
3. Maeckelbergh L, Colen S, Anné L. Upper arm compartment syndrome: a case report and review of the literature. Orthop Surg. 2013;5(3):229–32.

Block Failure and Rescue Block

26

Simon Bindelle

Case Scenario

A 55-year-old patient scheduled for a fifth meta-carpal fracture surgery under supraclavicular brachial plexus performed with 20 ml 0.5% Bupivacaine under ultrasound guidance. 30 min after the block performance, the patient complains of sharp pain at the surgical site during skin incision.

1. **What are the possible causes of block failure in this patient?**

The causes of block failure can be grouped into six categories.

Patient factors

- Comorbidities such as obesity, arthritis, and diabetes may lower success rates because positioning, access, nerve location, and identification can be challenging. ASA score >2 is an independent risk factor for block failure.
- Patient anxiety during surgery is common and can sometimes lead to less successful regional anaesthesia. Language barriers may worsen patient anxiety and interfere with the efficacy of block testing.
- Female sex has been significantly associated with block failure
- A history of substance abuse has been identified as a factor in block failure.

- In some rare cases, patients can resist local anaesthetics (multi-systemic disorders such as Ehler-Danlos syndrome and channelopathies involving voltage-gated sodium channels).

Experience of the operator

- Regional anaesthesia is practical; the clinician's expertise influences success rates. Sufficient exposure and teaching are required to progress in the learning curve.
- The most common mistakes when novice operators perform US-guided blocks are:
  - Needle advancement without visualization of the tip.
  - Unintentional probe movement.
  - Inadequate equipment preparation.
  - Poor ergonomics.

Inappropriate block

- Of course, a detailed knowledge of anatomy is mandatory to choose the appropriate block for each type of surgery. Communication with the surgeon is crucial to knowing the exact extent of the surgery.
- In this specific case (fifth metacarpal ORIF), a supraclavicular block may not have been the most suitable option because this block has a higher degree of ulnar sparing. This may lead to block failure as the ulnar nerve is responsible for the innervation of the fifth digit.

S. Bindelle (✉)
Groupe santé CHC, Liège, Belgium

Tourniquet use

- An arm tourniquet can cause a certain degree of discomfort to the patient, especially for durations above 20 min.
- Tourniquet pain has a double component: local pressure and muscle ischaemia.
- Blocking the intercostobrachial nerve can reduce discomfort due to local pressure, but does not affect muscle ischaemia pain. The musculocutaneous nerve should be blocked when performing an axillary block to reduce arm tourniquet pain.

Anatomical variation

- The innervation area of the peripheral nerve block may vary between patients, and innervation territories may overlap. It is, therefore, also recommended that the adjacent nerves involved be blocked. A more proximal approach is usually more likely to block all branches when compared to a more distal approach.[1]

Selection of local anaesthetic

- The choice of a local anaesthetic agent and the concentration used must be appropriate. A local anaesthetic with a short duration of action may cause discomfort in more prolonged procedures. A local anaesthetic with a prolonged onset will increase the time needed for an effective block. Lower concentrations of local anaesthetics are suitable for postoperative analgesia but may not provide surgical anaesthesia.

2. **When will you say that a block failure has occurred and what factors govern a block success?**
   - The precise definition of a failed block may vary. Commonly accepted criteria to define a failed block include:
     - Conversion to general anaesthesia after surgical incision

[1]https://resources.wfsahq.org/atotw/regional-anaesthesia-for-awake-hand-surgery-block-failure-andtrouble-shooting-issues.

- Use of IV opioids after surgical incision
- Rescue peripheral nerve block
- Surgeon infiltration of local anaesthetic into the surgical site

Failure frequency depends on the definition used and how it is measured. The rates range from 6% to 20%.

Determining factors for block success:
- Proper identification of the nerve or plexus;
- Needle placement close to the nerve;
- Visualization of LA spread around the nerve;
- Use of an adequate dose of LA;
- "The right dose of the right drug at the right place"

3. **What are the different types of block failure?**

Block failure is classified as:
- Complete failure: No sensory or motor blockade in the targeted area
- Partial failure: Some numbness, but inadequate for surgery
- Secondary failure: Initial success, but the block wears off before surgery completion.

4. **What are the key steps in assessing block success?**

Block success is assessed using:
- Sympathetic changes (temperature difference between limbs)
- Sensory blockade (loss of cold, touch, or pain perception)
- Motor blockade (loss of movement in specific myotomes).

5. **Discuss the management plan in case of a block failure.**

The two key components are:
- Techniques to reduce the chance of failure occurring
- Methods to manage failure if it occurs.

Table 26.1 Sensory territory, motor testing and landmarks for distal upper limb peripheral nerve blocks

Nerve tested	Cutaneous innervation	Test for motor block	Landmarks for the distal block
Musculocutaneous nerve	Lateral forearm	Elbow flexion	Axilla—between coracobrachialis and biceps brachii muscles
Radial nerve	Posterior forearm, dorsum of the hand, and radial side of the thumb	Wrist and elbow extension, forearm supination	Above the elbow—at the posterolateral aspect of the humerus
Ulnar nerve	The anterior aspect of the ulnar 1½ fingers (little finger and half of the ring finger) and the medial palmar skin Dorsal aspect of the ulnar 1½ fingers and medial aspect of the dorsum of the hand	Finger abduction, thumb adduction, fourth and fifth digit flexion	Mid-forearm—medial to the ulnar artery
Median nerve	Palmar and distal dorsal aspects of the lateral three-and-a-half digits and adjacent palm	Wrist flexion, forearm pronation, thumb flexion, second and third digit flexion	Above the elbow—medial or posterior to the brachial artery

Adapted from Pack E, Smith M. Regional anaesthesia for awake hand surgery: block failure and troubleshooting issues. Anaesthesia Tutorial of the Week. 2021;Tutorial 441 and Sehmbi H, Madjdpour C, Shah U, Chin K. Ultrasound-guided distal peripheral nerve block of the upper limb: a technical review. J Anaesth Clin Pharmacol. 2015;31:296–307

To reduce failure rates, the efficacy of the block should be assessed in the block room before transferring the patient to the theatre. This may include temperature, pain, soft touch, and motor block assessment. More time should be allowed before surgery if the block is not dense enough. If one of the nerves within the plexus is spared when testing the block, distal rescue blocks can be a valuable addition to the initial plexus block to complete the anaesthesia (Table 26.1).

6. What is a "rescue block," and when should it be used?

A rescue block is an additional nerve block performed when the primary block is incomplete or has failed. It should only be performed if the local anaesthetic systemic toxicity (LAST) risk is within safe limits.

7. How will you manage a block failure before the operation has begun?
- Allow adequate time for the onset of the block and reassess
- If the block is inadequate, check the remaining maximum dose of LA permissible.

- If sufficient LA dose still remaining, options available are
  - Repeat block
  - Perform rescue block (where the block is ineffective on sensorimotor testing)
- If LA maxima are reached, options available are
  - Are there contraindications to GA? if not, proceed with GA and systemic analgesia; if contraindications exist, then abandon the elective procedure and reschedule

8. How will you manage a block failure after the operation has begun?

The following options can be used intraoperatively in case of patient discomfort due to a block failure:
- Local anaesthetic supplementation by the surgeon at the surgical site.
- Distraction techniques: music, virtual reality headset, hypnosis.
- IV sedation in case of anxiety, tourniquet discomfort, or positional discomfort.
- In case of tourniquet discomfort, intermittent deflation can be discussed with the

surgical team. Alternatively, IV analgesia with opioids or ketamine.
- Conversion to a general anaesthetic if the previous options did not work.
- Abandoning the procedure as a last resort

9. What are the consequences of a block failure

Consequences of block failure include:
- Longer surgery duration.
- More frequent intraoperative analgesics administration.
- Increased incidence of unplanned hospitalizations.
- Prolongation of PACU length of stay.

10. What are the key considerations for managing a failed peripheral nerve catheter (PNC)?

A systematic approach is essential, including checking equipment and considering alternative pathologies. If a continuous nerve catheter fails, troubleshooting includes:
- Checking catheter depth and securing it properly
- Reassessing infusion pumps and tubing
- Scanning for local anaesthetic spread
- Considering catheter repositioning or replacement.

11. What is the role of adjuncts like dexamethasone or clonidine in reducing the incidence of block failure?

Adjuncts like dexamethasone prolong block duration, while clonidine enhances analgesia. However, they do not significantly reduce block failure rates.

Questions
1. What are the common patient-related factors contributing to block failure?
2. How does patient selection affect the success of regional anaesthesia (RA)?
3. How does obesity affect PNB success, and what mitigation strategies can be employed?
4. What are the risk factors for block failure?
5. What are the landmarks for the upper limb's most common distal nerve blocks?
6. What are the options to troubleshoot a failed block?
7. Are there any objective methods of assessing block success?
8. How does tourniquet pain impact PNB success, and what strategies can mitigate this?
9. What are the common myotomes tested for upper and lower limb block?
10. What are the medicolegal implications of patients perceiving pain during surgery?

Suggested Reading

1. Pack E, Smith M. Regional anaesthesia for awake hand surgery: block failure and troubleshooting issues. Anaesthesia Tutorial of the Week. 2021;Tutorial 441. Available at: https://resources.wfsahq.org/atotw/regional-anaesthesia-for-awake-hand-surgery-block-failure-and-troubleshooting-issues. Accessed 1 Aug 2022.
2. Picard L, Belnou P, Debes C, Lapidus N, Sung Tsai E, Gaillard J, Sautet A, Bonnet F, Lescot T, Verdonk F. Impact of regional block failure in ambulatory hand surgery on patient management: a cohort study. J Clin Med. 2020;9(8):2453.
3. Moreno-Martínez D, Perea-Bello A, Díaz-Bohada J, García-Rodriguez D, Echeverri-Mallarino V, Valencia-Peña M, Osorio-Cardona W, Silva-Enríquez P. Factors associated with failed brachial plexus regional anesthesia for upper limb surgery. Colomb J Anesthesiol. 2016;44(4):292–8.
4. Sites B, Spence B, Gallagher J, Wiley C, Bertrand M, Blike G. Characterizing novice behavior associated with learning ultrasound-guided peripheral regional anesthesia. Reg Anesth Pain Med. 2007;32(2):107–15.
5. Bottomley T, Gadsden J, West S. The failed peripheral nerve block. BJA Educ. 2023;23(3):92–100.
6. Sehmbi H, Madjdpour C, Shah U, Chin K. Ultrasound guided distal peripheral nerve block of the upper limb: a technical review. J Anaesthesiol Clin Pharmacol. 2015;31(3):296–307.

Neurotoxicity of LA and Adjuvants

27

Venkat Duraiswamy

Case Scenario

A 37-year-old male underwent an ORIF of the left clavicle under GA, Interscalene block, & Superficial cervical plexus. He presented back to the hospital with the c/o, unable to abduct the shoulders, and numbness over the shoulders.

1. What is the incidence of nerve injuries?

The incidence of nerve injuries may vary from <3:100 with the single-shot nerve block to 0.4–2% with peripheral nerve catheters. Most of the injuries are minor, and permanent injuries are rare. Most of the injuries fully recover within a year. Long-term neurological injury is extremely rare, with an estimated incidence ranging from 0.024% to 0.04%.

2. What are the risk factors for nerve injury?

Perioperative nerve injury is a complex phenomenon and can be caused by several clinical factors.

(a) Anaesthetic risk factors
- Regional block technique
- Long bevel needles have a high chance of causing nerve puncture; short bevel needle injuries are generally more severe.
- Interfascicular injection
- High-opening injection pressure
- Local anaesthetic-induced neurotoxicity

(b) Surgical factors

Surgery can stress anatomical structures and mechanically induce traction, transaction, compression, contusion, ischaemia, and stretching nerves. Additional risk factors include positioning and the use of a tourniquet.

(c) Patient factors

Pre-existing neuropathies like diabetic peripheral neuropathy, multiple sclerosis, GBS, post-polio syndrome, peripheral vascular diseases, vasculitis, cigarette smoking, and hypertension.

3. What are the drugs that cause Neurotoxicity?

All LAs have neurotoxic effects. The degree of neurotoxicity is concentration, dose, and time-dependent. LAs have vasoconstrictor properties and can theoretically damage nerves through ischaemia.

Lignocaine, tetracaine, Bupivacaine, Ropivacaine, Adrenaline, and Midazolam worsen LA neurotoxicity.

Preservatives added to steroids, such as benzyl alcohol and propylene glycol.

In high doses, dexmedetomidine (>1 µg/kg) causes vasoconstriction, which increases the intraneural LA concentration, potentiating the neurotoxic effects.

4. How do Local anaesthetics induce Neurotoxicity?

V. Duraiswamy (✉)
East Surrey Hospital, Surrey, UK

The degree of neurotoxicity of LA is concentration, dose, and time-dependent.

At the cellular level, the neurotoxicity of local anaesthetics is caused by the effect of
1. Intrinsic caspase-pathway
2. PI3K-pathway
3. MAPK pathway

The vasoconstrictive effect of local anaesthetics can aggravate nerve damage via ischaemia, and this damage can be aggravated further with adjuvant adrenaline. Adrenaline also extends the exposure of nerves to local anaesthetics, putting nerves at greater risk of ischemic damage (Fig. 27.1).

5. **What are the neurological complications of Lignocaine?**

All the neurological complications reported are due to 5% Lignocaine, which is not in clinical use now. Spinal lignocaine is implicated in the syndrome of transient neurologic symptoms (previously referred to as transient radicular irritation), manifested by pain or dysesthesia in the buttocks or legs after recovery from anaesthesia.

Also, Cauda equina syndrome and Persistent lumbosacral neuropathy were caused by 5% Lignocaine.

6. **How do you manage nerve injuries?**

Please attach the RA UK nerve injury algorithm.

Fig. 27.1 Cellular mechanism of LA toxicity

Ischaemia and reperfusion
↓
Oxidative injury
↓
Neuronal damage, initiation of apoptosis by affecting Schwann cells

Fragmentation of DNA
↓
Disrupts the membrane potential in mitochondria
↓
Uncoupling of oxidative phosphorylation
↓
Release of cytochrome C
↓
Initiation of the caspase pathway
↓
Apoptosis

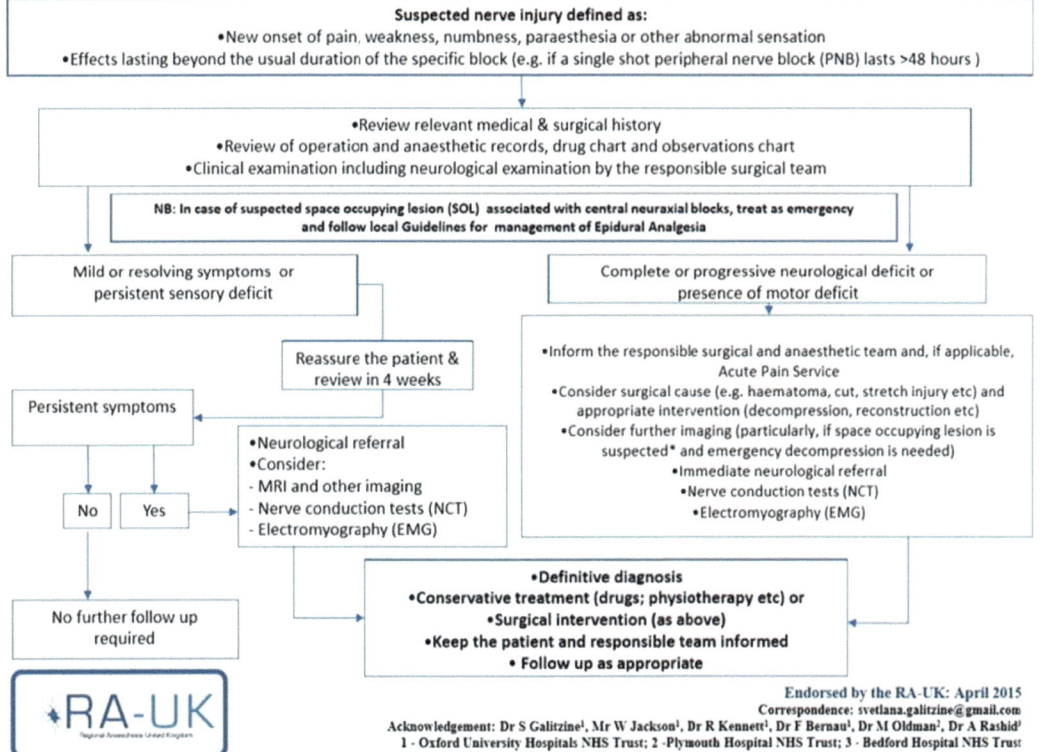

Algorithm for management of nerve injury associated with regional anaesthesia

Suspected nerve injury defined as:
• New onset of pain, weakness, numbness, paraesthesia or other abnormal sensation
• Effects lasting beyond the usual duration of the specific block (e.g. if a single shot peripheral nerve block (PNB) lasts >48 hours)

• Review relevant medical & surgical history
• Review of operation and anaesthetic records, drug chart and observations chart
• Clinical examination including neurological examination by the responsible surgical team

NB: In case of suspected space occupying lesion (SOL) associated with central neuraxial blocks, treat as emergency and follow local Guidelines for management of Epidural Analgesia

Mild or resolving symptoms or persistent sensory deficit

Complete or progressive neurological deficit or presence of motor deficit

Reassure the patient & review in 4 weeks

Persistent symptoms

• Inform the responsible surgical and anaesthetic team and, if applicable, Acute Pain Service
• Consider surgical cause (e.g. haematoma, cut, stretch injury etc) and appropriate intervention (decompression, reconstruction etc)
• Consider further imaging (particularly, if space occupying lesion is suspected* and emergency decompression is needed)
• Immediate neurological referral
• Nerve conduction tests (NCT)
• Electromyography (EMG)

No   Yes

• Neurological referral
• Consider:
  - MRI and other imaging
  - Nerve conduction tests (NCT)
  - Electromyography (EMG)

No further follow up required

• Definitive diagnosis
• Conservative treatment (drugs; physiotherapy etc) or
• Surgical intervention (as above)
• Keep the patient and responsible team informed
• Follow up as appropriate

Endorsed by the RA-UK: April 2015
Correspondence: svetlana.galitzine@gmail.com
Acknowledgement: Dr S Galitzine[1], Mr W Jackson[1], Dr R Kennett[1], Dr F Bernau[1], Dr M Oldman[2], Dr A Rashid[3]
1 - Oxford University Hospitals NHS Trust; 2 -Plymouth Hospital NHS Trust; 3 - Bedford Hospital NHS Trust

Questions

1. What are the typical presenting symptoms of transient neurologic symptoms?
2. What is the mechanism of transient neurologic dysfunction following spinal anaesthesia with lignocaine?
3. What is the mechanism of cauda equina syndrome following spinal anaesthesia?
4. What is the management of transient neurologic symptoms?
5. What is the management of cauda equina syndrome?
6. What adjuvants are safe for use in neuraxial anaesthesia for paediatric patients?
7. Is adrenaline a safe adjuvant for neuraxial anaesthesia?

Suggested Reading

1. NYSORA.
2. Verlinde M, Hollmann MW, Stevens MF, Hermanns H, Werdehausen R, Lirk P. Local anesthetic-induced neurotoxicity. Int J Mol Sci. 2016;17:339. https://doi.org/10.3390/ijms17030339.
3. Lirk P, Brummett CM. Regional anaesthesia, diabetic neuropathy, and dexmedetomidine: a neurotoxic combination? Br J Anaesth. 2019;122(1):16–8.
4. Kim EJ, Kim HY, Ahn JH. Neurotoxicity of local anesthetics in dentistry. J Dent Anesth Pain Med. 2020;20(2):55–61.

Spinal Anaesthesia Induced Hypotension

28

Joselo D. Macachor and Ashutosh Joshi

Introduction

Definitions of spinal induced hypotension vary, and thus the reported incidence of hypotension ranges from 0% to more than 50% in nonpregnant patients [1]. The maintenance of venous return is paramount to maintaining normotension under spinal anesthesia. Resistance vessels dilate (supplied by the T1–T12 preganglionic sympathetic fibers), and blood volume is redistributed depending on posture and gravity. In the head-up position, blood pools into the lower extremities and the splanchnic circulation. The height of the block determines the extent of hypotension—a block below L2 has no effect on arterial pressure. The sympathetic block extends two to six segments above the sensory block, implying that if there is a sensory blockade to cold at T4, it is likely that the whole of the sympathetic outflow (T1–T12) will be blocked. In this scenario, cardioaccelerator fibers from T1 to T4 will not provide the compensatory tachycardia of low volume states.

1. **What is the pathophysiology of spinal hypotension syndrome?**

Reflexes

The decreased venous return to the heart is sensed by stretch receptors in the right atrium, leading to decreased heart rate (Bainbridge reflex). With normal, or even mild-moderate volume deficits, increased heart rate and cardiac output can compensate for this vasodilation. With severe volume deficits (profound haemorrhage, dehydration), stretch receptors in the ventricular walls are stimulated by this empty chamber and devastatingly activate the Bezold-Jarisch reflex (BJR), inducing a triad of bradycardia, hypotension and apnea [2]. Age-related changes in the elderly worsen systolic function, diastolic relaxation, and neurohumoral responses.

Supine Hypotensive Syndrome

The supine hypotensive syndrome is most marked in pregnant patients. From the 20th week of gestation onwards, the dextro-rotation of the gravid uterus may occlude the inferior vena cava in the supine parturient, by pressing against the vertebral column, resulting in decreased venous return, hypotension, and decreased uterine blood flow. Initially, the obstruction causes an increased systemic vascular resistance (SVR) and higher-pressure readings in the upper half of the body, but 50–90% of parturients will experience hypotension after spinal anaesthesia, defined as:

J. D. Macachor · A. Joshi (✉)
Department of Anaesthesia, Khoo Teck Puat Hospital, Singapore, Singapore
e-mail: Macachor.joselo@nhghealth.com.sg;
Ashutosh.Joshi@nhghealth.com.sg

© The Author(s), under exclusive license to Springer Nature Switzerland AG 2026
S. Phillips et al. (eds.), *Regional Anaesthesia*, https://doi.org/10.1007/978-3-032-05165-3_28

1. SBP less than 90 mmHg
2. SBP less than 80% of baseline, and/or,
3. Greater than 25% decrease in SBP from baseline

Other mechanisms to explain spinal-induced hypotension are:

- Skeletal muscle paralysis
- Ascending medullary vasomotor block (high spinal)
- Diaphragmatic paralysis and respiratory insufficiency, especially with excessive sedation
- Preexisting autonomic dysfunction
- Heart block

2. **How can we prevent this?**

No one measure is sufficiently effective to prevent hypotension. Correcting absolute blood volume deficits and prompt vasoconstriction is the most logical strategy. One must be aware of predictors for hypotension, such as obesity, preeclampsia, diabetes, autonomic neuropathy, and prolonged fasting. Preexisting hypovolemia before central neuraxial sympathetic blockade and change in patient position (Trendelenburg to supine or sitting) can lead to cardiovascular collapse and precipitate a cardiac arrest.

A standard sequence of atropine, ephedrine, and epinephrine can be used for bradycardia.

Spinal anaesthesia techniques to limit vasodilatation—low dose strategies

1. Restrict block height to what is necessary. For example, a hemorrhoidectomy requires only a block up to S2, a hysterectomy up to T7 level.
2. Perform unilateral spinal anaesthesia. Place the patient on the side to be operated on for 20 min until a predominantly unilateral block is established, using small doses of bupivacaine between 3.5 and 8 mg.
3. Mix local anesthetic with fentanyl—this reduces the local anesthetic dose and improves the quality of analgesia with lower doses.
4. Use a spinal catheter and start injecting fractions of local anesthetic every 15 min, until a sufficient block height is achieved

5. Consider combined spinal-epidural anaesthesia, which has its advantages: the flexibility to augment the block height by increasing local anesthetic volume or by the technique of Epidural volume extension (EVE). EVE starts with a low-dose intrathecal local anesthetic injection followed by epidural saline injection, compressing the subarachnoid space and pushing the spinal solution upwards, however, this expansion technique is not reliable [3]. Block duration can be extended by giving aliquots before the block recedes.

Mechanical lower extremity compression, head-down tilt

1. Tilt the patient in a slight head-down tilt to increase venous return
2. Apply an Esmarch bandage from ankle to mid-thigh—this decreases hypotension incidence from 83 to 16% in obstetrics
3. Relieve vena caval compression: displace the uterus by adopting a full-left lateral position or using a uterine displacement device, such as a wedge under the hips. Manual uterine displacement with left lateral tilt lowers hypotension risk.

3. **What is the role of fluids in the management of spinal hypotension syndrome?**

Fluids

Correct hypovolemia. But balance this against the risk of excessive fluid administration and pulmonary edema.

Timing of fluid management

Fluid loading "fills the tank" made functionally empty by acute vasodilation. There is a difference between:

1. Preloading—defined as a 1–2 L bolus of IV fluid 10–20 min before spinal anaesthesia.
2. Coloading—IV fluids are administered immediately after the induction of spinal anaesthesia as the sympathetic block sets in and is completed within 5 min.

Crystalloids versus colloids

Dextran and gelatin may cause an allergic reaction. Hydroxyethyl starch (HES) is linked to

Table 28.1   Management of spinal-induced hypotension

Atropine	Antimuscarinic, HR increase	Small doses (5 µg/kg) prevent SAIH Caution with high-risk cardiac patients
Ephedrine	Indirectly increases endogenous norepinephrine release	Dose not to exceed 15 mg during elective cesarean section. Consider if both hypotensive and bradycardic [3]
Phenylephrine 100 µg IV bolus 0–100 µg/min infusion rate; initiate at between 25–50 µg/min immediately after spinal induction	Direct-acting a1 adrenergic agonist	The effect on cardiac output depends on the starting conditions of the return function Prophylactic phenylephrine infusion immediately before spinal reduces hypotension Titrate down the infusion with bradycardia or reactive hypertension
Norepinephrine Infusion range 0.07–0.08 µg/kg/min	Potent a-adrenergic Weak B-adrenergic	Prophylactic administration needs further study
Caffeine, theophylline	B-sympathomimetic	More data needed
Ondansetron	Serotonin receptor antagonist Blocks 5-HT3 receptors	More data needed

SAIH spinal anaesthesia-induced hypotension

renal failure and mortality in the critically ill, but not in cesarean delivery patients. Judicious use of small-volume expanders is known to reduce the degree of precipitous fall in blood pressure in patients with vasoactive hypertension with low intravascular volume, such as pre-eclampsia.

4. **How sedation affects spinal hypotension syndrome**.

Judicious sedation use. The patient who can communicate gives ample warning of vasovagal reaction (dizziness, lightheadedness). For anxiolysis, reduce midazolam and propofol doses by 40–75% during spinal anaesthesia. Regional anaesthesia by itself causes deafferentation. 'Affective dyspnea' is a phenomenon that can occur from high spinal levels with intercostal paresis, with patients feeling an inability to breathe. At the same time, diaphragmatic function is still intact, and ventilation is unhindered. Reserve opioids for discomfort or pain. Consider end-tidal carbon dioxide monitoring with a side-stream capnography to warn of hypoventilation and apnea.

5. **How the use of inotropic drugs help improve this? What will be your drug of choice and why?**

The commonly used drugs are summarized in Table 28.1.

Ephedrine
Ephedrine is the conventionally used vasoconstrictor. Vasopressors rapidly reverse the physiologic changes induced by spinal anaesthesia. Coronary, cerebral, and muscle blood flow increases, while renal and splanchnic blood flow decreases. With long-term Angiotensin converting enzyme (ACE) inhibitors, the effect of ephedrine is diminished from norepinephrine depletion from storage (action is indirect and preganglionic).

Phenylephrine
Obstetric anaesthesia guidelines favor phenylephrine over ephedrine for cesarean sections because phenylephrine has a better uteroplacental blood flow (UPBF) profile. Fetal acidosis occurs if hypotension lasts more than 2 min. Variable rate infusions offer finer blood pressure

control and greater hemodynamic stability. They reduce the number of interventions to maintain blood pressure.

Other vasopressors

Methoxamine and metaraminol have predominantly alpha-1 effects. Atropine pretreatment may be deleterious in coronary disease, but small doses (5 μg/kg) may help patients with low baseline heart rates. Norepinephrine, 5 μg/ml infusion, is as effective as phenylephrine in controlling blood pressure, albeit with less bradycardia and maintained cardiac output.

Serotonin favours the BJR (a vagally mediated reflex) but is stifled by 5HT3 antagonists (ondansetron). (Table 28.1, Fig. 28.1).

6. **What are recent updates in the management of spinal hypotension syndrome?**

Preloading is of questionable benefit because

1. Crystalloid solutions immediately redistribute from intravascular to interstitial space, such that only 28% of lactated Ringer's remain in the intravascular space after 30 min

2. Volume load stretches the right atrium, releasing atrial natriuretic peptide (ANP), which causes peripheral dilatation, fluid excretion, and eventually decreases the intravascular volume.

Colloid loading failed to show improvement over crystalloid loading. Clinical management has moved from a fluid-based strategy towards vasopressor-based prophylaxis support through fluid co-loading.

The current debate is on whether phenylephrine infusions or boluses should be given. Treatment strategy depends on context—Personnel (staffing and trained assistance), preoperative volume status, and resources (rich or deficient—supplies, monitors, infusion pumps, institutional practice standards) [7]. Examples include:

1. reactive (early and aggressive fluid loading plus vasopressors) when the BP drops significantly

2. preventive (titrated phenylephrine infusion rates with crystalloids) at the cost of reactive hypertension

Algorithm for low BP

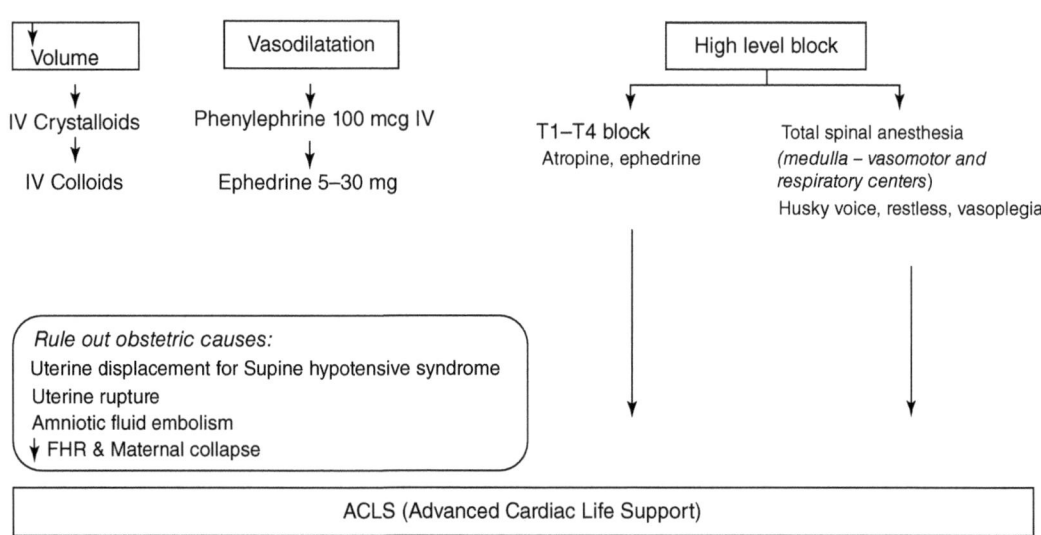

Fig. 28.1 Algorithm for management of spinal-induced hypotension

Questions

1. What are the risk factors for post-spinal hypotension?
2. Which vasopressor used to treat post-spinal hypotension has the most favourable profile of fetal acid-base status following birth?
3. Compare phenylephrine and norepinephrine for treating post-spinal hypotension.
4. What are effective non-pharmacological preventive strategies for post-spinal hypotension?
5. What are the early symptoms and signs of high spinal anaesthesia and total spinal anaesthesia? How do you manage a case of total spinal anaesthesia?
6. How does subdural injection result in high or total spinal anaesthesia?
7. What is the mechanism of ondansetron in the prevention of post-spinal hypotension? How do you administer this drug for this purpose?
8. What are the presenting features and diagnostic investigations for amniotic fluid embolism?

Suggested Reading

1. Tarkkila P. Complications associated with spinal anaesthesia. In: Finucane BT, editor. Complications of regional anaesthesia [Internet]. New York: Springer New York; 2007. p. 149–66. Available from: http://link.springer.com/10.1007/978-0-387-68904-3_9.
2. Pellegrini JE. Treatment and prevention of spinal-induced hypotension in the cesarean section patient: what does the evidence say? Annu Rev Nurs Res. 2017;35:159–78.
3. Lee JE, George RB, Habib AS. Spinal-induced hypotension: incidence, mechanisms, prophylaxis, and management: Summarizing 20 years of research. Best Pract Res Clin Anaesthesiol. 2017;31:57–68.
4. Chooi C, Cox JJ, Lumb RS, Middleton P, Chemali M, Emmett RS, et al. Techniques for preventing hypotension during spinal anaesthesia for caesarean section. Cochrane Database Syst Rev. 2020;7:CD002251.
5. Ferré F, Martin C, Bosch L, Kurrek M, Lairez O, Minville V. Control of spinal anaesthesia-induced hypotension in adults. Local Reg Anesth. 2020;13:39–46.
6. Butwick AJ, Goodnough LT. Transfusion and coagulation management in major obstetric hemorrhage. Curr Opin Anaesthesiol. 2015;28:275–84.
7. Bishop DG, Rodseth RN, Dyer RA. Recipes for obstetric spinal hypotension: the clinical context counts. S Afr Med J. 2016;106:861–4.

Vertebral Canal Haematoma

29

Sioned Phillips

Case Scenario

A patient undergoing liver resection who has had a thoracic epidural inserted for perioperative analgesia now complains of localised back pain over the epidural insertion site. It is 6 h post-completion of surgery.

1. **What is the differential diagnosis of back pain following an epidural?**

Causes of back pain after an epidural:

- Traumatic insertion/bruising.
- Infection/epidural abscess.
- Epidural/vertebral canal haematoma.
- Surgical insult.
- Exacerbation of pre-existing back pain.
- Positioning related.

2. **Enumerate the clinical signs and symptoms of a VCH.**
   - Neurological deficit outlasting the expected duration of the block.
   - Motor block more profound than expected during epidural utilisation.
   - Bowel and bladder dysfunction.
   - Motor weakness, which is not always bilateral.

- In severe cases, complete paralysis of affected limbs and autonomic dysfunction.
- Signs and symptoms typically progress rapidly in patients.
- Acute severe back pain with radiation has been described as a classical symptom, but NAP 3 has warned that this is not a universal sign, with lower limb weakness or numbness being more common.
- Fevers may suggest an epidural abscess, which seems to present in a more delayed fashion than VCH

3. **What is the incidence of VCH following central neuraxial block?**

Spinal Anaesthesia:

- No cases of VCH attributed to spinal anaesthesia were noted in the NAP 3 audit out of 360,000 spinal anaesthetics.
- Historically, the incidence of VCH after spinal anaesthesia has been quoted as <1:220,000.

Epidural Anaesthesia:

- The NAP 3 audit recognised that, while rare, VCHs occurred in patients receiving a perioperative epidural.

S. Phillips (✉)
Department of Anaesthesia, Frimley Park Hospital, Camberley, UK
e-mail: sioned.phillips@nhs.net

- When focusing only on these perioperative epidurals, the incidence of VCH causing permanent harm is 5.1 in 100,000 or 1 in 19,500.
- Thus, perioperative epidural provision is a relatively high risk for VCH when compared to spinal anaesthesia.
- Of note, in NAP 3, no VCH cases were reported in obstetric patients undergoing neuraxial blockades.

4. **What is the pathophysiology of VCH?**
   - Dorsal venous plexus commonly implicated.
   - Risk factors as described below conspire to increase the risk of bleeding and/or increase the pressure effect of resultant haematoma on the spinal cord.

5. **What are the Risk factors for VCH?**
   - Increasing age.
   - Female gender.
   - Orthopaedic surgery
   - Disorders of coagulation (Physiological or iatrogenic)
   - Difficult neuraxial insertion (Multiple attempts, bloody tap)
   - Abnormalities of the vertebral column or blood vessels therein. (e.g. Lumbar stenosis, ankylosing spondylitis or other anatomical abnormalities)
   - Reduced renal function (predisposing to more significant than anticipated anticoagulant activity).
   - Emergency operations.

6. **Discuss the management plan for this patient.**
Stop any epidural medication administration pending review. This helps rule out any contribution from the local anaesthetic towards neurological issues.
Review the patient's history:
   - Operation notes and anaesthetic notes—coagulopathy, surgical insult, difficult epidural insertion, timing of anticoagulants, presence of high-risk factors?

- Any pre-existing history that might explain these symptoms, such as prior back injury potentially exacerbated by surgery?
- What is the timeframe for the development of these symptoms? Classically, it is rapidly progressive in the case of VCH. It may occur before or after catheter removal.
- Motor weakness beyond the expected duration of the block is particularly concerning and could be expected to be at or below the level of the epidural insertion.

Perform and document a thorough neurological examination:
   - Power of lower limbs
   - Tone
   - Sensation
   - Reflexes.
   - Signs of meningism
   - Examination of the back for tenderness or overlying erythema.
   - Review the complete vital signs, particularly concerning temperature (typical in epidural abscess).

Investigations:
   - Guided by history and examination.
   - Blood: Coagulation, FBC, CRP −/+ blood culture
   - Imaging of the spine: MRI gold standard, with high sensitivity and specificity. MRI scans are superior to CT as they help define the hematoma's extent, volume, and precise location. They are the most sensitive and specific imaging modality available.
   - Non-contrast CT or CT myelography is preferred if MRI is unavailable or the patient cannot get an MRI. They can show space-occupying lesions that are most amenable to surgical management. Myelography was previously the modality of choice before MRI.

CT findings:
   - The hematoma is usually visualised as a biconvex-shaped hyperdense lesion within the spinal canal, lying adjacent to the vertebral body.
   - The lesion will be sharply demarcated and separated from the less dense spinal canal.

- However, an epidural haematoma is a neurosurgical emergency. As such, if suspected, it should be discussed with the local neurosurgical centre, which can arrange an urgent MRI after transfer to their centre.
- Non-contrast or CT myelography is the preferred imaging modality if MRI is unavailable.

Management:
- Urgent cessation/reversal of any anticoagulation.
- Urgent MRI imaging is the investigation of choice—high sensitivity and specificity.
- Discussion with a neurosurgeon to consider the evacuation of haematoma should be undertaken as soon as feasible.

Prevention:
- Where feasible, avoid neuraxial procedures in individuals on anticoagulants, post-thrombolysis, or at increased risk of bleeding.
- It is crucial to be cognisant of and adhere to current regional anaesthesia and anticoagulation guidelines, such as ESRA guidelines. This commitment to following guidelines is a key part of ensuring patient safety.
- If not already in place, document the safe window for epidural catheter removal and consider implementing ward-based guidelines or educational sessions in your institution.

Outcome Estimation
- Epidural haematoma is a neurosurgical emergency.

- Urgent surgical decompression is the treatment of choice.
- Recovery post-surgery is dependent on the degree of pre-operative deficit and the interval between the onset of symptoms and surgical decompression.
- Best outcomes are seen when surgery occurs within 8 h of symptoms.
- Recovery beyond this is rare but not impossible.

Questions
1. What are the risk factors for an epidural hematoma?
2. Your hospital does not offer 24-h MRI imaging; what other imaging could be considered?
3. How will you manage this problem?

Suggested Reading

1. Cook TM, Counsell D, Wildsmith JAW. Major complications of central neuraxial block: report on The Third National Audit Project of the Royal College of Anaesthetists. Br J Anaesth. 2009;102(2):179–90. https://doi.org/10.1093/bja/aen360.
2. Nelson A, Benzon HT, Jabri RS. Diagnosis and management of spinal and peripheral nerve hematoma. NYSORA Website. Retrieved from https://www.nysora.com/topics/complications/diagnosis-management-spinal-peripheral-nerve-hematoma/. Accessed on 8/4/2024.
3. Moen V, Dahlgren N, Irestedt L. Severe neurological complications after central neuraxial blockades in Sweden. Anaesthesiology. 2004;1010:950–9.
4. Kietaibl S, et al. Regional anaesthesia in patients on antithrombotic drugs: joint ESAIC/ESRA guidelines. Eur J Anaesthesiol. 2022;39:100–32.
5. Hadzic A. Hadzic's textbook of regional anaesthesia and acute pain management—self assessment and review. New York: McGraw Hill; 2019. p. 367–70.

Infection with Regional Anaesthesia

30

Venkat Duraiswamy

Case Scenario

A 70-year-old was admitted with a history of falls; CT Traumagram showed posterior four to nine rib fractures. The patient has a history of type 2 Diabetes Mellitus and is currently on immunosuppressants (Methotrexate) for Rheumatoid Arthritis. An ESP catheter was inserted under aseptic conditions for rib fracture pain management. Two days later, the patient developed a low-grade fever, and the CRP was high; there was redness and swelling around the ESP catheter.

1. What is your differential diagnosis?

After a thorough examination and review of the investigations, my differentials are

- ESP Catheter-related infections
- Chest infection
- open wound infection

2. What are the key points for the management of this patient?

- A complete examination of the patient and review of blood results to r/o other causes of infection
- Remove the catheter immediately
- Discuss with microbiology for appropriate antibiotics
- Surgical review for drainage of the abscess

3. A 26-year-old lady presents with fever, back pain, and paraesthesia of the lower limbs 5 days after a labour epidural. How do you manage this patient?

I will take a thorough history and examination, particularly the back and neurological examination. Review the anaesthetic chart for details about epidural issues, such as difficulty in insertion and sterile precautions.

A multi-disciplinary approach with input from obstetrics, anaesthetics, spine/neurosurgeon, and infectious diseases is crucial for comprehensive patient care.

Requires an MRI for diagnosis.

Timely diagnosis of Lumbar/thoracic spinal epidural abscess, early surgical treatment, anti-infection management, and rehabilitation exercise are essential for the full recovery of lower limb muscle strength. If any signs of infection occur, an in situ epidural catheter should be removed immediately, and the appropriate imaging and consultation (e.g., neurologist or infectious disease specialist) should be initiated promptly.

4. What is the incidence of infection with the peripheral nerve block?

The infection risk for single-shot PNB is negligible. Bacterial colonisation of peripheral nerve catheters ranges from 7.5% to 57%, but the risk of infection is low, from 0% to 3%.

V. Duraiswamy (✉)
East Surrey Hospital, Surrey, UK

One study reported the incidence in paediatrics as 0.01%–0.03%, and another reported the incidence of cutaneous infection as 0.05%.

However, it is not just block site infections that the anaesthetist needs to be aware of, but the risk of transmission of blood-borne diseases such as human immunodeficiency virus (HIV), hepatitis B virus (HBV) and hepatitis C virus (HCV) between patients due to contaminated equipment (e.g. USS probe). These viruses can survive on dry, inanimate surfaces for more than 1 week, and infection may take months to manifest clinically, making it difficult to ascribe to the PNB.

5. What are the risk factors for infection?

The risk of infection is increased in patients with the following:

- critical care unit admission,
- trauma
- Diabetes mellitus
- immune compromise
- male sex
- The absence of antibiotics

It can be minimised by removing the catheter within 48–72 h of placement.

6. What are the signs and symptoms of infection?

Local symptoms include discharge at the insertion site, redness, swelling or local pain.

Systemic symptoms such as fever and lethargy. The findings of the investigation include raised CRP and WBC count.

Meningitis is more common after spinal anaesthesia, whereas epidural abscess is more common after epidural anaesthesia.

Early signs and symptoms of post-procedure infection (e.g., back pain, fever, headache, erythema at insertion site) may be followed by later signs (e.g., stiff neck, radiating pain, photophobia, loss of motor function, confusion). While meningitis and epidural abscess are both complications of the neuraxial block, the risk factors and causative organisms are disparate. For example, Staphylococcus is the organism most associated with epidural abscesses; often, these infections occur in patients with impaired immunity. Conversely, meningitis follows a dural puncture typically caused by alpha-hemolytic streptococci, with the organism's source being the proceduralist's nasopharynx.

7. What is the source of infection?

The aetiology of infectious complications often needs to be clarified. Potential aetiologies can be classified as Intrinsic or Extrinsic.

Intrinsic factors are generally related to the underlying health of the patient and include risk factors such as:

- IV drug abuse
- Trauma
- Malignancy
- Diabetes mellitus
- Pregnancy
- Immunocompromised
- Hematogenous spread from a remote site of infection

Staphylococcus Aureus is the most commonly isolated bacteria, followed by Streptococci, Escherichia coli, and Pseudomonas aeruginosa.

Extrinsic include sources of bacteria:

- Invasion of skin bacteria through the needle puncture site
- Contaminated syringes
- Catheter hubs
- Local anaesthetics
- Breaches in aseptic techniques

The most frequently detected microorganism on the skin surface is Staphylococcus epidermidis (65%–70%) of skin flora, whereas Staphylococcus aureus (1%–2%) of skin flora is the most prevalent microorganism in epidural infection. This discrepancy suggests that S. aureus may be more resistant to disinfectants.

8. How do you prevent infection?

- A thorough hand washing dramatically reduces the risk of cross-contamination and should occur before performing any regional anaesthetic technique (Table 30.1).
- Skin disinfection with 0.5% chlorhexidine. Both chlorhexidine and alcohol are neurotoxic and should be allowed to dry thoroughly before the needle is inserted.

Table 30.1 Recommendations for the aseptic preparation of a patient for the procedure

	Single-shot PNB	Continuous catheter PNB	Single-shot neuraxial block	Continuous neuraxial catheter	Long-term implanted device/catheter (e.g. intrathecal pump)
Skin disinfection (i.e. 0.5% chlorhexidine with 70% alcohol)	+	+	+	+	+
Sterile procedure drape (field)	(+)	+	+	+	+
Sterile gloves	+	+	+	+	+
Sterile gown		+	+	+	+
Mask	+	+	+	+	+
Hair cover	+	+	+	+	+
Prophylactic antibiotics	−	−	−	−	+ single dose
Filter on injection/infusion system	−	+		+	NA
Tunnelling of a catheter		+ (to prevent dislocation)		+ If used for more than 3 days	

Adapted from German DEGUM and Belgian BARA guidelines
+ strongly recommended, (+) consider, − not recommended, *NA* not applicable, *PNB* peripheral nerve block

(Chlorhexidine 2% offers no substantial added anti-bacterial benefit over the 0.5% but increases the risk of neurotoxicity)

- Continuous catheter placement warrants a complete aseptic technique.
- A dedicated single-use sterile transducer covering the probe and cable is recommended to reduce interpatient transmission of infection. (Adherent film dressing, e.g. Tegaderm, is not endorsed by either published guidelines or equipment manufacturers)
- The transducer and cable disinfection should be performed between each patient using wipes, foam, or other approved agents with antibacterial, antiviral, and antifungal properties.
- A sterile gel is recommended as a conductive medium in preference to a multidose dispenser.

Questions

1. What is the complication of accidental contamination of intrathecal drugs with chlorhexidine or betadine?
2. What is the recommended technique of asepsis before spinal anaesthesia?
3. What are the recommendations for anaesthesiologists for sterile precautions for a superficial nerve block?
4. What are the signs of epidural abscess, and how do you manage a suspected case of epidural abscess?
5. What are the recommendations for the culture of a continuous catheter in a suspected case of infection?
6. Can the aetiology of epidural abscess be conclusively attributed to a previous neuraxial intervention?

Suggested Reading

1. Hebl JR. The importance and implications of aseptic techniques during regional anesthesia. Reg Anesth Pain Med. 2006;31(4):311–23.
2. Walker BJ, et al. Complications in pediatric regional anesthesia: an analysis of more than 100,000 blocks from the Pediatric Regional Anesthesia Network. Anesthesiology. 2018;129:721–32.
3. Topor B, et al. Best practices for safety and quality in peripheral regional anaesthesia. BJA Educ. 2020;20(10):341–7.
4. NYSORA Compendium of Regional Anaesthesia.

Simon Bindelle

Case Scenario

A patient is scheduled for a hallux valgus repair on his right foot under general anesthesia and a popliteal block. The anaesthetist confirms the surgical marking on the right leg and then asks the patient to turn into a prone position to perform a popliteal block. The assistant preps the site while the anaesthetist answers a phone call. When the block is done, and the patient turns onto his back, the anaesthetist realizes his mistake as he just blocked the left leg.

1. What is the incidence of wrong side block?

Wrong-site procedures are regarded as "never events" as they are preventable and can have serious consequences for patients. However, if preventative measures have been implemented, these events should not happen.

The incidence of wrong-site blocks is uncertain as they are likely under-reported, but it is thought to be about ten times higher than that of wrong-site surgery. The 5th National Audit Project (NAP5) Activity Project estimated the incidence of wrong-site blocks to be around 1 in 6250.

2. Enumerate the risk factors associated with wrong-site nerve blocks

Risk factors can be divided into four main categories: Procedural, patient, practitioner, and organisational (Table 31.1).

The five most common risk factors are:

- Time pressure
- Personnel factors
- Surgical mark not visible
- Communication issues
- Distractions during the procedure

3. Enumerate the strategies to reduce wrong-side blocks (Table 31.2).

In the UK, the Nottingham group launched a safety initiative in 2010 called "Stop before you block," aiming to reduce the incidence of wrong-site blocks. It emphasized the importance of a stop-moment before nerve block performance. An updated approach was published in 2018 as a standard operating policy (SOP). The block process is deconstructed into three separate steps: Preparation, Stop, and Block (Fig. 31.1).

S. Bindelle (✉)
Groupe santé CHC, Liège, Belgium

Table 31.1 Risk factors for wrong site block

Category	Possible scenarios
Procedure	Position change (prone) Change in the position of the equipment Inappropriate marking for surgery The timeout not done properly Distraction like alarm, phone, background noise
Patient	Unable to communicate (anesthesia/sedation, language issues, lack of capability due to altered higher mental function) Similar name One-sided procedure Multiple procedures at the same time
Surgical team	Change of surgeon Lack of communication Pressure to increase the number of cases Fatigue WHO checklist not done An inexperienced person handling
Organization	Lack of system/policy Change in the scheduling of the operations Regional blocks given outside the OT in the procedure room

Table 31.2 Strategies to prevent errors for wrong site blocks

Strategy	Possible intervention
Marking for procedure	A proper mark on the block site, in addition to marking by the surgeon
Timeout	Should be done
Nerve block checklist	Should be done by a proceduralist and one more person
Aids	Posters, signs, and stickers Simulation before giving a block
Team	Educate everyone involved and have a plan with good team dynamics
Audit	Regular audit to check for compliance with protocols for patient safety

Fig. 31.1 Stop before you block, adapted from RA-UK NHS

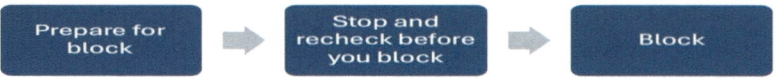

4. What are the risks of a wrong-sided block?

Wrong-site nerve blocks (WSNBs) carry several risks, including:

- Local Anaesthetic Toxicity:
- Contribution to Wrong-Site Surgery
- Neurological Injury: There is a risk of nerve damage or other neurological complications.
- Direct and Indirect Costs to the Patient: These costs may include increased length of hospitalisation, additional medical expenses, prolonged immobility, and inadequate physiotherapy.
- Phrenic Nerve Palsy: potentially requiring artificial ventilation.
- Psychological Trauma: Patients may experience psychological distress and reduced confidence in the healthcare system.
- Opportunity Cost: This includes harm or inconvenience due to cancellation of the intended procedure.
- Other complications: Infection, vascular injury, haematoma, respiratory depression.

Beyond the immediate physical risks, wrong-site blocks can diminish healthcare quality and erode patient satisfaction and confidence in the healthcare system.

5. **How is the process of a wrong-sided nerve block investigated?**

The process of investigating wrong-site nerve blocks (WSNBs) involves several key steps to identify the root causes and contributing factors and prevent future occurrences.

Key aspects of the investigation process include:

- Data Collection and Analysis: includes reviewing event reports to identify steps in the operative procedure that contributed to or could have prevented the error.
- Root Cause Analysis (RCA).
- Identifying Contributing Factors: time pressure, personnel factors, lack of site-mark visibility, inadequate communication, last-minute schedule changes, or patients with similar names.
- Systematic Review: Systematic literature reviews are conducted to aggregate information on the incidence, patient consequences, and conditions contributing to WSNBs, as well as evidence-based prevention methods.
- Surveys and Audits
- Learning from Errors: Sharing lessons learned from wrong-site blocks & reporting incidents is crucial to prevent future incidents.
- Multidisciplinary Approach:

- "Work-as-done" analysis: Analysing what happens in practice, rather than relying on prescribed procedures, can highlight discrepancies and inform safer processes.
- Focus on system factors: Investigations should look beyond individual blame and focus on system-level factors contributing to errors.

Questions

1. Which actions can be taken to reduce the incidence of wrong-site blocks?
2. What are the medico-legal concerns in case the wrong side is blocked?
3. How can you reduce the incidence of nerve injury?
4. What is a root cause analysis?

Suggested Reading

1. Kwofie K, Uppal V. Wrong-site nerve blocks: evidence review and prevention strategies. Curr Opin Anaesthesiol. 2020;33(5):698–703.
2. Salg.ac.uk. SALG | Stop before you block. 2022 [online]. Available at: https://www.salg.ac.uk/salg-publications/stop-before-you-block/. Accessed 17 May 2022.
3. Pandit J, Matthews J, Pandit M. "Mock before you block": an in-built action-check to prevent wrong-side anaesthetic nerve blocks. Anaesthesia. 2016;72(2):150–5.

Post Dural Puncture Headache

Muditha Mawathage

PDPH Management

Case Scenario

A woman, 30 years old, experiences a headache 24 h after delivery, having had epidural analgesia for labour.

1. **What is the differential diagnosis of headache in the postoperative period? Understanding the various causes of non procedural puncture headaches following dural puncture is crucial for accurate diagnosis and effective management (Table 32.1).**

Table 32.1 **Causes** of nonprocedural puncture headache following dural puncture

Benign	Serious
Nonspecific headache.	Meningitis
Exacerbation of chronic headache	Subdural hematoma
Hypertensive headache	SAH
Pneumocephalus	Preeclampsia/eclampsia
Sinusitis	Dural venous sinus thrombosis

2. **Enumerate the clinical signs and symptoms of post-dural puncture headache (PDPH)**

- History of known or possible dural puncture
- Delayed onset of symptoms, but **within 48 h**, rarely >5 days (65% within 24 h, 92% within 48 h) (within 1 h—if associated with pneumocephalus) [1]
- Headache
  - **Postural nature**—worsening within 15 min with standing/sitting & improving within 15 min with recumbency (orthostatic headache)
  - always **bilateral**
  - frontal (25%), occipital (25%) or both
  - dull, aching, throbbing, or pressure-type**Associated symptoms**
  - Nausea (majority), vomiting
  - Pain & stiffens in—neck, shoulders
  - Auditory symptoms (frequently unilateral)—hypoacusis, tinnitus, hyperacusis, vestibular disturbances (dizziness, vertigo)
  - Visual symptoms—diplopia, blurred vision, photophobia, accommodation difficulties
  - Cranial nerve palsies—80% associated with diplopia

M. Mawathage (✉)
Frimley Park Hospital, Frimley, UK
e-mail: muditha.mawathage1@nhs.net

S. Phillips et al. (eds.), *Regional Anaesthesia*, https://doi.org/10.1007/978-3-032-05165-3_32

3. **What is the incidence of PDPH?**

Spinal anesthesia

- $\leq 1\%$ incidence with expert techniques and fine noncutting needles [1]
- 1.7% incidence in obstetric patients when 27G Whitacre needles [1]
- Continuous spinal catheters are associated with a lower incidence compared to single-dose spinal techniques when using similar-gauge needles

Epidural anesthesia

- Known accidental dural puncture (ADP)—1.5% risk in obstetric anaesthesia, 52–80% may develop PDPH [2]
- Unknown dural puncture (DP)—25% incidence of PDPH
- Diagnostic lumbar puncture
- 10% incidence

4. **What is the pathophysiology of PDPH?**

- Not well understood
- CSF is produced mainly in the choroid plexus at a rate of 0.35 ml/min and reabsorbed via arachnoid villi
- Total volume 150 ml, half of the volume extracranial
- Normal lumbar opening pressures
  - 5–15 cmH2O in supine position
  - 40–50 cmH2O in an upright position
- With DP → sudden loss & persistent leak of CSF through the meninges → CSF hypotension → loss of intracranial support → brain to sag in upright position → traction and pressure on the pain-sensitive structures within the cranium (dura, cranial nerves, bridging veins, and venous sinuses) & cerebral vasodilation (mainly venous)
- Associated nerve pathways
  - Frontal pain—ophthalmic branch of the facial nerve
  - Occipital pain—CN IX & X
  - Neck & shoulder pain—Cervical nerves C1–C3
  - Nausea—CN X
  - Visual disturbances—CN III, IV, and VI
  - Blindness—CN II
  - Auditory disturbances—CN VIII

5. **What are the risk factors for PDPH?**

- Patient characteristics such as young age, female gender, history of headaches, and pregnancy. Other risk factors like history of headache, smoking, and depression have a moderate to low level of certainty.
- Procedure and equipment → large gauge, cutting needles, inserting cutting needles with the bevel perpendicular to the long axis of the spine, a more significant number of dural punctures, paramedian vs midline approach.
- Level of neuraxial block, patient position, and skills of the operator

6. **Enumerate the treatment strategies for PDPH**

- Spontaneous resolution usually occurs within 5–12 days (59% within 4 days, 80% within 1 week)
- Supportive measures include
  - Reassurance
  - Bed rest
  - Quiet environment
  - Avoid dehydration (oral ± IV fluid)
  - Regular multimodal oral analgesics—acetaminophen and NSAIDs should be offered to all
  - Antiemetics
  - Stool softeners (to avoid straining and worsening CSF leak)
  - Abdominal binders (insufficient evidence)
  - Other pharmacologic treatments described include (methylxanthines, caffeine (200 mg over 24 h and maximum 900 mg/24 h), sumatriptan, corticosteroids, ACTH or cosyntropin, neostigmine, piritramide, methergine, and gabapentinoids)
  - Encourage mobilisation, thromboembolic deterrent stockings, and consideration of low-molecular-weight heparin prophylaxis if immobile.
  - Neuroimaging should be done if any focal neurological deficit, visual changes, altered consciousness, or seizures are present

7. **Mention nerve blocks and interventions that may be given to manage PDPH.**

Nerve blocks (currently insufficient evidence to recommend the treatment of obstetric PDPH)
- Greater occipital nerve block (GONBs)—block pain transmission to the trigeminal nucleus caudalis, reducing central sensitisation, which 'switches off' the headache
- Sphenopalatine ganglion blocks (SPGBs)—block parasympathetic flow to cerebral vasculature, reducing cerebral vasodilatation
- Epidural interventions
  - Crystalloids
  - Dextran
  - Hydroxyethyl starch
  - Gelatin
  - Fibrin glue
  - Blood patch—gold standard

8. **How will you give an Epidural blood patch?**
   - Indication: severe symptoms/ failure, worsening or recurrence of symptoms after pharmacologic measures, patient preference, no contraindication
   - Optimum timing: Maximum benefit after 48 h of dural puncture, <48 h—more significant requirement of repeat EBP
   - Investigations: PDPH is a clinical diagnosis. Urgent investigations may be considered if the headache changes in nature, neurological signs develop, the consciousness level reduces, the headache is atypical, or when two epidural blood patches have been unsuccessful.

9. **Epidural blood patch procedure**
   - Take written informed consent and explain the risks involved
   - Risks of the procedure include repeat dural puncture, back pain (mainly acute, no evidence for progressing to chronic back pain), and neurological complications
   - Two anesthetists, ideally one consultant, should be present

- Plan the procedure in the operation theater
- Ensure full asepsis
- Turn the patient into a lateral decubitus position
- Establish IV access
- Insert Epidural needle into the epidural space at or below the level of the previous dural puncture (Blood injected during an epidural blood patch spread predominantly cranially)
- Second anaesthetist draws at least 20 ml of venous autologous blood using an 18G needle under strict aseptic conditions
- Inject the blood into the epidural space (ideally at or one space below) until the patient complains of pressure or pain (in the back, buttocks, or head) or the entire 20 ml (no more than 30 ml)
- Keep the patient in the supine position for 1–2 h
- Current insufficient evidence for routine blood culture
- Advise on discharge:
    No heavy weight bearing, air travel, or Valsalva manoeuvres for the next 24–48 h
    Continue oral analgesics, stool softeners, ± cough suppressants as required.
    Contact details of anaesthetist if there are worsening or recurrence of symptoms
- Follow-up and documentation: verbal and written advice information should also be given to the woman's general practitioner and community midwife

10. **What factors determine the success rate of an Epidural blood patch?**

Multiple factors are likely to affect the success of an epidural blood patch. Although success rates of over 90% have been reported in older observational studies, more recent evidence suggests that complete and permanent relief of symptoms following a single epidural blood patch is only likely to occur in up to one-third of cases where headache follows a dural puncture with an epidural needle. Complete or partial relief may be seen in 50–80%, requiring a second blood patch. There is insufficient evidence regarding the optimum timing of repeat EBP and the effect of epidural blood patch on the success of subsequent neuraxial blockade.

11. **What measures may be used to prevent PDPH?**

Questions

1. What procedural factors are associated with the reduction of PDPH?
2. What measures may be used to prevent PDPH?
3. What is the role of an intrathecal catheter after inadvertent dural puncture?
4. What is the role of prophylactic epidural blood patch in reducing PDPH
5. Evidence for needle design factors in lowering incidence of PDPH
6. What are contraindications for EBP?
7. What are the other consequences of untreated intracranial hypotension?

8. When should EBP be performed under radiologic guidance?
9. What is the role of routine blood cultures before EBP?
10. Would subsequent epidural anaesthesia or analgesia be a contraindication in a patient with EBP?
11. What are the long-term complications of PDPH?

Suggested Reading

1. Hadzic A. Headache after neuraxial anaesthesia. In: Hadzic A, editor. Hadzic's text book of regional anaesthesia and acute pain managment. New York: McGraw-Hill; 2017. p. 481.
2. Sabharwal A, Stocks G. Postpartum headache: diagnosis and management. Contin Educ Anaesth Crit Care Pain. 2011;11(5):181–5.
3. OAA. Treatment of obstetric post-dural puncture headache. Obstetric Anaesthetists' Association. December 2018. https://www.oaa-anaes.ac.uk/assets/_managed/cms/files/Guidelines/New%20PDPH%20Guidelines.pdf.
4. Royal College of Anaesthetists and Association of Anaesthetists of Great Britain and Ireland. Risks associated with your anaesthetic. Section 10: Headache after a spinal or epidural injection. 2015.

John Bailes

Case Scenario

A 70-year-old gentleman with a medical background of moderate COPD and ischaemic heart disease undergoes right shoulder arthroscopic surgery. He receives an interscalene nerve block before proceeding with a general anaesthetic. In the recovery room, he complains of dyspnoea, and his oxygen saturation is recorded at 84% on 5 L oxygen.

1. **What is the most likely diagnosis in this case?**

It is well documented that pain in the immediate postoperative phase after shoulder surgery can be severe. Interscalene nerve blocks have been used widely as part of multimodal analgesic strategies to counteract this. One of the most common complications of the interscalene block is phrenic nerve palsy because it passes very close to the C5 nerve root along its course. This, in turn, results in ipsilateral hemidiaphragmatic paresis. This is of concern in high-risk patients, where a reduction in lung function caused by hemidiaphragmatic paresis can precipitate respiratory decompensation.

2. **What is the differential diagnosis of the present scenario?**

Differential diagnosis of dyspnoea and respiratory distress after interscalene brachial plexus block:

Phrenic nerve palsy
Iatrogenic pneumothorax
Atelectasis
Pneumonia
Pulmonary embolism

3. **What are the signs and symptoms of phrenic nerve palsy**

Acute
  Shortness of breath (dyspnoea)
  Hypoxaemia
  Signs of respiratory distress—accessory muscle use/tachypnoea
  Anxiety
Chronic
  Recurrent pneumonia
  Intermittent anxiety
  Orthopnoea
  Daytime somnolence
  Dyspnoea on exertion

J. Bailes (✉)
Frimley Park Hospital, Frimley, UK
e-mail: bailesjohn@doctors.org.uk

S. Phillips et al. (eds.), *Regional Anaesthesia*, https://doi.org/10.1007/978-3-032-05165-3_33

4. **Discuss management/Treatment plan:**

History
Consider the following points after taking a focused and detailed history of the patient's symptoms.
Review anaesthetic chart:
- When was the block performed? Phrenic nerve palsy is usually transient but can become a permanent lesion.
- How much local anaesthetic was injected? Interscalene volumes >20 mL will almost certainly cause phrenic nerve palsy.
- Were there any technical difficulties? Making direct trauma to the phrenic nerve more likely.

Examination
Complete set of observations, noting SpO2.
Examine the thorax, looking specifically for
- Asymmetrical respiration pattern with decreased expansion on the affected side
- Tracheal deviation is rare but has been reported
- Increased dullness to percussion in the lower zone of the affected side
- Absent breath sounds in the lower zone of the affected side
- Lower than usual oxygen saturations. These are usually preserved in healthy individuals. However, it can drop significantly with concurrent cardiorespiratory co-morbidity.

Diagnose and assess the severity of phrenic nerve palsy:
- Pulmonary function tests. These tests will show a global reduction in lung function from baseline or versus predicted values. Unilateral phrenic nerve palsy can reduce peak expiratory flow rates between 15% and 42%.
- Chest x-ray. It may show elevation of the ipsilateral diaphragm and loss of lung volume.

- Diaphragmatic ultrasound scan (USS). This has been shown to have 93% sensitivity and 100% specificity for diagnosing phrenic nerve dysfunction.
- Arterial blood gas analysis (ABG) will show the impact of the hemidiaphragmatic paresis on the effectiveness of gas exchange.

Management
Supportive measures:
- Titrate oxygen to physiological SpO2
- Non-invasive ventilation—Continuous positive airway pressure (CPAP) or BiPAP (Bilevel Airway pressure) may be needed
- Endotracheal intubation if no improvement, with progressive hypoxia or hypercarbia
- Monitored in a high dependency area until the local anaesthetic wears off and symptoms resolve.

5. **How long does the phrenic nerve palsy usually last?**

Transient phrenic nerve palsy, caused by the spread of local anaesthetic, will last depending upon the type and mass of local anaesthetic are injected. The incidence of transient phrenic nerve palsy depends upon several factors, although it has been widely reported that with interscalene block at volumes of 20 mL and above, the incidence will be 100%.

6. **What strategies are there to reduce the chance of phrenic nerve palsy when performing brachial plexus nerve blocks?**

- Reduce local anaesthetic volume. Evidence shows that using a maximum volume of 10 mL or even 5 mL reduces phrenic nerve palsy but retains the analgesic benefit of the interscalene nerve block.
- Reduce local anaesthetic concentration. Multiple studies have shown that reducing the concentration of local anaesthetic reduces the incidence of phrenic nerve

palsy. However, care should be taken here, as some studies also showed reduced analgesic benefit.

- Change the site of injection. There is evidence that injecting extrafascially or lower down at the C7 nerve root reduces phrenic nerve palsy.
- Perform an alternative nerve block. Examples include performing a superior trunk block, infraclavicular block, combining suprascapular + axillary nerve blocks or local infiltration analgesia (LIA) by surgeons.

7. **Which patient risk factors would make you concerned about causing transient phrenic nerve palsy?**

- Respiratory co-morbidity whereby a 25–30% reduction in lung function may cause decompensation. Examples include:
  - obstructive lung disease, e.g., COPD
  - restrictive lung disease, e.g., Idiopathic Pulmonary Fibrosis
  - cancer of the lung, e.g., lung adenocarcinoma
- High BMI
- Pre-existing contralateral phrenic nerve palsy

The concern for causing transient phrenic nerve palsy is higher if a combination of these factors exists.

Suggested Reading

1. Querney J, Singh SI, Sebbag I. Tracheal deviation with phrenic nerve palsy after brachial plexus block. Anaesth Rep. 2021;9(1):2637–3726.
2. Wiesmann T, Feldmann C, Müller HH, Nentwig L, Beermann A, El-Zayat BF, et al. Phrenic palsy and analgesic quality of continuous supraclavicular vs. interscalene plexus blocks after shoulder surgery. Acta Anaesthesiol Scand. 2016;60(8):1142–51.
3. Boon AJ, Sekiguchi H, Harper CJ, Strommen JA, Ghahfarokhi LS, Watson JC, et al. Sensitivity and specificity of diagnostic ultrasound in the diagnosis of phrenic neuropathy. Neurology. 2014;84(14):1264–70.
4. El-Boghdadly K, Chin KJ, Chan VWS. Phrenic nerve palsy and regional anesthesia for shoulder surgery: anatomical, physiologic, and clinical considerations. Anaesthesiology. 2017;127(1):173–91.
5. Boussuges A, Gole Y, Blanc P. Diaphragmatic motion studied by M-mode ultrasonography: methods, reproducibility, and normal values. Chest. 2009;135(2):391–400.
6. Lloyd T, Tang Y-M, Benson MD, King S. Diaphragmatic paralysis: M mode ultrasound for adult diagnosis. Spinal Cord. 2006;44(8):1362–4393.
7. Urmey WF, Talts KH, Sharrock NE. One hundred percent of hemidiaphragmatic paresis is associated with interscalene brachial plexus anesthesia, as diagnosed by ultrasonography. Anaesth Analg. 1991;72(4):498–503.

Management of Patients on Anticoagulants

34

Nicolas Smal

Case Scenario

A 75-year-old female is sent to your preoperative clinic by the thoracic surgeon. She is scheduled for a right open pneumonectomy for a pulmonary adenocarcinoma. Her medical history includes smoking, hypertension, chronic atrial fibrillation, and chronic kidney disease (CKD) staged 3a.

Her treatment consists of amiodarone 200 mg/day, bisoprolol 2.5 mg BID, rivaroxaban 20 mg/day, and she sometimes takes 1 g of aspirin for headaches. Her blood tests are unremarkable except for her glomerular filtration rate (GFR), which is 48 ml/min/1.73 m².

For this surgery, your local protocol suggests a general anaesthesia with epidural analgesia. Despite ultrasonography guidance, the epidural puncture is complex, and blood is aspirated through the needle during the procedure. You eventually manage to site the catheter before surgery, which is functional. After the surgery, you discuss the need for thromboprophylaxis. The surgeon and you both agree to use a "low" (prophylactic) antithrombotic dose for at least 72 h because the surgery was bloody and complicated.

1. **What is the accepted interval from the rivaroxaban dose before a neuraxial procedure?**

According to guidelines, the recommended time is 72 h before the neuraxial procedure when taking a direct Xa inhibitor (DXA). However, there is a difference between ESAIC/ESRA and ASRA guidelines. In the ESAIC/ESRA, time can be modulated depending on the dose regimen of drugs ("high dose" or "low dose") or level of kidney disease. A prophylactic (once-a-day dose) is typically a low dose, and a treatment dose given twice a day is a high dose. Also, in patients with renal disease, a low dose may behave like a high dose due to reduced clearance, and one needs to be extra cautious. For specific dosages, you may refer to the table in the ESRA or ASRA guidelines.

2. **Is there a difference in time intervals because of ultrasound guidance?**

ESAIC/ESRA guidelines recommend using ultrasound guidance for patients on antithrombotic drugs, but ultrasound guidance does not influence time intervals.

3. **Can a bleeding risk score modify intervals before regional anaesthesia procedures for patients on antithrombotic drugs?**

No, a bleeding risk scoring system exists, but it is not helpful.

N. Smal (✉)
Department of Anaesthesia, CHC Groupe Santé,
Liege, Belgium
e-mail: nicolas.smal@chc.be

© The Author(s), under exclusive license to Springer Nature Switzerland AG 2026
S. Phillips et al. (eds.), *Regional Anaesthesia*, https://doi.org/10.1007/978-3-032-05165-3_34

4. **Is there a need for preoperative bridging?**

No bridging for DXA. There are no specific rules for anticoagulation bridging before regional anaesthesia. However, it may be considered in high-risk cases on an individual basis. Also, when in doubt, a superficial block (vascular structures can be compressed by direct pressure in case of inadvertent bleeding) under ultrasound guidance may be considered. General recommendations from the European Heart Rhythm Association must be followed.

5. **Should rivaroxaban levels be tested before the neuraxial procedure?**

Following ASRA guidelines, DXA must be tested if the time to neuraxial puncture is less than 72 h. Still, an acceptable level of residual DXA activity to proceed with neuraxial block remains to be determined. ESAIC/ESRA guidelines recommend testing DXA levels when a "high" dose of DXA is used, and in case of renal impairment, less than 30 ml/min/1.73 m^2 GFR in case of neuraxial block.

6. **Should she take aspirin on the days before surgery?**

The neuraxial procedure can be performed under "low" dose aspirin (<200 mg) if the risk-benefit analysis is in favour. In case of a "high" dose, the last dose should be at least 3–5 days.

7. **How do you explain the risks of anticoagulants and epidurals to the patient?**

To improve monitoring, the patient should be warned about potential spinal haematoma and asked to report any related symptoms.

8. **What would you do if she took a vitamin K antagonist (VKA)?**

Time from last drug dose to neuraxial procedure depends on the drug:

    acenocoumarol 3 days

    warfarine/fluindione 5 days

    phenprocoumone 7 days.

An International Normalized Ratio (INR) must be performed before surgery and has to be <1.5.

Preoperative bridging with low molecular weight heparin (LMWH) at "high" (anticoagulant) regimen is often required. Time from last "high" dose LMWH to neuraxial procedure is 24 and 48 h in case of renal impairment less than 30 ml/min/1.73 m^2 GFR. A preoperative antiXa testing (target: <0.1 IU/ml) may be considered if renal impairment is less than 30 ml/min/1.73 m^2 GFR and in older, frail, or very low body weight patients.

9. **Which postoperative antithrombotic treatment would you use, and what time from epidural procedure to the first antithrombotic dose?**

DXA and dabigatran.

VKA (following ASRA guidelines, ESAIC/ESRA guidelines advise to bridge with LMWH), unfractionated heparin (UFH) or LMWH—all these drugs at "low" (prophylactic) dose. The first "low" dose of UFH/LMWH is allowed if five half-lives of the drug have passed. In this case, a bloody tap during the procedure is an argument to delay the first dose by 24 h. You will need a pre-procedure platelet count because treatment will be >4 days, and there is a risk of heparin-induced thrombocytopenia (HIT).

10. **What if the patient has a medical history of Heparin-induced thrombocytopenia (HIT)?**

Fondaparinux is the drug of choice in this medical situation. Unfortunately, the catheter is not allowed during a fondaparinux treatment. A peripheral regional anaesthesia technique should be encouraged instead (Such as serratus anterior plane block or erector spinae plane block).

11. **How long can you use a catheter in a patient with anticoagulants?**

Pragmatically, you can keep a catheter if antithrombotic treatment is at a "low" dose.

12. **What specific concern do you have for a patient on prophylactic dose anticoagulants with an epidural catheter, and how will you monitor for this?**

Spinal or epidural hematoma (SHE) is an uncommon but devastating complication of neuraxial puncture. Early signs or symptoms include new or increased back pain, progressive leg weakness or paraesthesia, bladder or bowel disturbances, and sensory loss unrelated to the block. In patients receiving a continuous local anaesthetic infusion, the unexpected progressive motor block should increase the level of suspicion, avoiding attributing the increasing motor and sensory blockade to the action of the local anaesthetic agent. These patients should be examined frequently to detect new or progressive neurologic symptoms. No specific duration is recommended, but monitoring is as frequent as 4–6 h.

The local anaesthetic dose should be at a low concentration to allow monitoring for SHE. For UHF/LMWH, antiXa monitoring is not helpful when the drug regimen is "low".

13. **Is the addition of a nonsteroidal anti-inflammatory drug (NSAID) a good idea?**

NSAID is safe around neuraxial procedures. However, if associated with another antithrombotic drug (here LMWH/UFH), COX-2 inhibitors should be favoured. In this case, NSAID use could worsen renal damage and cause LMWH accumulation.

14. **Are there safety rules for removing a perineuraxial catheter?**

The time from the last drug intake to catheter removal is 4–6 h for "low" dose UHF (IV or SC) and 12 h for "low" dose LMWH. A platelet count should be done before catheter removal because of the HIT risk (treatment > 4 days). There is no need to perform an anti-Xa level when using a low-dose regimen and GFR is >30 ml/min/1.73 m^2. Neurologic monitoring should be extended 24–48 h after catheter removal.

15. **How long should the last dose of rivaroxaban have elapsed to a superficial nerve block? Would you test rivaroxaban activity?**

Superficial nerve block is allowed under any antithrombotic treatment at any dose. Next, the drug intake time is kept the same. ESAIC/ESRA guidelines recommend making a risk-benefit analysis for P2Y12 inhibitors. Ultrasound guidance should be used in these cases.

16. **Is an infraclavicular block allowed in a patient on anticoagulants with an emergency procedure of the upper limb?**

Deep/spinal block-induced bleeding can lead to severe complications. Indeed, compression to avoid/stop haemorrhage is often difficult or impossible, and surgery is needed to manage these situations. On the other hand, a consequence of superficial block-induced bleeding with superficial hematoma is of less clinical significance. Thus, deep/spinal nerve blocks can be considered "high-risk procedures". In contrast, superficial nerve blocks are "low-risk procedures" (This classification is dynamic and can also vary depending on the operator's experience or the available equipment). (Table 34.1) The infraclavicular block is a "deep" and should be managed like an epidural block.

Second Scenario

You meet at your antenatal clinic a 34-year-old woman. She is 35 weeks pregnant, G4P3. In her medical history, you notice three deliveries with epidural analgesia, morbid obesity (BMI > 45), superficial venous thrombosis during the first pregnancy, and an incidental cerebral aneurysm with endovascular treatment (stent). The third-trimester blood sample is standard, and the pregnancy is going well. Her treatment consists of iron, folic acid, gingko, and clopidogrel 75 mg/day. She wants epidural analgesia, and you agree with her because of her morbid obesity.

After a quick call with her neurologist and obstetrician, you decide to plan a labour induction and interrupt clopidogrel before. The neu-

Table 34.1 Nerve blocks classification

Type of block	Deep	Superficial
Consequences of bleeding	Significant and may be disastrous	Not much clinical significance
Management of bleeding	Difficult as the site may be non-compressible	Easy as the location is, it's compressible
Management	Need to customise the antithrombotic drugs to reduce the risk of bleeding	Need not withdraw antithrombotic drugs for bleeding
Example	Stellate ganglion, infraclavicular, epidural, paravertebral, lumbar plexus etc.	Occipital, peribulbar, interscalene, supraclavicular, intercostal, erector spinae, ilioinguinal, femoral, adductor canal, sural

Adapted from ESRA guidelines 2022

rologist tells you that the stent is at high thrombotic risk and asks you to find a prophylactic solution.

Questions

1. **What are the differences between obstetric patients and the non-pregnant population who are on anti-thrombotic treatment and regional anaesthesia?**

The rules are the same for pregnant and non-pregnant populations. In selected parturients at high risk for a thrombotic event who take UFH/LMWH/VKA and require an unplanned or urgent intervention for maternal or fetal indication, the risk of general anaesthesia may be greater than the risk of neuraxial anaesthesia. In these cases, a deviation from guidelines may be considered after multidisciplinary discussion and individual risk-benefit analysis.

2. **You decide to bridge clopidogrel with "low" dose aspirin, and you know that neuraxial procedures are allowed if benefit-risk analysis is in favour. What time from the last clopidogrel intake to the neuraxial puncture?**

P2Y12 inhibitors must be discontinued before the neuraxial procedure. Clopidogrel 5–7 days, ticlopidine 10 days, prasugrel 7–10 days and ticagrelor 5–7 days. Seven days seems safer in this case as bridging can increase bleeding risk.

3. **Do you need a drug level test or a test to measure the activity of the drug before a neuraxial procedure?**

No monitoring can be recommended for platelet inhibitors in any situation.

A platelet count is needed if aspirin is a "high" dose.

4. **You remember ginkgo could have an anti-thrombotic effect; what do you tell her about that?**

Herbal medications are not a reason to cancel a procedure. However, there needs to be more studies about their association with antithrombotic drugs. In this case, you can discontinue it. Time to normal hemostasis after discontinuation is 7 days for garlic, 36 h for ginseng, and 24 h for ginkgo.

Suggested Reading

1. Horlocker TT, Vandermeulen E, Kopp SL, Gogarten W, Leffert LR, Benzon HT. Regional anesthesia in the patient receiving antithrombotic or thrombolytic therapy: American Society of Regional Anesthesia and Pain Medicine evidence-based guidelines (Fourth Edition). Obstet Anesth Dig. 2019;39(1):28–9.
2. Kietaibl S, Ferrandis R, Godier A, Llau J, Lobo C, Macfarlane AJ, et al. Regional anaesthesia in patients on antithrombotic drugs: joint ESAIC/ESRA guidelines. Eur J Anaesthesiol. 2022;39(2):100–32.

Richard Wand

Case Scenario

You have anaesthetised a fit 26-year-old male for an anterior cruciate ligament reconstruction. The patient has been given a general anaesthetic maintained with sevoflurane. An ultrasound-guided adductor canal block using 15 ml of 0.25% levobupivacaine was given. After an hour and 15 min, the systolic blood pressure increased, and the patient started spontaneously breathing with an elevated respiratory rate.

1. **What is the differential diagnosis of the present scenario?**
   - Acute surgical pain
   - Awareness of anaesthesia
   - Inadequacy of muscle relaxants
   - Vasopressor use
   - Equipment error
   - Tourniquet pain

   In this case, the symptoms can be explained by arterial tourniquet pain.

2. **What are the local effects of a tourniquet?**

   The application of a tourniquet typically results in progressive compression effects on the tissue directly beneath it. These effects are directly related to the pressure and duration of the tourniquet application, leading to specific local effects.

(a) Muscular effects: As muscles are deprived of arterial blood supply without sufficient venous drainage, aerobic metabolism initially persists, consuming oxygen and substrates and producing carbon dioxide and water as the primary metabolites. Without arterial perfusion, oxygen supply falls, and metabolism progressively switches to anaerobic pathways, producing lactic acid as a byproduct. This and elevated intracellular carbon dioxide levels result in tissue acidosis. Within 1 h, morphological changes in the mitochondria become visible, and by 2 h, microvascular injury begins to occur. Muscles directly under the tourniquet may also develop local fibre necrosis due to the compression. Once released, these changes cause an increase in vascular permeability and can result in a swollen, still painful limb after the operation that may persist for up to 6 weeks.

(b) Neuronal effects: Within 15–45 min, a combined sensory and motor conduction block may develop, which is usually easily reversible on tourniquet release. Directly under the tourniquet, high pressures can compress myelinated nerve fibres, causing the nerves to bulge at the tourniquet boundaries. This results in the displacement of the nodes of the Ranvier and stretching of the fibres under the tourniquet. This is likely responsible for the

R. Wand (✉)
Wexham Park Hospital, Slough, UK

conduction block; changes can persist for 6 months.

3. What are the local effects of a tourniquet?

Systemic tourniquet effects can occur during inflation and deflation and are related to the location, pressure, and duration of the tourniquet used.

(a) Cardiovascular:
- Inflation leads to a transient increase in preload and afterload, increasing blood pressure.
- Blood pressure often progressively rises during the case known as 'Tourniquet-induced hypertension'. The mechanism is unknown but likely secondary to tourniquet pain, causing sympathetic nervous system activation.
- On release, rapid redistribution occurs, and the venous return of toxic metabolites and carbon dioxide causes vasodilation, resulting in a hypotensive response.

(b) Respiratory
- Consequently, stored carbon dioxide is subsequently washed back into the systemic circulation, causing an increase in end-tidal CO2 in the ventilated patient and a compensatory increase in minute volume when spontaneously breathing. Due to size differences, these changes are more incredible with lower limb tourniquets (0.7–2.4 kPa) than upper limb tourniquets (0.1–1.6 kPa).

(c) Neurological
- Transient Increases in carbon dioxide may increase cerebral blood flow and result in raised intracranial pressure, which is of particular significance in polytrauma patients.

(d) Temperature
- Progressively increases while the tourniquet is applied and is reduced on its release.

(e) Haematological

- A hypercoagulable state may develop while the tourniquet is applied, but there is no evidence of increased incidence of venous thromboembolism intra-operatively.

(f) Metabolic
- A slight increase in potassium (0.3 mmol/L) during tourniquet release is often noted, as is a transient rise in lactate.

4. What are the complications of the tourniquet application?

- Nerve damage: Tourniquet-induced nerve damage has an incidence of 0.024%, with the sciatic and radial nerves being most affected. This is thought to be related to direct nerve pressure and ischaemic time.
- Post-tourniquet syndrome. This is the development of a swollen, still, weak limb with the potential for some degree of rhabdomyolysis, lasting approximately 6 weeks.
- Cutaneous skin injury from poor tourniquet positioning.
- Catastrophic vascular injury can occur when the tourniquet is directly applied over heavily atherosclerotic vessels, which may cause the plaque to rupture.
- Intraoperative bleeding may still occur if systolic blood pressure is significantly elevated or the tourniquet is misused.

5. Why does pain occur on application of a tourniquet?

Tourniquet pain occurs post inflation of tourniquet. Generally, it starts as a progressive dull aching pain, often despite adequate anaesthesia. When used for awake procedures under regional anaesthesia alone, it can be severe enough to warrant conversion to general anaesthesia even when a documented adequate block was performed.

The potential risks associated with tourniquet pain, including nerve damage and cutaneous skin injury, should be a cause for concern. This underscores the need for us to be vigilant and proactive in managing this aspect of patient care.

- Maybe due to unmyelinated slowly conducting C-fibres, which are less effectively blocked by regional anaesthetic techniques and show more resistance to local anaesthetics.
- Continuous stimulation of cutaneous C-fibres at the site of the tourniquet. In the dorsal horn, the inhibitory postsynaptic effects of larger nerve fibres may be blocked by anaesthetic agents; therefore, their expected inhibitory effects are also blocked, resulting in unopposed stimulation of these C-fibres.
- In spinal anaesthesia, C-fibres have returned to function earlier than larger A-fibres so that that tourniquet pain may be the first sign of the density of the block reduction.
- In the upper limb, the medial aspect of the arm is innervated by the lateral cutaneous branches of the second intercostal brachial nerves. These do not originate from the brachial plexus, are purely sensitive, and are often missed by brachial plexus blocks alone.

6. **What strategies can be used to treat pain?**
   - Minimise tourniquet pressure
   - Minimise tourniquet time
   - Larger neuraxial doses of anaesthetic agents
   - Topical local anaesthetic technique to the tourniquet site
   - For upper limb surgery, blockade of the intercostal brachial nerve and the brachial plexus reduces the incidence and onset time of tourniquet pain.

Techniques:
   - Local Anaesthetic injection in the nerve pathway using superficial nerve anatomy (along the axillary vein in the midaxillary line);

- Local Anaesthetic injection with US guidance and thus selective Intercostobrachial nerve blockade.
- IV lidocaine 1.5 mg/kg bolus before tourniquet inflation has been shown to reduce hypertension for lower limb procedures.
- Paracetamol and NSAIDs
- Systemic opioids
- Low-dose ketamine
- It's important to note that while several strategies exist to treat tourniquet pain, a comprehensive treatment strategy has yet to be established. This presents a challenge for us as medical professionals: to continue our research and develop more effective ways to manage this issue.
- Early release of the tourniquet

7. **What is the maximum recommended tourniquet time?**
Most recommendations are for no more than 120 min in a healthy adult. If this time has been exceeded, an audible reminder should be given every 10 min. There is very rarely justification for tourniquet time over 150 min.

8. **What pressure should be used to inflate a tourniquet?**
   - The British Society of Orthopaedics recommends,
   - <16 years old, limb occlusion pressure + 50 mmHg
   - >16 years old upper limb, systolic blood pressure + 50–100 mmHg
   - >16 years old lower limb, systolic blood pressure + 70–130 mmHg

9. **What should you do if it is an anticipated lengthy procedure?**
   - Discuss maximum tourniquet time pre-operatively. Release the tourniquet when time reaches. Allow a minimum of 15 min before re-application.

Questions

1. What is the pain mechanism due to a tourniquet under a functional regional block?
2. What are complications related to prolonged tourniquet use under anaesthesia?
3. What is the recommended minimum dermatomal blockade level for knee surgery under a tourniquet?
4. What are the metabolic changes following tourniquet release?
5. What nerve block can prevent tourniquet pain in a lower limb surgery?

Suggested Reading

1. Deloughry J, Griffiths R. Arterial tourniquets. Contin Educ Anaesth Crit Care Pain. 2009;9(2):56–60.
2. Dickson M, White H, Kinney W, Kambam JR. Extremity tourniquet deflation increases end-tidal pCO2. Anesth Analg. 1990;70:457–8.
3. Siamdoust S, Zaman B, et al. Comparison of the effect of intercoastobrachial nerve block with and without ultrasound guidance on tourniquet pain after axillary brachial plexus block: a randomised clinical trial. Anesth Pain Med. 2023;12(2):e134819.
4. Kumar K, Railton C, et al. Tourniquet application during anaesthesia. What we need to know. J Anaesthesiol Clin Pharmacol. 2016;32(4):424–30.
5. Sun Y, Zhao J, et al. A single injection of lidocaine to reduce tourniquet hypertension in ambulatory arthroscopic patients under general anaesthesia: randomised double-blind, placebo-controlled trial. BJS Open. 2023;7(2):zrad014.
6. British Orthopaedic Association. The safe use of the intraoperative tourniquets. British Orthopaedic Association; 2021.

Interscalene Block

36

Sioned Phillips

Level of Difficulty Difficult

Anatomy & Surface Anatomy

The brachial plexus is formed by the ventral rami of C5–T1 nerve roots (Fig. 36.1).

The C5–C7 roots travel superficially between the anterior and middle scalene muscles (interscalene groove).

The C5 & C6 roots combine to form the upper trunk of the brachial plexus, and the C7 root continues as the middle trunk. Both trunks supply sensation to the shoulder, distal clavicle, and upper arm.

In most individuals, the roots (C5–7) will lie at a depth of 1–3 cm and often lie on top of one another within the interscalene groove.

In the elderly, the scalene muscles can be challenging to delineate, leading to difficulty identifying the interscalene groove. Identification of nerve roots and vertebral level can therefore be done by tracing roots proximally and determining the corresponding transverse process (Fig. 36.2): C5 & C6 transverse processes have a bifid appearance owing to both anterior and posterior tubercles (C5 more prominent posterior tubercle; C6 larger anterior tubercle). C7 has only a posterior tubercle (easy to identify).

There may be anatomical variation with nerve roots travelling within the anterior or middle scalene muscle and even passing anterior to them.

Important Anatomical Structures

The Vertebral artery is found anterior medial to the plexus and must be avoided. Other arteries within the area of interest are the branches of the Thyrocervical trunk, the inferior thyroid, the superior scapular artery, and the transverse cervical artery. Colour Doppler imaging helps identify these structures.

At the cricoid level, the Phrenic nerve lies superficial to the interscalene groove; it then lies anterior to the anterior scalene muscle as it descends within the neck.

The dorsal scapular and long thoracic nerves pass through the middle scalene muscle and can be damaged depending on the approach to the brachial plexus.

S. Phillips (✉)
Department of Anaesthesia, Frimley Park Hospital, Camberley, UK
e-mail: sioned.phillips@nhs.net

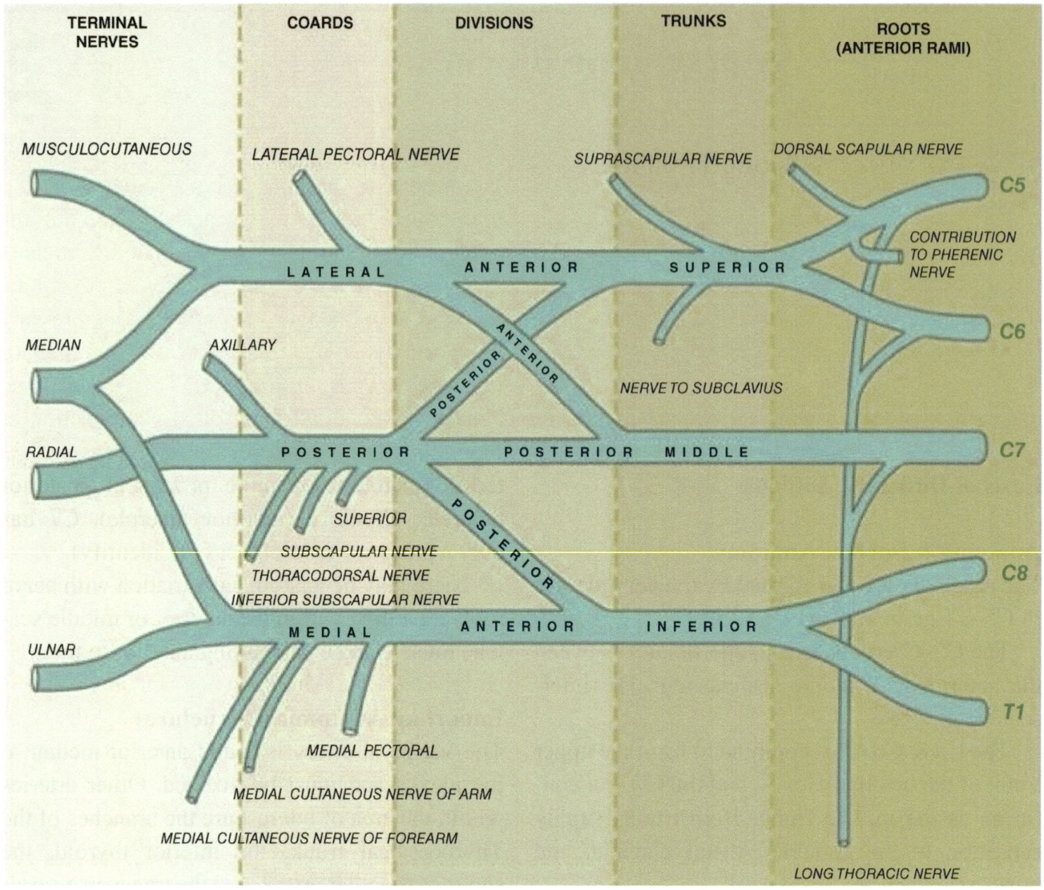

TERMINAL NERVES
COARDS
DIVISIONS
TRUNKS
ROOTS (ANTERIOR RAMI)
MUSCULOCUTANEOUS
LATERAL PECTORAL NERVE
SUPRASCAPULAR NERVE
DORSAL SCAPULAR NERVE
C5
CONTRIBUTION TO PHERENIC NERVE
LATERAL
ANTERIOR
SUPERIOR
ANTERIOR
POSTERIOR
C6
MEDIAN
AXILLARY
NERVE TO SUBCLAVIUS
RADIAL
POSTERIOR
POSTERIOR
MIDDLE
C7
SUPERIOR
POSTERIOR
SUBSCAPULAR NERVE
THORACODORSAL NERVE
INFERIOR SUBSCAPULAR NERVE
C8
MEDIAL
ANTERIOR
INFERIOR
ULNAR
T1
MEDIAL PECTORAL
MEDIAL CULTANEOUS NERVE OF ARM
MEDIAL CULTANEOUS NERVE OF FOREARM
LONG THORACIC NERVE

Fig. 36.1 Brachial plexus

Ant.med.
Post.lat.
Scm
ASm
C5
C6
MSm
IJ. V
C7
Car. A
Ve. V
Ve. A
C7 TP
LCm

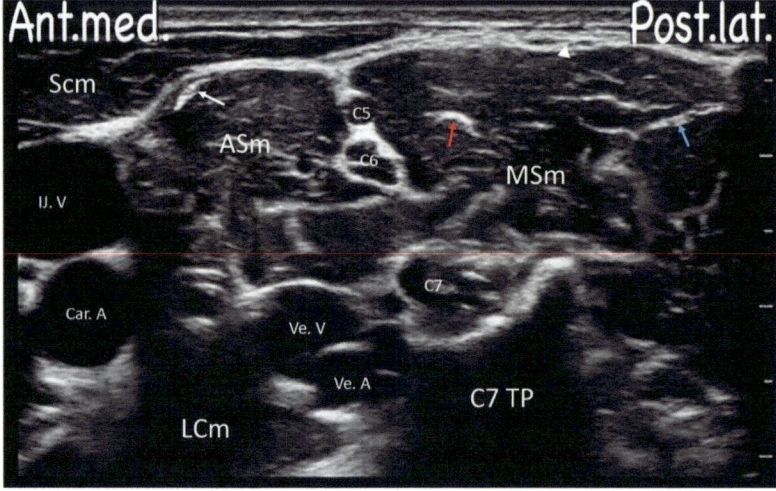

Fig. 36.2 Ultrasound of the brachial plexus in the interscalene region showing sternocleidomastoid muscle (Scm), anterior scalene muscle (ASm), middle scalene muscle (MSm), longus colli muscle (LCm), internal jugular vein (IJ. V), carotid artery (Car. A), vertebral artery (Ve. A), vertebral vein (Ve. V), cervical nerve roots (C5, C6, C7), and C7 transverse process (C7 TP), with anterior-medial (Ant.med.) and posterior-lateral (Post.lat.) orientations. Red and blue arrows mark relevant structures for nerve identification

Surface Landmarks

Cricoid, sternomastoid, external jugular vein, interscalene groove

Indications

Anaesthesia & Analgesia for shoulder surgery
Acromioclavicular, proximal arm and humeral surgery
Clavicle (Lateral 2/3—in combination with superficial cervical plexus)
Manipulation of the dislocated shoulder.

Contraindications

Absolute

Patient refusal
Contralateral phrenic nerve palsy
Contralateral recurrent laryngeal nerve palsy

Relative

Severe respiratory disease (phrenic nerve palsy may worsen respiratory function)

Advantages over Other Techniques

The interscalene block will cover multiple nerves that innervate the shoulder. Some of these can be blocked individually. However, a single shot interscalene block will provide better anaesthesia/analgesia to the shoulder, encompassing all nerves that innervate the shoulder joint.

Nerves Blocked

An interscalene block will block the brachial plexus at the nerve roots (C5/C6/C7) or the upper (C5/6) and middle trunks (C7). This will lead to the blockade of the:

Suprascapular nerve
Axillary nerve
Lateral pectoral nerve
Dorsal scapular nerve
Nerve to supraspinatus
Nerve to infraspinatus

The local anaesthetic often spreads to block C4 and the supraclavicular nerve (a branch of the cervical plexus).

Techniques

Landmark techniques

Winnie's Approach

Patient supine, head away from the side to be blocked.

Landmarks are the posterior border of the SCM, the interscalene groove, and the cricoid cartilage.

The interscalene groove can be found by palpating the posterior border of SCM, then moving laterally and posterior to identify the interscalene groove. To make the interscalene groove more prominent, ask the patient to sniff or take a deep breath.

The needle insertion site is the interscalene groove at the level of C6 (Cricoid cartilage).

Aim the needle at the contralateral elbow.

Do not insert the needle more than 25 mm.

Endpoints for appropriate nerve stimulation are below (muscle responses acceptable).

Meier's Approach

Patient supine, head away from the side to be blocked.

Landmarks are the posterior border of the SCM, the interscalene groove, and the thyroid cartilage.

The interscalene groove can be found by palpating the posterior border of the SCM.

The needle insertion site is the interscalene groove at the level of C4 (Thyroid cartilage). Aim the needle caudad and lateral at a 30° angle. The brachial plexus is found at 30–40 mm with this trajectory.

Endpoints for appropriate nerve stimulation are below (muscle responses acceptable).

Ultrasound Techniques

Scanning protocol

Either:

Identify the trachea at the cricoid level (C6), then scan from medial to lateral to identify the thyroid gland, carotid artery, and internal jugular vein. The sternocleidomastoid (SCM) is superficial to these vessels. Deep to the lateral border of

SCM, the anterior and middle scalene muscles lie within the interscalene grooves and the brachial plexus.

Or

Identify the subclavian artery at the supraclavicular fossa. Lateral to the subclavian artery will lie the trunks and divisions of the brachial plexus (a bunch of grapes appearance). The brachial plexus may also lie posterior or superior to the subclavian artery. Scan cephalad following the nerves proximally within the neck until the roots lie between the anterior and middle scalene muscles. At the interscalene brachial plexus block level, the nerves are seen as round or oval hypoechoic structures.

Structures to Identify
Anterior scalene muscle
Middle scalene muscle
C5 nerve root
C6 nerve root
Upper trunk of brachial plexus

Common carotid artery
Internal jugular vein
Transverse process of C5
Transverse process of C6
Sternocleidomastoid
C7 nerve root

Block Performance
Position/Ergonomics: The patient should be in the semi-recumbent position with their head turned to the contralateral side of the block. If using the US, then the machine is best placed.
   Probe: Linear transducer 8–14 mHz
   Settings: Multibeam resolution
   Depth: 2–3 cm
   Needle size: 22 g short bevel, 50 mm insulated stimulating needle

Needling Technique
The posterior lateral to anterior medial passes through the middle scalene muscle in the plane.

Out of plane, cephalad to caudad. Caution as the needle is not as well visualised.

Optimal Needle Tip Position
Close to C5, C6 nerve root

Drug Choice
Surgical anaesthesia: 15–20 ml of 0.5% bupivacaine or 0.75% ropivacaine.
Analgesia: 5–10 ml of 0.25% bupivacaine or 0.375% ropivacaine. Note that this volume will not spread to the superficial cervical plexus, which may require a separate injection.

Optimal current if nerve stimulation is used: 0.2–0.5 mA
   Muscle responses acceptable: Biceps, deltoid (C5, C6)
      Triceps (C7,C8)
      Other motor responses may be elicited; this can be used to help redirect the needle.

- Contraction of the diaphragm- phrenic nerve-moves the needle position posteriorly.
- Shoulder/scapular movement- dorsal scapular nerve- move needle more anterior
- Scapular movement- nerve to lavator scapulae- move needle more anterior and caudad
- Trapezius muscle contraction- accessory nerve- move needle more caudad and anterior

Testing Block Success
Inability to perform shoulder abduction- deltoid muscle, innervated by C5, C6
Inability to perform elbow flexion- biceps muscle- innervated by C5, C6
Failure to perform elbow extension- triceps muscle- innervated by C7, C8

Side Effects
Horner's Syndrome (ipsilateral ptosis, miosis, and enopthalmia)
Phrenic nerve blockade
Recurrent laryngeal nerve blockade

Complications Specific to the Block

Vertebral artery puncture

Intrathecal injection

Epidural injection

Pneumothorax

Continuous Regional anaesthesia Techniques

The out-of-plane approach is better suited for catheter insertion as the catheter has less muscle to traverse.

Indication

Mainly shoulder arthroplasty, however, there are indications for a single-shot block where post-operative pain is expected to be a significant problem.

Catheter

Multi-orifice catheter

Regime

2 ml/h 0.125% bupivacaine

+/− bolus's of 5 ml

Suggested Reading

1. Polcaro L, Charlick M, Daly DT. Anatomy, Head and Neck: Brachial Plexus. [Updated 2023 Aug 14]. In: StatPearls [Internet]. Treasure Island (FL): StatPearls Publishing; 2026 Jan-. Available from: https://www.ncbi.nlm.nih.gov/books/NBK531473/.
2. Raju P, Coventry D. Ultrasound-guided brachial plexus blocks. Continuing Education in Anaesthesia, Critical Care and Pain, 14, 185–91.
3. Owen RL, VanderWielen BA, Amundson AW, Johnson RL. Tale of two approaches to ultrasound-guided inter-scalene brachial plexus block: a pro-con. Reg Anesth Pain Med. 2025 Jun 24:rapm-2025-106624. https://doi.org/10.1136/rapm-2025-106624.
4. Madison SJ, Humsi J, Loland VJ, Suresh PJ, Sandhu NS, Bishop MJ, Donohue MC, Nie D, Ferguson EJ, Morgan AC, Ilfeld BM. Ultrasound-guided root/trunk (interscalene) block for hand and forearm anesthesia. Reg Anesth Pain Med. 2013 May-Jun;38(3):226–32.

Axillary Block

37

Anju Gupta and Louise Frost

Level of Difficulty Intermediate.

Anatomy and Surface Anatomy
The cords of the brachial plexus branch into their terminal nerves as they pass through the axilla. (Fig. 37.1). The cords and their relevant terminal nerves are described below:

Medial:
> Median nerve
> Ulnar nerve
> Medial cutaneous nerve of the arm
> Medial cutaneous nerve of the forearm
> Medial pectoral

Posterior:
> Radial
> Axillary
> Upper subscapular
> Lower Subscapular
> Thoracodorsal

Lateral:
> Musculocutaneous
> Median nerve (lateral root)
> Lateral pectoral

At the level of the base of the axilla and proximal upper arm, the nerves of the axillary block run close to the brachial artery, where they can be easily visualised on ultrasound.

Indications
Anaesthesia/analgesia to the hand and forearm.

Contraindications

Absolute:
> Patient refusal

Relative:
> Coagulopathy
> Local infection

Advantages over Other Techniques
No risk of some of the complications associated with more proximal brachial plexus blocks, such as pneumothorax, Horner's syndrome, or phrenic nerve blockade.

Ability to quickly provide direct compression in the event of puncturing a blood vessel. Patient does not lose the motor power in the shoulder unlike the other proximal blocks.

Principal Nerves Blocked
> Musculocutaneous
> Radial
> Median
> Ulnar

A. Gupta
Anesthesiology Pain and Critical Care, All India Institute of Medical Sciences, New Delhi, India

L. Frost (✉)
Department of Anaesthesia, Waikato Hospital, Hamilton, New Zealand
e-mail: louise.frost@doctors.net.uk

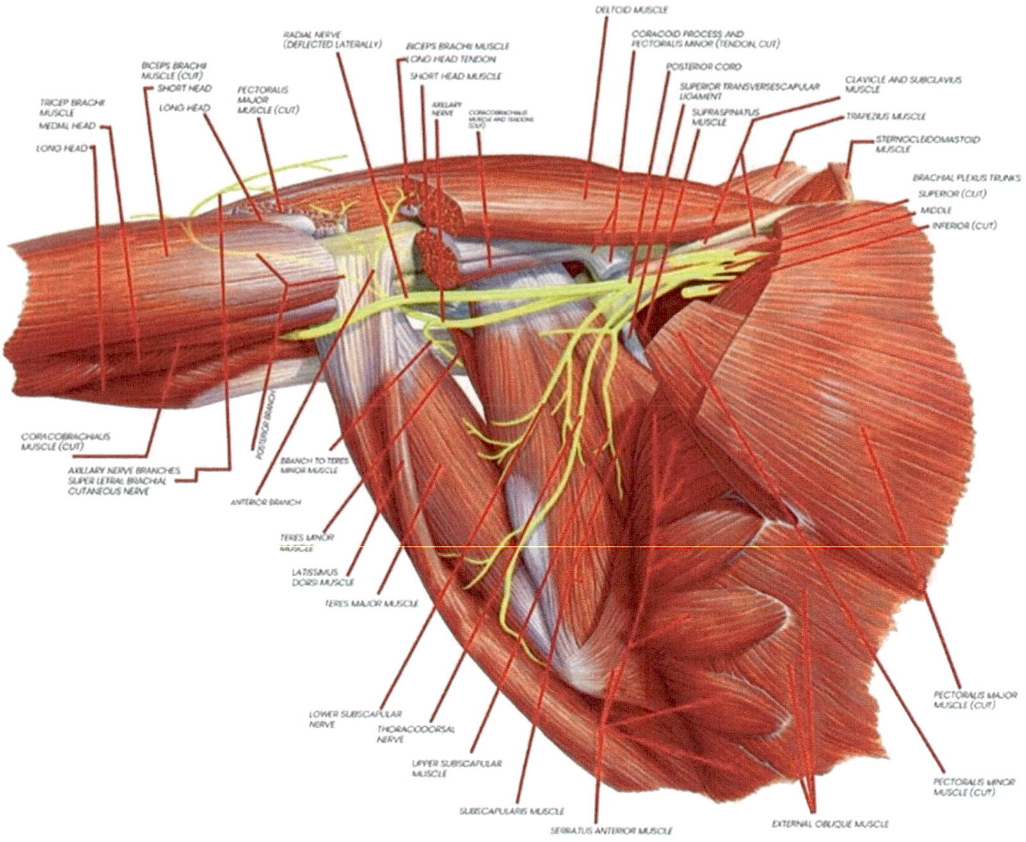

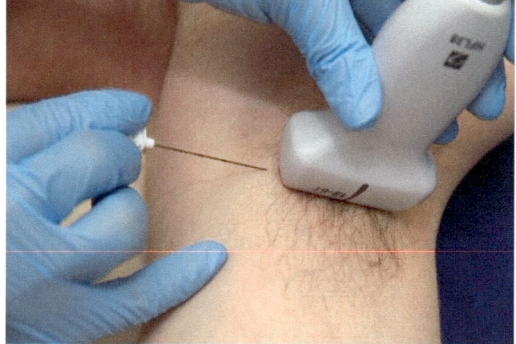

Fig. 37.1 Brachial plexus at the level of axilla

Positioning

Supine, with arm abducted to 90 degrees at the shoulder, positioned on a flat surface. The elbow should be flexed if a nerve stimulator is used. The operator seated near the patient's head, needling cephalad-caudad (Fig. 37.2).

Anatomical Block Techniques.

Ultrasound Techniques

- Scanning protocol:
  - The axilla and arm should be prepared to allow each nerve to be identified by tracing distally before performing the block.
  - The probe should be placed transversely across the axilla at the level of the anterior axillary fold (insertion of pectoralis major)
- Structures to identify:
  Identify the pulsatile brachial artery, using minimal pressure to visualise and note the

Fig. 37.2 Ergonomics and needling direction for Axillary brachial plexus block

locations of the surrounding veins, which can vary in number and location around the artery (Fig. 37.3).

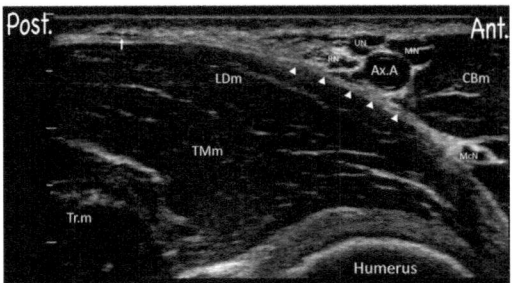

Fig. 37.3 Ultrasound image for axillary brachial plexus block showing the conjoined tendon of Latissimus Dorsi muscle (LDm), teres major muscle (TMm), triceps muscle (Tr.m), humerus, radial nerve (RN), ulnar nerve (UN), median nerve (MN) around the axillary artery (Ax.A). Musculocutaneous nerve (McN) is embedded in the cora-cobrachialis muscle (CBm). Arrowheads—fascia over conjoined tendon, arrow—intercostobrachial nerve

Locate and identify each nerve as follows:

Musculocutaneous

Typically found anteriorly and slightly distant to the artery, moving between the biceps and coracobrachialis, or within the muscle itself. Echogenic, often oval and "fish-like" in appearance. When traced proximally, it slides towards the artery and can sometimes be seen to join with the median nerve. In approximately 16% of the population, the median and musculocutaneous nerves have yet to diverge in the axilla, and so can be blocked together as a single entity.

Radial

Often the most difficult nerve to visualize at this level, the radial sits deep and posterior to the artery ("4–6 o'clock") on the conjoined tendon of latissimus dorsi and teres major. Visualisation may be improved by tilting the ultrasound beam towards the axilla. Scanning distally, the radial moves deeper and away from the artery before descending into the spiral groove.

Median

This is often large and superficial, lying adjacent to the artery at a "10–12 o'clock" position. Its identity is quickly confirmed as the only nerve to remain with the artery with distal scanning. The medial cutaneous nerve of the forearm may at times be visu-

alised as a smaller structure adjacent to the median nerve in the proximal views.

Ulnar

Commonly found in a 1–3 o'clock position. Scanning distally, the ulnar nerve moves posteriorly and away from the artery, often passing deep to a vein, before running superficially on the triceps side, moving towards the medial epicondyle.

Block Performance

- Position/Ergonomics
  When a patient is positioned superficially, the elbow of the arm holding the probe can be stabilised by resting next to the patient's head. The arm performing the needling can rest on the surface supporting the patient's arm (Fig. 37.2).
- Probe: Linear probe, high frequency, e.g., 14–6 MHz, or higher if available.
- Settings: Nerve
- Depth: 2–4 cm, depending on body habitus
- Needle size: 50 mm, short bevelled
- Needling technique: In-plane, targeting nerves above and below the brachial artery. Nerves may be blocked in any order, though blocking deeper structures first may avoid some distortion of the anatomy of areas yet to be blocked by local anaesthetic.
- Optimal needle tip position: Below and above each target nerve, visualising good spread of local anaesthetic around the nerve.
- Drug choice: Dependent on the requirements of block onset and duration. Lidocaine 1–2% with adrenaline may provide anaesthesia of up to 4 h duration, bupivacaine 0.25–0.5% may last over 8 h.
- Volume- approximately 3–5 ml per nerve, although 20–40 ml of total volume may be used for the block, depending on operator experience- adjust the dosage to avoid toxicity.
- Optimal current if NS used- Start at current 1 mA, frequency 2 Hz, pulse width 0.1 millisec. At maximal motor response, reduce current towards 0.5 mA. If movement is still present at 0.2 mA, consider intraneural placement. The motor response should disappear immediately on injection of local anaesthetic

due to increased needle-nerve distance as the fluid displaces the nerve.

- Muscle responses acceptable
  - *Musculocutaneous Nerve:* elbow flexion
  - *Median:* index/middle finger flexion
  - *Ulnar:* thumb adduction, little finger flexion, thumb/little finger opposition
  - *Radial:* thumb/finger extension
- Testing block success- motor deficits in the following movements:
  - *Mucocutaneous-* elbow flexion
  - *Median-*index/middle finger flexion
  - *Ulnar-* Thumb to little finger opposition
  - *Radial-* finger/wrist extension
- Pearls
  - If the musculocutaneous nerve is distant from the artery, it may be blocked as a separate injection point. This allows you to optimise your ultrasound view of the other nerves and use a second insertion site closer to the artery. This can avoid the problem of insufficient needle length for the more distant structures.
  - Angle probe into the axilla to improve views of the conjoined tendon and often the radial nerve.
- Side effects- nil specific to block
- Complications- intravascular injection, aspirate carefully and injection in small aliquots. Easing pressure off of the probe can help to identify the axillary veins, which can be variable in number.
- The intercostobrachial nerve can be difficult to visualise on ultrasound. It may be blocked by a linear subcutaneous injection of local anaesthetic to the axilla.

Continuous Techniques
Indication
For extended analgesia following complex elbow, forearm or hand surgery

Using a similar needling technique, catheter insertion aims to leave the catheter tip within the fascial sheath. It is typically inserted in a plane, aiming to place the catheter below the artery to maximise the chance of radial nerve coverage if required. Infraclavicular catheters may be preferable over axillary catheters as they may have a lower prevalence of catheter colonisation/infection and catheter dislodgement.

Catheter
Multi-orifice catheter
Regime
5 mls/h 0.125% bupivacaine
+/− bolus's of 8 mls

Questions
1. Which nerves in the subcutaneous plane of the axilla are relevant to axillary block and should be targeted?
2. What are the techniques to block intercostobrachial nerve?
3. Which nerve is most frequently spared in axillary nerve block and what are the techniques to improve its coverage?
4. What precautions should be taken to avoid local anaesthetic toxicity in axillary block?
5. If ulnar nerve is spared with axillary brachial plexus block, what rescue block can be helpful for hand surgery?

Suggested Reading

1. Hazdic Textbook of RA Copyright 2017. McGraw-Hill Education.
2. Nicholls B, Conn D, Roberts A. The Abbott pocket guide to practical peripheral nerve blockade. Abott Laboratories Ltd; 2003.
3. Townsley P, et al. A pocket guide to regional anaesthesia. RA-UK; 2019.
4. Ellis, Lawson. Anatomy for anaesthetists. 9th ed. Wiley Blackwell Publishing; 2014.

Namita Sharma and Chetan Mehra

Level of Difficulty Moderate/Easy

Anatomy & Surface Anatomy

The femoral nerve is the largest branch of the lumbar plexus. It arises from the dorsal divisions of the L2, L3, and L4 ventral rami within the psoas major and deep to the fascia iliaca. It emerges from the lateral border of the psoas major. It descends within the groove formed between the psoas and iliacus muscles, passing below the inguinal ligament to enter the anterior compartment of the thigh within the femoral triangle. It lies posterolateral to the femoral vessels outside the femoral sheath, superior to the iliacus and beneath the fascia iliaca.

Immediately after passing below the inguinal ligament, the femoral nerve divides into anterior and posterior divisions, providing cutaneous, muscular, articular and vascular branches. The anterior division provides motor supply to the sartorius and pectineus muscles and sensory innervation to the skin of the anterior and medial thigh. The posterior division provides motor innervation to the quadriceps femoris muscle (rectus femoris, vastus lateralis, vastus intermedius, and vastus medialis) and sensory innervation to the medial aspect of the leg down to the medial malleolus via the saphenous nerve. The hip joint receives some of its sensory supply from the nerve to the rectus femoris, whilst the nerves to the three vasti contribute to the sensory innervation of the knee joint.

Important Anatomical Structures
Surface Landmarks

Anterior superior iliac spine (ASIS), pubic tubercle, inguinal ligament, inguinal crease, femoral artery

Indications
Analgesia

- Fractured neck/shaft of femur
- Knee surgery, e.g., total knee arthroplasty, anterior cruciate ligament repair
- Quadriceps tendon repair
- In combination with a sciatic or popliteal block: above or below-knee amputation

Anaesthesia

- Anterior thigh surgery, e.g., skin graft or muscle biopsy
- Superficial surgery on the medial aspect of the leg below the knee
- In combination with a sciatic or popliteal block: complete anaesthesia of the lower leg, ankle, and foot

N. Sharma (✉)
Ashford and St Peter's Hospital, Chertsey, UK

C. Mehra
Department of Anaesthesia, Indraprastha Apollo Hospital, New Delhi, Delhi, India

S. Phillips et al. (eds.), *Regional Anaesthesia*, https://doi.org/10.1007/978-3-032-05165-3_38

Contraindications

Absolute

- Patient refusal
- Allergy to local anaesthetics
- Inflammation or infection over the injection site

Relative

- Anticoagulation or bleeding disorders
- Previous ilioinguinal surgery (e.g., prosthetic femoral artery graft)
- Pre-existing peripheral neuropathies
- Risk of compartment syndrome (e.g., tibial fractures)

Advantages Over Other Techniques

- The femoral nerve is relatively easily identified on ultrasound lateral to the femoral artery.
- Iliopsoas and the fascia iliaca can be identified even in obese or elderly subjects.

Nerve Territories Blocked

A femoral nerve block will lead to anaesthesia of the anterior-medial aspect of the thigh and knee and the medial border of the leg and medial malleolus. Affected muscles include sartorius, quadriceps femoris, iliopsoas, and pectineus. The femoral nerve also innervates the anterior aspect of the hip joint, the anterior aspect of the femur and the anteromedial aspect of the knee joint.

Block Performance

Position/Ergonomics: Patient supine, with the target limb abducted 10°–20° and externally rotated. The operator should stand on the ipsilateral side. Probe placement: Transverse across the upper thigh, just below the inguinal ligament (Fig. 38.1).

    Probe: Linear transducer 8–14 MHz

    Settings: Multibeam resolution

    Depth: 2–5 cm

    Needle size: 22 G, short bevel, 50–80 mm insulated stimulating needle

Needling Technique

Identify the femoral artery and vein medially, with the femoral nerve seen just lateral to the artery and underneath the fascia iliaca. Optimise the image of the femoral nerve using caudal or cranial tilt of the probe. The needle is advanced through the subcutaneous tissue, fascia lata, and fascia iliaca.

In plane: Lateral to medial, below the inguinal crease.

Out of plane: Caudal to cephalad, below the inguinal crease, lateral to the femoral artery.

Optimal Needle Tip Position

Lateral and inferior to the nerve, below the fascia iliaca. Hydro-dissection can move the needle during block performance to ensure LA surrounds the nerve.

Fig. 38.1 Ultrasound of the femoral region showing the femoral artery (Fem. A), femoral vein (Fem. V), femoral nerve (Fem. N), sartorius muscle (Sm), pectineus muscle (Pm), iliopsoas muscle (IPm), with medial (Med.) and lateral (Lat.) orientations

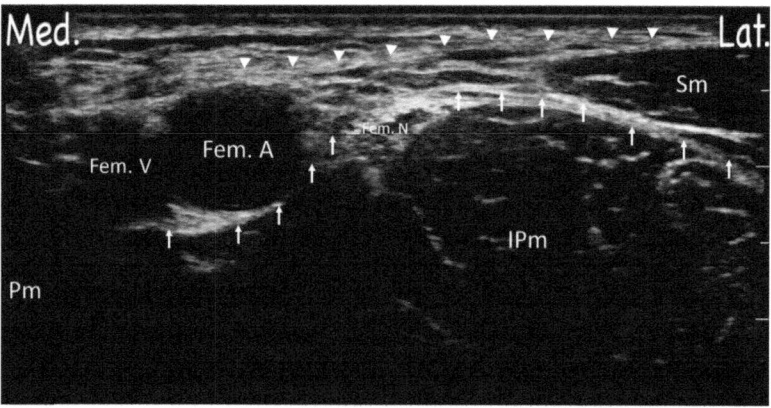

Drug Choice

For surgical anaesthesia: Lidocaine 1.5–2%, Ropivacaine 0.5–0.75% or Bupivacaine 0.5%, depending on the duration of surgery.

For post-operative analgesia: Ropivacaine or Bupivacaine 0.25%.

Volume: 10–20 ml

Optimal current if nerve stimulation is used: Commence at 1 mA.

Muscle Responses Acceptable

The needle's position is adequate when quadriceps muscle contractions (patellar twitch) are elicited with a current output between 0.3 and 0.5 mA.

Other motor responses may be elicited, which can be used to help redirect the needle:

- Local twitch due to direct stimulation of iliopsoas or pectineus: needle insertion too deep, withdraw 1 cm and redirect.
- Sartorius muscle twitch: needle tip is superficial and medial to the target; redirect the needle laterally and/or deeper 1–3 mm.

Testing block success: Quadriceps muscle weakness (knee extension), anaesthesia of the anterior-medial aspect of the thigh and medial aspect of the lower leg.

Clinical Pearls

- The femoral nerve is often a flattened oval or triangular hyperechoic structure lateral to the femoral artery.

- To ensure no branches are missed, the block should be performed as proximally as possible and before the division of the femoral artery.
- Despite being a large nerve, it can sometimes be challenging to identify. If this is the case, a fascia iliaca block can be performed instead.

Side Effects

Quadriceps muscle weakness may delay postoperative physiotherapy and mobilisation, which is undesirable following procedures such as Total Knee arthroplasty.

Complications

- Haematoma
- Vascular puncture
- Difficulty weight-bearing, leading to falls

Continuous Techniques

Indications: Pain management after major femur or knee surgery, above or below knee amputation.

Catheter: Multi-orifice catheter

Regime(s):

- 10 ml/h
- 5 ml/h background infusion with a 15 ml patient-controlled bolus every 4–6 hours

Suggested Reading

1. Gray H. Gray's anatomy: the anatomical basis of clinical practice. Amsterdam: Elsevier.

Adductor Canal Block

Namita Sharma and Chetan Mehra

Level of Difficulty Easy

Introduction

The adductor canal block (ACB) has emerged as a precise and effective analgesic technique following knee surgery since its inception in 2009. It offers a comparable level of analgesia to the femoral nerve block while preserving the strength of the quadriceps, a testament to its precision and efficacy.

Several approaches have been described to block the saphenous nerve from the inguinal region to the medial malleolus.

Anatomy

- **Relevant nerve supply of the knee**
  The knee is innervated by the femoral nerve (via the saphenous nerve and branches to three vasti muscles), the posterior branch of obturator nerve, and the genicular branches of tibial and common peroneal nerves.

N. Sharma (✉)
Ashford and St Peter's Hospital, Chertsey, UK

C. Mehra
Department of Anaesthesia, Indraprastha Apollo Hospital, New Delhi, Delhi, India

The nerve to the vastus medialis has sensory and motor components. It shows a high degree of innervation to the knee joint capsule through intramuscular, extramuscular, and deep genicular nerves. The saphenous nerve innervates via the superficial infrapatellar and posterior branches. It also contributes to the origin of the deep genicular nerves. The obturator nerve has been seen to play a small and largely inconsistent role.

- **Adductor canal**
  The adductor canal, a crucial intermuscular space housing the neurovascular structures of the thigh, extends from the apex of the femoral triangle (Scarpa's triangle) to the adductor hiatus. This anatomical continuity between the femoral triangle and popliteal fossa compartments is significant for the procedure.
  It is conical in shape and triangular in cross-section. The average canal length in men and women is reportedly 8.5 and 10.5 cm, respectively.

  Proximal Border of Adductor Canal: The AC begins at the apex of the femoral triangle. This is where the medial border of the sartorius muscle crosses the medial border of the adductor longus muscle.
  Distal Border: The AC ends at the adductor hiatus, the largest of five fibrous openings within the adductor magnus muscle. The superficial femoral artery passes distally through the adductor hiatus to be renamed as the popliteal artery.

Anterolateral Border: Vastus medialis muscle

Posteromedial Border: Adductor longus and adductor magnus muscles (sometimes referred to as the floor of the adductor canal)

Medial Border: Vasto-adductor membrane (sometimes called the "roof" of the Adductor Canal). Vasto-adductor membrane (VAM) is an aponeurotic sheath sandwiched between the sartorius muscle and the actual adductor canal.

- **True Adductor Canal versus Subsartorial Space**

  The adductor canal is deep into the sartorius muscle, and the span of the sartorius muscle determines its limits. The space between the vastoadductor membrane and the sartorius muscle is called the subsartorial space. However, the distinction is important because the true AC and the sub-sartorial space (superficial to the vastoadductor membrane) contain distinct groups of nerves.

- **Femoral Triangle** (Scarpa's triangle)

  It is an anatomic space with the inguinal ligament forming the proximal border; the medial border of sartorius forming the lateral border; the medial border of adductor longus forming the medial border; the iliopsoas, pectineus, adductor longus, and adductor brevis muscles forming the floor. The intersection between the medial borders of the sartorius and adductor longus muscles forms the apex of the femoral triangle.

- **Subsartorial plexus**

  The sub-sartorial space lies superficial to the vasto-adductor membrane and deep to the sartorius muscle. It houses the subsartorial plexus, which is formed by the contributions from four nerves, namely, the medial cutaneous nerve of the thigh (a branch of the femoral nerve), the saphenous nerve (a branch from the femoral nerve), the cutaneous branch of the anterior division of the obturator nerve, along with the nerve to vastus medialis.

- **Surface Landmarks of the Adductor Canal**

  The adductor canal can be located using surface landmarks and ultrasound. It was initially reported that the midpoint between the anterior superior iliac spine (ASIS) and the patellar base corresponds to the proximal end of the adductor canal. However, it has been demonstrated that the midpoint between the two landmarks localises the femoral triangle. Instead, the adductor canal can be more reliably localized a few centimetres from the original midpoint location.

- **Contents of the Adductor Canal**

  The adductor canal houses the superficial femoral artery, the femoral vein, and the saphenous nerve. Additionally, the nerve to vastus medialis, medial femoral cutaneous nerves, and articular branches of the obturator nerve traverse the canal, although their exact locations remain debatable.

Indications for Adductor Canal Block

1. Post-operative analgesia for knee surgeries is a component of multi-modal analgesia, such as total knee arthroplasty and arthroscopic cruciate ligament reconstruction.
2. Saphenous vein stripping/harvesting.
3. Supplement for medial foot/ankle surgery combined with sciatic nerve block.

Contraindications

Absolute

- Patient refusal

Relative

- Allergy to a local anaesthetic agent
- Patient on anticoagulants (refer to ESAIC/ESRA 2022 guidelines)
- Infection at the site of injection

Advantages Over Other Techniques

- Advantage over femoral nerve block:
  Using ACB over FNB helps avoid quadriceps weakness and reduces the time required to attain an independent ambulatory status, thus aiding faster recovery and rehabilitation.
- Advantage over epidural anaesthesia/analgesia:

ACB avoids bilateral lower limb anaesthesia, prevents significant hemodynamic compromise or urinary retention, and can be used in patients with spine abnormalities.

Techniques of Adductor Canal Block
- **Peripheral Nerve Stimulator-guided technique**:
  The landmark for needle insertion is approximately four finger breadths (7–8 cm) above the adductor tubercle on the medial condyle of the femur in the groove (Jobert's fossa), between the sartorius and the vastus medialis muscle.
  A peripheral nerve stimulator can stimulate extramuscular branches of the nerve to the vastus medialis. The needle is inserted in the groove between the vastus medialis and sartorius and directed perpendicular to the skin with slight posterior angulation until the contraction of the vastus medialis muscle is elicited, followed by LA injection.
- **Ultrasound-guided technique**
  Ultrasound Anatomy
  The sartorius appears as a trapezoid-shaped muscle on cross-section. The adductor longus is replaced by the adductor magnus while scanning distally on the medial side of the adductor canal. The femoral vein (compressible), femoral artery (pulsatile), and saphenous nerve can be identified at a depth of 2–3 cm (Fig. 39.1).

Ultrasound techniques
Scanning Protocol:
Place the transducer anteromedially at the junction between the middle and distal third of the thigh and identify the proximal and distal ends of the adductor canal. The proximal end of the adductor canal can be determined at the level at which the medial border of the sartorius mus-

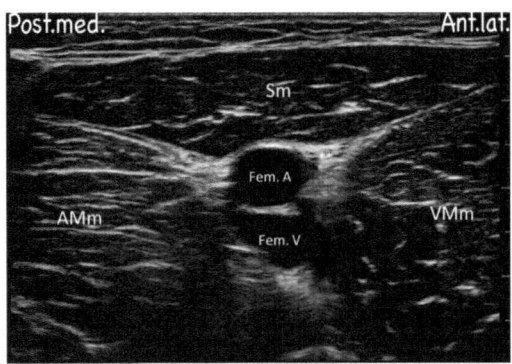

Fig. 39.1 Ultrasound of the adductor canal showing the femoral artery (Fem. A), femoral vein (Fem. V), sartorius muscle (Sm), adductor magnus muscle (AMm), vastus medialis muscle (VMm), with posterior-medial (Post. med.) and anterior-lateral (Ant.lat.) orientations

cle crosses the medial border of the adductor longus muscle. The level at which the femoral artery passes through the adductor hiatus to become the popliteal artery is identified as the distal end of the adductor canal (Fig. 39.1).

Both proximal and distal injection sites within the adductor canal have been described.

A pure saphenous nerve block can be performed at the most distal level, where the femoral artery still lies immediately deep into the sartorius muscle, thus minimizing the motor deficit of the vastus medialis.

Block Performance
Position/Ergonomics: The patient lies supine, with the thigh abducted and externally rotated to allow access to the medial thigh.

Probe: A linear, high-frequency transducer (8–10 MHz) with a sterile sleeve and gel is used generally. A curvilinear transducer may be needed for a more extensive patient.

Settings: Multibeam resolution

Depth settings: 7–10 cm depending upon the patient's habitus

Needle size: 22 G short bevel, 50–100 mm insulated stimulating needle

Needling Technique

The needle is inserted in-plane in a lateral to medial orientation and advanced towards the femoral artery. An out-of-plane needling approach, in which the needle passes through the belly of the sartorius muscle, can also be used. Saline hydrodissection can help visualize the needle tip.

Optimal Needle Tip Position

The needle tip should finally lie just anterolateral to the femoral artery, deep to the sartorius muscle, and local anaesthetic should be injected to spread around the artery, as confirmed with ultrasound visualization. Visualization of the nerve is not mandatory for block performance.

Nerve to Vastus Medialis Blockade with Adductor Canal Block

The nerve to Vastus Medialis blockade has been cited as a possible cause of motor weakness following the adductor canal block. The nerve runs lateral to the femoral vessels and saphenous nerve after emerging from the femoral nerve. The nerve to the vastus medialis travels within its fascial sheath, separate from the adductor canal. It then divides into a sensory branch (posteromedial) and one to four muscular branches (anterolateral) that enter the vastus medialis muscle to supply motor innervation (Table 39.1). The location of the muscular branch is found slightly below the mid-thigh level.

Hence, the block performed at the proximal end of the adductor canal may be the optimal injection location as it would block the saphenous nerve and the sensory branches of the nerve to vastus medialis while sparing its motor fibres.

Therefore, an adductor canal block executed proximal to the adductor canal would anaesthetize the nerve to the vastus medialis and the saphenous nerve and should be called a femoral triangle block.

Drug Choice

Local anaesthetic volume: 10–15 ml
Surgical anaesthesia: 0.25% Bupivacaine/0.375% Ropivacaine
Analgesia: 0.2% Ropivacaine

Table 39.1 The nerves likely to get blocked depending on the location of the block

	Level of Adductor Canal Block (Anatomical correlation)	Nerves are likely to be blocked
1	Femoral triangle (Mid-thigh)	Saphenous nerve and NVM
2	The proximal end of the Adductor canal	Saphenous nerve and sensory branches of NVM (motor fibres of NVM spared)
3	Distal Adductor canal	Saphenous nerve

Testing Block Success

The sensory deficit on the medial side of the leg spans from the medial side of the knee to the medial malleolus.

Potential Complications

Puncture of the femoral vessels, causing a hematoma

Direct impalement of the saphenous nerve leading to neuralgia

Continuous Regional Analgesia Techniques

A single injection of an adductor canal block provided a mean duration of nearly 10.5 h of pain relief. For extended post-operative analgesia, a continuous perineural catheter insertion can be performed.

Both in-plane and out-of-plane techniques can be used for catheter insertion.

The catheter can then be secured by tunnelling into subcutaneous tissues.

Indication

Total knee arthroplasty, arthroscopic reconstructive surgeries.

Catheter

A multi-orifice catheter helps evenly distribute local anaesthetic within the adductor canal and plane where the nerve to vastus medialis lies.

Regime

5 ml/h 0.125% Bupivacaine or 0.2% Ropivacaine, with a provision of patient-controlled perineural boluses of 5 ml of the same solution.

Points to Understand

1. Continuum of the femoral triangle, adductor canal, adductor hiatus, and popliteal fossa

The adductor canal is not a closed space. It communicates with the femoral triangle proximally and the adductor hiatus distally. The injected local anaesthetic drug in the adductor canal has been seen to spread to the femoral triangle, even as far as the popliteal fossa.

Thus, these characteristics of the ACB influence the degree of pain relief and muscle weakness (Fig. 39.1).

2. Sciatic nerve weakness with adductor canal block

An extension of local anaesthetic distally to bathe the peroneal and tibial nerves has also been observed. This drug spread appears to occur through the adductor hiatus, the accessory hiatus, and/or in the intermuscular plane of the adductor magnus, resulting in some sensory block of the sciatic nerve and/or its branches in the popliteal fossa (especially if ACB is performed at the level of the adductor hiatus).

Post-procedure advice/precautions

Adductor canal blocks performed proximally or using larger volumes can lead to weakness in the quadriceps. Hence, patient education and assisted ambulation (with or without a knee brace) should be encouraged post-surgery.

Suggested Reading

1. Manickam B, Perlas A, Duggan E, Brull R, Chan VW, Ramlogan R. Feasibility and efficacy of ultrasound-guided block of the saphenous nerve in the adductor canal. Reg Anesth Pain Med. 2009;34:578–80.
2. Burckett-St Laurant D, Peng P, Girón Arango L, Niazi AU, Chan VW, Agur A, et al. The nerves of the adductor canal and the innervation of the knee: an anatomic study. Reg Anesth Pain Med. 2016;41:321–7.
3. Bendtsen TF, Moriggl B, Chan V, Borglum J. The optimal analgesic block for total knee arthroplasty. Reg Anesth Pain Med. 2016;41:711–9.
4. Panchamia JK, Niesen AD, Amundson AW. Adductor canal versus femoral triangle: let us all get on the same page. Anesth Analg. 2018;127(3):e50.
5. Wong WY, Bjørn S, Strid JM, Børglum J, Bendtsen TF. Defining the location of the adductor canal using ultrasound. Reg Anesth Pain Med. 2017;42(2):241–5.
6. Thiranagama R. Nerve supply of human vastus medialis. J Anat. 1990;170:193–8.
7. Kietaibl S, Ferrandis R, Godier A, Llau J, Lobo C, Macfarlane AJ, Schlimp CJ, Vandermeulen E, Volk T, von Heymann C, Wolmarans M, Afshari A. regional anaesthesia in patients on antithrombotic drugs: Joint ESAIC/ESRA guidelines. Eur J Anaesthesiol. 2022;39(2):100–32.
8. Ishiguro S, Yokochi A, Yoshioka K, Asano N, Deguchi A, Iwasaki Y, et al. Technical communication: anatomy and clinical implications of ultrasound-guided selective femoral nerve block. Anesth Analg. 2012;115:1467–70.
9. Singh SK, Roy R, Agarwal G, Pradhan C. Peripheral nerve stimulator (PNS) guided adductor canal block: a novel approach to regional analgesia technique. Anaesth Pain Intensive Care. 2017;21(3):340–3.
10. Guntz E, Herman P, Debizet E, Delhaye D, Coulic V, Sosnowski M. Sciatic nerve block in the popliteal fossa: description of a new medial approach. Can J Anesth. 2004;51:817–20.
11. Kim MK, Moon HY, Ryu CG, Kang H, Lee HJ, Shin HY. The analgesic efficacy of the continuous adductor canal block compared to continuous intravenous fentanyl infusion with a single-shot adductor canal block in total knee arthroplasty: a randomized controlled trial. Korean J Pain. 2019;32:30–8.
12. Jæger P, Zaric D, Fomsgaard JS, Hilsted KL, Bjerregaard J, Gyrn J, et al. Adductor canal block versus femoral nerve block for analgesia after total knee arthroplasty: a randomized, double-blind study. Reg Anesth Pain Med. 2013;38:526–32.
13. Gautier PE, Hadzic A, Lecoq JP, Brichant JF, Kuroda MM, Vandepitte C. Distribution of injectate and sensory-motor blockade after adductor canal block. Anesth Analg. 2016;122:279–82.
14. Deloach JK, Boezaart AP. Is an adductor canal block simply an indirect femoral nerve block? Anesthesiology. 2014;121:1349–50.
15. Chen J, Lesser JB, Hadzic A, Reiss W, Resta-Flarer F. Adductor canal block can result in motor block of the quadriceps muscle. Reg Anesth Pain Med. 2014;39:170–1.
16. Andersen HL, Andersen SL, Tranum-Jensen J. The spread of injectate during saphenous nerve block at the adductor canal: a cadaver study. Acta Anaesthesiol Scand. 2015;59:238–45.
17. Gautier PE, Lecoq JP, Vandepitte C, Harstein G, Brichant JF. Impairment of sciatic nerve function during adductor canal block. Reg Anesth Pain Med. 2015;40:85–9.
18. Cowlishaw P, Kotze P. Adductor canal block – or subsartorial canal block? Reg Anesth Pain Med. 2015;40:175–6.

Popliteal Sciatic Nerve Block

Namita Sharma and Chetan Mehra

Level of Difficulty Intermediate

Functional Anatomy

The sciatic nerve consists of two separate trunks: the tibial and common peroneal nerves. A common epineural sheath envelops the two nerves at their outset in the pelvis. The sciatic nerve diverges into its two components at a variable distance (usually 50–120 mm proximal to the popliteal crease) while descending towards the knee.

The tibial nerve (the larger of the two divisions) continues vertically through the popliteal fossa and terminates as the medial and lateral plantar nerves. Its collateral branches give rise to the cutaneous sural nerves, muscular branches to the muscles of the calf, and articular branches to the ankle joint.

The common peroneal nerve descends along the head and neck of the fibula. It gives articular branches to the knee joint and cutaneous branches that form the sural nerve. Its terminal branches are the superficial and deep peroneal nerves.

Indications

The sciatic nerve block at the popliteal level anesthetizes the leg distal to the hamstring muscles. It can provide surgical anaesthesia for procedures below the level of the knee, including corrective foot surgery, foot debridement, short saphenous vein stripping, repair of the Achilles tendon, toe amputation, and midfoot amputation.

If the medial aspect of the lower leg and foot is required to be anaesthetised, then a femoral nerve or saphenous nerve block needs to be used in conjunction to cover this area.

Contraindications

Previous popliteal surgery (e.g., presence of a vascular graft), popliteal tumor, local infection, pre-existing sciatic neuropathy

Advantages Over Other Techniques

Easy to master, relatively constant landmarks, can be performed using surface landmarks, a peripheral nerve stimulator, and ultrasound. Less hemodynamic alterations. It can be performed with the patient in the supine, lateral, or prone position.

Nerves Blocked (Distribution of Anaesthesia)

Popliteal blockade results in anaesthesia of the entire distal two-thirds of the lower extremity, except the medial aspect of the leg (which is supplied by the saphenous branch of the femoral nerve).

Equipment

Marking pen and surface electrode (for PNS guided technique)

5–10 cm long, short-bevel, insulated stimulating needle (depending upon the approach used)

N. Sharma (✉)
Ashford and St Peter's Hospital, Chertsey, UK

C. Mehra
Department of Anaesthesia, Indraprastha Apollo Hospital, New Delhi, Delhi, India

Peripheral nerve stimulator

Ultrasound machine with a high-frequency linear probe

Techniques

1. Intertendinous (Posterior) Approach

- **Patient position:**
  The patient lies in the prone or lateral position with the ipsilateral foot positioned on rest or placed off the surface of the table, to allow observation of the evoked motor responses of the foot or toes when used along with a peripheral nerve stimulator.
- **Ergonomics:**
  The operator stands on the ipsilateral side of the patient to observe the evoked motor responses while simultaneously performing the block.
- **Anatomic Landmarks**
- **Margins** of the popliteal fossa are marked as follows
  1. Biceps femoris tendon forms the lateral side
  2. Semitendinosus and semimembranosus tendons form the medial side
  3. The intercondylar line forms the base of the popliteal fossa crease (line A)

  These landmarks can be accentuated by asking the patient to flex the knee joint against resistance, which allows easy palpation of the tendons.

A perpendicular line (line B) is drawn cranially from the mid-point of the popliteal fossa crease, and a point X is marked at a distance of 5–7 cm on this line. The popliteal artery pulsation can be appreciated here. The point of needle entry is marked 1 cm lateral to point X.

(a) Peripheral Nerve Stimulator Guided Technique

A 5 cm insulated nerve block needle is inserted either perpendicular or directed slightly cranially at the marked point X.

The nerve stimulator should be initially set to deliver 1.0 mA current (2 Hz, 100 s). Sciatic nerve (tibial or common peroneal components) is typically stimulated at a depth of 1–3 cm from the skin surface.

Evoked Motor Responses are acceptable.

Plantar flexion and/or inversion—Tibial Nerve stimulation

Dorsi flexion and/or eversion—Common Peroneal Nerve stimulation

Optimal current if nerve stimulation is used

The needle position is accepted when evoked motor response is elicited with current intensity of 0.3–0.5 mA.

Troubleshooting

- Local twitch of biceps muscle due to direct stimulation of biceps femoris indicates the too-lateral placement of the needle: Withdraw the needle and redirect 5°–10° medially.
- Local twitch of semitendinosus/semimembranosus muscles due to direct stimulation of these muscles can happen due to too medial placement of the needle: Withdraw the needle and redirect 5°–10° laterally.
- Vascular puncture due to puncture of popliteal vessels can occur due to medial placement of the needle; redirect the needle laterally.

Drug Choice

Surgical anaesthesia: 15–20 ml of 0.5% bupivacaine or 0.75% ropivacaine.

Analgesia: 15–20 ml of 0.125% bupivacaine or 0.2% ropivacaine.

A local anaesthetic solution is injected in small aliquots, with repeated negative blood aspiration.

Testing Block Success and Block Dynamics

Sensory deficit below the knee level (baring the medial strip of skin supplied by the saphenous nerve). The motor deficit is confirmed by weakness in the movement of the ankle or toes.

2. Lateral Approach

The main advantage of the lateral approach to the popliteal block is that the patient does not need to be positioned in the prone position as with the posterior approach. The patient's position is a key factor in the success of the procedure.

- **Patient position:**
  The patient lies in the supine position with the Knee flexed at 90° without any external rotation at the hip joint. Any deviation from this angle changes the relationship of the sciatic nerve to the femur and biceps femoris muscle.
- **Ergonomics:**
  The operator should preferably be seated, facing the side to be blocked. The bed height should be adjusted so that the performer can simultaneously monitor both the patient and the responses to nerve stimulation.
- **Anatomic Landmarks:**
  Surface landmarks are appreciated on the lateral aspect of the thigh, just cranial to the popliteal fossa crease and marked as follows:
  1. Popliteal fossa crease
  2. Vastus lateralis muscle
  3. Biceps femoris muscle

The needle insertion site is marked at a point 8 cm above the popliteal fossa crease in the groove between the vastus lateralis and biceps femoris muscles.

Knee flexion helps identify the popliteal fossa crease, biceps, and vastus lateralis muscles.

Peripheral Nerve Stimulator Guided Technique

The sciatic nerve is positioned between the biceps and semitendinosus muscles.

Due to the delicate nature of the sciatic nerve, caution and precision are paramount in the technique. The needle is inserted in a horizontal plane between the vastus lateralis and biceps femoris muscles and advanced to contact with the femur. It is then redirected and advanced posteriorly up to 30° to stimulate the nerve.

Frequent needle manipulations with a slightly posterior redirection (5°–10° posterior angulation) may be needed to locate the sciatic nerve. This is a normal part of the procedure and should not cause concern.

During block performance, the common peroneal nerve stimulation is usually obtained first.

Time because the nerve is positioned laterally and more superficial than the tibial nerve.

Nerve depth: 5–7 cm

Troubleshooting

- Reassess anatomic landmarks and ensure the leg is not externally rotated in the hip joint.
- Direct stimulation of the biceps femoris muscle indicates too shallow placement of the needle: advance the needle deeper.
- Direct stimulation of the vastus lateralis muscle indicates an anterior placement of the needle: redirect the needle posteriorly.

Ultrasound Guided Popliteal Sciatic Nerve Block

Concept of The Paraneural Sheath and the Fascial Compartments Surrounding the Sciatic Nerve at the Popliteal Fossa:

A paraneural sheath has been suggested as a hyperechoic fascial layer between the outer surface of the sciatic nerve (an epineurium) and the epimysium of the surrounding muscles while scanning the sciatic nerve using ultrasound. The paraneural sheath is distinct from the epineurium, better delineated after the local anaesthetic injection, and envelopes the sciatic nerve and the common peroneal and tibial nerves separately. The authors classified the fascial compartments as the "subepimyseal perineural compartment" and the "subparaneural compartment" surrounding the sciatic nerve and acting as conduits for local anaesthetic spread during a popliteal SNB.

To facilitate atraumatic paraneural penetration, finding the groove between the two components at the bifurcation level is suggested because ultrasound differentiation between the paraneural sheath and epineurium at the pre-bifurcation level can be difficult.

- **Scanning protocol:**
  Transducer position: Transverse over the popliteal crease posteriorly or on the lateral aspect of the thigh, and then slide cranially while identifying relevant anatomical landmarks.
  The transducer position and the ultrasound image for the lateral and posterior approaches remain the same. The sciatic nerve and/or tib-

ial and common peroneal nerves are viewed on the short axis (Fig. 40.1).

- **Structures to identify:**

Identify the popliteal artery (pulsatile, hypoechoic) or popliteal vein (compressible, hypoechoic) in the centre of the superficial. The vein lies more posterior than the artery.

The tibial nerve is identified immediately posterior to the vessels, appearing as a distinct hyperechoic circle with internal hypoechoic fascicles (honeycombing pattern). The transducer is then moved in a proximal direction to identify the common peroneal nerve, which appears as a smaller hyperechoic circle joining the tibial component from the lateral aspect of the screen. Alternate dorsiflexion and plantar flexion of the foot (sea-saw sign) can improve ultrasonographic identification of sciatic nerve components.

The transducer is finally adjusted at the point of bifurcation of the sciatic nerve into tibial and common peroneal nerve divisions.

The ultrasound beam's depth, gain, and direction should be adjusted to better visualize the nerves, as they offer anisotropy.

Block Performance

Position/Ergonomics: The patient lies in the supine position for the lateral approach and prone or lateral decubitus position for the posterior approach.

When the sciatic nerve is blocked with the lateral approach in the supine position, the lower limb must be sufficiently elevated to enable adequate space around the knee joint for the transducer to be applied.

Probe: A linear high-frequency transducer (8–12 MHz) with gel and a covering sheath.

A curved transducer might be needed in a very obese patient.

Settings: Musculoskeletal

Depth: The sciatic nerve is typically visualised at a 2–4 cm depth.

Needle size: 10 cm short bevel, insulated nerve block needle

Needling Technique

Lateral approach—in-plane
Posterior approach—out-of-plane

Optimal Needle Tip Position

The needle is advanced to pierce the perineurium of the sciatic nerve. A tactile and visual "popping" sensation may be felt as this tissue is breached.

Local anaesthetic spread is noted circumferentially around the sciatic nerve within a common epineural sheath of tibial and common peroneal nerves. Local anaesthetic spread proximally and distally to the injection site around both nerve divisions can be seen with the proximal and distal translation of the transducer.

This drug spread typically results in the separation of TN and CPN during and after the injection.

Alternatively, separate blocks of the Tibial Nerve and Common Peroneal Nerve can be made.

The sub-paraneural spread of local anaesthetic is considered the ultrasound endpoint.

If nerve stimulation is used (0.5 mA, 0.1 ms), the needle tip's contact with the sciatic nerve usually causes a motor response in the calf or foot.

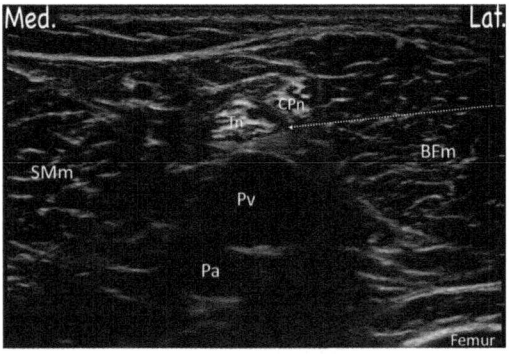

Fig. 40.1 Ultrasound-Guided Anatomy for Sciatic Nerve Block at the Popliteal Fossa. Visualization of the sciatic nerve bifurcating into the tibial (Tn) and common peroneal (CPn) nerves, with adjacent structures including the popliteal vein (Pv), popliteal artery (Pa), and surrounding muscles

Key Points

- **Lateral approach**

The needle is inserted in an in-plane manner, around 3–4 cm away from the edge of the transducer, to improve its alignment with the faceplate of the transducer and thus produce a better image.

- **Posterior Approach**
  An out-of-plane needle insertion technique is used, and the needle tip is targeted just distal to the bifurcation of the sciatic nerve into the tibial and common peroneal nerves. The procedure for the lateral approach remains the same as described.
- Note that although the image appears the same, there is a 180° difference in patient orientation.
- Different depths and angles of the divisions of the sciatic nerve cause anisotropy and difficulty in capturing both nerves perpendicular in the same image. The traceback approach along the tibial nerve at the popliteal crease augments the popliteal venous flow by squeezing the calf, allowing for easier identification of the TN.

Medial Approach to Popliteal Sciatic Nerve Block

Patients are supine, with the hip and knee on the operated side flexed and the thigh externally rotated at approximately 45°.

The popliteal vessels and the tibial nerve are identified first by positioning a linear transducer in the popliteal fossa. The transducer is then slid proximally and placed at the level of the SN bifurcation to locate the tibial nerve and the common peroneal nerve. A 100 mm insulated needle is then inserted in-plane with the transducer toward the SN bifurcation from the medial side of the thigh. When using a medial approach, the needle tip may be closer to the tibial nerve than the common peroneal nerve. Avoidance of lower limb elevation or position change is advantageous for this approach.

Different leg positions (gapped, figure of four, or using a sandbag under the ankle) have been used to obtain enough space to perform the supine block. However, the knee is unsteady in these positions, and an assistant, towels, or special equipment is usually required to gain the position. To bypass these requirements and the unsteadiness of the knee, Taha et al. It was suggested to rest the lateral aspects of the thigh, knee, leg, and foot on the bed. This can be achieved by using the figure-of-four position

with a slight knee flexion, with or without a minor ipsilateral pelvic tilt. They described (a) a scanning technique for the medial aspect of the thigh, using a curvilinear transducer and an out-of-plane needle insertion technique; (b) a scanning technique for the posterior aspect of the thigh, using a linear transducer and an in-plane needle insertion technique for the popliteal sciatic nerve block.

Recently, Ultrasound guided CAPS (Crosswise Approach to Popliteal Sciatic) block has been described by Mistry et al. which is a supine lateral approach and involves a lateral-to-medial, transverse approach, targeting the sciatic nerve 5–10 cm above the popliteal crease. A linear or curvilinear ultrasound probe is placed on the lateral distal thigh, scanning across the leg in short axis to identify the femur, biceps femoris muscle, and the sciatic nerve. Nerve is approached in an out-of-plane manner, with minimal adjustments of the ipsilateral leg.

Continuous Catheter Technique
Indication

Reconstructive lower limb surgeries below the level of the knee, including complex ankle surgeries, where post-operative pain is expected to be a significant problem post-operatively.

- **Technique**
  A perineural catheter can be inserted using either a lateral or posterior technique. The block needle is advanced slowly with a slight cranial direction while seeking a plantar or dorsiflexion of the foot or toes.
  The catheter is advanced for 5 cm beyond the needle tip. The catheter is checked for inadvertent intravascular placement by negative aspiration test for blood and tunnelled subcutaneously to avoid accidental dislodgement.

Advantages of the lateral approach for continuous catheter techniques:

(a) The biceps femoris muscle tends to stabilize the catheter and decrease the chance of dislodgment, compared with the subcutaneous tissue of the popliteal fossa in the prone approach.

(b) If the knee is to be flexed and extended, the side of the thigh is less mobile than the back of the knee.

(c) Access to the catheter site is more convenient with the lateral approach compared with the prone approach.

Advantages of posterior (out-of-plane) approach for continuous catheter techniques:

(a) The catheter has less muscle to traverse, so patient discomfort is less.

Catheter

A kit for catheter placement with 80–100 mm introducer needle

Regime

Initial bolus dose: 10–15 ml 0.25% Bupivacaine

Continuous infusion: A low basal infusion rate (e.g., 5 ml/h) associated with a provision of PCA boluses (e.g., 2.5 ml—lockout of 30 min) of 0.125% plain bupivacaine, or 0.2% plain ropivacaine.

Potential Complications

Complications after a popliteal block are uncommon. These include:

- A hematoma can happen with multiple needle passes, a larger needle diameter
- Infection
- Nerve injury

Clinical Pearls

- Risk of fall when mobilising because of foot drop (tibial nerve blockade causing weakness in dorsiflexion), so the patient needs to wear a brace.
- Check for pressure points under plaster (sensory blockade)
- Popliteal fossa block anesthetizes the leg distal to the hamstring muscles, hence, it allows patients to retain knee flexion.

Suggested Reading

1. McCartney CJL, Brauner I, Chan VWS. Ultrasound guidance for a lateral approach to the sciatic nerve in the popliteal fossa. Anaesthesia. 2004;59(10):1023–5.
2. Buys MJ, Arndt CD, Vagh F, Hoard A, Gerstein N. Ultrasound-guided sciatic nerve block in the popliteal fossa using a lateral approach: onset time comparing separate Tibial and common peroneal nerve injections versus injecting proximal to the bifurcation. Anesth Analg. 2010;110:635–7.
3. Sinha A, Chan VWS. Ultrasound imaging for popliteal sciatic nerve block. Reg Anesth Pain Med. 2010;29:130–4.
4. Prasad A, Perlas A, Ramlogan R, Brull R, Chan V. Ultrasound-guided popliteal block distal to sciatic nerve bifurcation shortens onset time: a prospective randomized double-blind study. Reg Anesth Pain Med. 2010;35:267–71.
5. Guntz E, Herman P, Debizet E, Delhaye D, Coulic V, Sosnowski M. Sciatic nerve block in the popliteal fossa: description of a new medical approach. Can J Anesth. 2004;51:817820.
6. Taha AM, Ahmed AF. Supine ultrasound-guided popliteal block: a medial approach. Br J Anaesth. 2016;116:295296.
7. Gürkan Y, Sarisoy HT, Cağlayan C, Solak M, Toker K. "Figure of four" position improves the visibility of the sciatic nerve in the popliteal fossa. Agri. 2009;21:149–54.
8. Lim J, Cheng Y. A novel convenient way of performing medial approach to sciatic nerve block in the supine position. Reg Anesth Pain Med. 2021;70:A76–7.
9. Mistry T, Sonawane K, Keshri V, et al. Ultrasound-guided CAPS (Cross-Sectional Approach to Popliteal Sciatic) block: a novel technique for supine popliteal fossa block. Cureus. 2022;14(1):e20894.
10. Karmakar MK, Shariat AN, Pangthipampai P, et al. High-definition ultrasound imaging defines the paraneural sheath and the fascial compartments surrounding the sciatic nerve at the popliteal fossa. Reg Anesth Pain Med. 2013;38:447–51.
11. Andersen HL, Andersen SL, Tranum-Jensen J. Injection inside the paraneural sheath of the sciatic nerve: direct comparison among ultrasound imaging, macroscopic anatomy, and histologic analysis. Reg Anesth Pain Med. 2012;37:410–4.
12. Lin J-A, Lee Y-J, Lu H-T, Lin Y-T. Ultrasound standard for popliteal sciatic block: circular expansion of the paraneural sheath with the needle in-plane from lateral-to-medial in the 'reverse Sim's position'. Br J Anaesth. 2015;115:938–40.
13. Bruhn J, Van Geffen GJ, Gielen MJ, Scheffer GJ. Visualization of the course of the sciatic nerve

in adult volunteers by ultrasonography. Acta Anaesthesiol Scand. 2008;52:1298–302.

14. Tsui BC, Finucane BT. The importance of ultrasound landmarks: a 'traceback' approach using the popliteal blood vessels to identify the sciatic nerve. Reg Anesth Pain Med. 2006;31:481–2.

15. Auyong DB, Benonis JG, Gonzales J. Distal squeeze technique increases venous blood flow and allows for easy identification of veins with ultrasound. Reg Anesth Pain Med. 2010;35:314.

16. Schafhalter-Zoppoth I, Younger SJ, Collins AB, Gray AT. The 'seesaw' sign: improved sonographic identification of the sciatic nerve. Anesthesiology. 2004;101:808–9.

Erector Spinae Plane Block

41

Arunangshu Chakraborty and Amit Dixit

Level of Difficulty Basic

Anatomy

Erector spinae is a group of muscles comprising iliocostalis, longissimus, and spinalis, which runs from the base of the skull to the median crest of the sacrum (Fig. 41.1).

Erector spinae plane (ESP) block is a novel interfascial paraspinal plane block first described by Forero et al. in 2016, in which local anaesthetic (LA) is deposited over the transverse process, which is about 3 cm lateral to the spinous process, deep to the three columns of the erector spinae (ES) muscle. LA diffuses across interfascial planes and reaches paravertebral space via a costotransverse groove (Fig. 41.1). Block action is predominantly via dorsal rami and also at times via ventral rami (especially in the thoracic region).

A single-shot ESP provides the benefit of a multilevel thoracic paravertebral block (TPVB) without its risks. Since its introduction, it has become rapidly popular as a choice of technique for regional anaesthesia as well as interventional pain management.

A. Chakraborty (✉)
Sultan Qaboos Comprehensive Cancer Care
and Research Centre, Muscat, Oman

A. Dixit
Department of Anaesthesia, Ruby Hall Hospital,
Pune, India

While the endpoint for injection in the thoracic and lumbar level is the lateral edge of the transverse process, in the sacral level, the endpoint is the intermediate crest of the sacrum.

Surface Anatomy

ESPB can also be performed using the landmark technique. 3 cm away from the midline spinous process, a 23 G spinal needle is introduced perpendicular to the skin and body. The needle then passes through the skin, subcutaneous tissue, and erector spinae muscle. LA is deposited over the tip of the transverse process (bony anatomical landmark). Block may be performed at two levels can be done bilaterally or can be repeated depending on the indication for the block.

Indications

1. Thoracic: VATS and Open thoracic surgeries, fracture ribs, breast surgeries, open cardiac surgeries
2. Abdominal: Laparoscopic cholecystectomy, gastric bypass, PCNL, renal transplant, caesarean section, midline laparotomies.
3. Novel indications: ASIS bone graft, hip and femur surgery (e.g., at L4 level), refractory headache, chronic shoulder pain, chronic thoracic neuropathic pain, spine surgery as rescue block for breakthrough post-surgical pain.
4. Thoracic ESP block has been used for the management of back pain due to a wide variety of causes, such as radiculopathy and vertebral fracture.

Fig. 41.1 Anatomy relation of ESP muscle, transverse process, costotransverse groove, dorsal and ventral rami with their branches

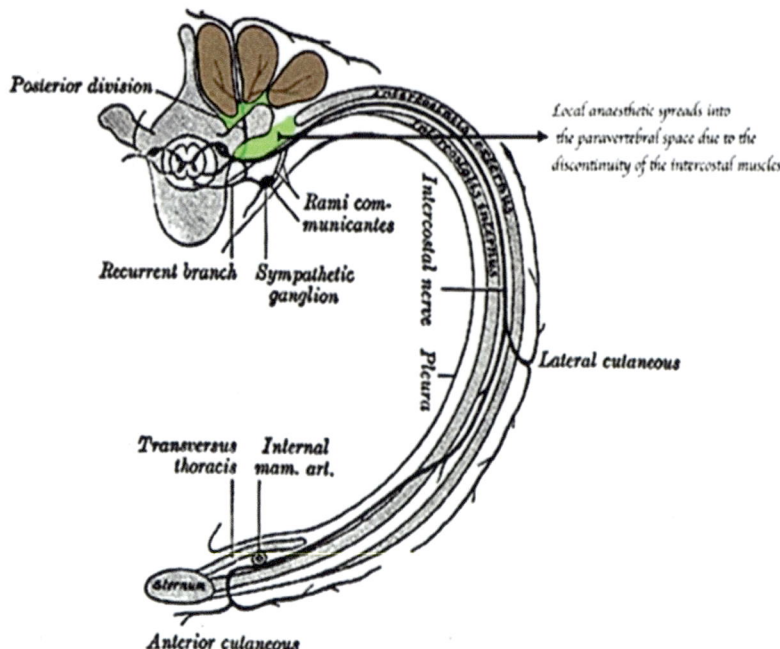

5. Sacral erector spinae block has been used for analgesia for perineal surgeries and radicular pain management.

Technique

Positioning: Prone, sitting, or lateral decubitus position.

Scanning technique

Structures to identify: transverse process, erector spinae muscle, rhomboid muscle (till T7), and trapezius muscle. Usually, ribs and pleura are not seen in this scan.

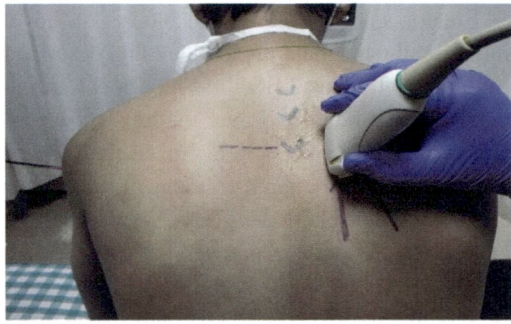

Fig. 41.2 Probe position parasagittal in-plane technique for Erector Spinae Plane Block

Block Position/Ergonomics

Patient sitting (most commonly), lateral or prone. The operator is standing behind the patient in a sitting position, machine is in front of the patient & operator (Fig. 41.2).

　Probes: Linear or curvilinear

　Settings: Nerve/MSK, general/penetration, compound imaging/multibeam

　Depth: 4–10 cm

　Needle size: 50–100 mm B-bevel nerve block stimulating needle/23 G spinal (80–90 mm)

Needling Technique

A high-frequency linear or curvilinear (in obese) probe is placed in the parasagittal or transverse plane. Both in plane and out-of-plane techniques can be used. The spinous process is first identified in the transverse imaging and then moves about 3 cm laterally till the transverse process can be imaged. LA is deposited at the edge of the transverse process (seen as a hyperechoic square pattern of the transverse process on USG).

Hydrodissection helps prevent inadvertent intramuscular injection in the erector spinae muscle. Block can be performed at any level, starting from the cervical region to the sacral level, depending on the indications. Multilevel injections or continuous ESP catheters, either unilateral or bilateral, can be used in selected cases for better quality of analgesia. Block action is checked after block completion.

Optimal Needle Tip Position

While the endpoint for injection in the thoracic and lumbar level is the lateral edge of the transverse process, in the sacral level, the endpoint is the intermediate crest of the sacrum.

Drug Choice and Volume

Single injection at T4/T5 or T8/T9 using a volume of 0.3 mg/kg produces adequate analgesia in isolated hemithorax and hemiabdomen, respectively. The usual concentration is 0.2–0.375% ropivacaine or 0.125–0.25% levobupivacaine/bupivacaine with or without 4 mg dexamethasone as an adjuvant can be employed. All interfascial plane blocks work well when combined with multimodal analgesia.

Clinical Pearls

- ESP is a versatile block that can be used from the cervical to the sacral level.
- ESP for breast surgery has the advantage of covering all the dermatomes in a single injection compared with thoracic paravertebral, where multiple injections have to be made.
- ESP retains all the benefits of TPVB while being free from the complications that come with TPVB.
- ESPB can be safely performed in patients with borderline (minimal) coagulation issues
- Chances of vascular puncture and hematoma formation are rare.
- ESPB is less likely to cause pneumothorax as compared to TPVB
- ESPB causes minimal haemodynamic changes, like hypotension, as compared to TPVB and Thoracic epidural

Side Effects

- Complications: They are rare as per case reports. Minimal hypotension or lower limb weakness due to the spread of LA in the epidural space has been reported.
- LAST
- Infection
- Hematoma

Continuous Techniques

The catheter can be inserted in the erector spinae plane blocks for the management of pain following complex breast surgeries, rib fractures, thoracotomies, and patients in chronic pain (Fig. 41.3).

18 G Tuohy needle is inserted below the erector spinae muscle at the edge of the transverse process using either in-plane caudocranial/carniocaudal direction or out-of-plane from lateral to medial direction. Hydrodissection should be done to create the fascial plane between the erector spinae muscle and the transverse process. The catheter is inserted 3–5 cm beyond the needle tip. The catheter can be secured with surgical glue and semi-permeable dressings.

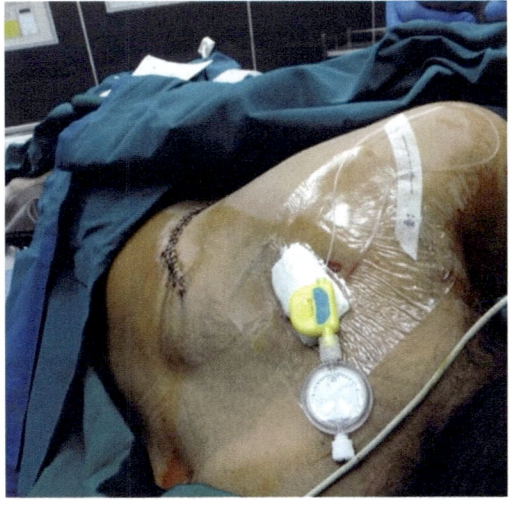

Fig. 41.3 Erector spinae continuous catheter in a case of breast surgery with latissimus dorsi flap

Suggested Regime

- 20–30 ml 0.25% levobupivacaine or 0.375% ropivacaine 8th hourly
- Infusion of 0.125% levobupivacaine or 0.2% ropivacaine at the rate of 5–12 ml/h.
- Patient controlled regional anaesthesia (PCRA)- 4 ml/h infusion, 20–30 ml 0.125% levobupivacaine or 0.2% ropivacaine bolus with 4 h lock out

Contraindications

1. Patient refusal
2. Allergy to drugs used
3. Local site infection

Recent Modifications

Thoracolumbar Interfascial Plane (TLIP) Block. The TLIP block is another paraspinal fascial plane block, which was described earlier to ESPB and is similar to ESPB, albeit with a different injection endpoint and technique.

Anatomy

TLIP is a modification of the ESPB block, first described by Hand and colleagues in 2015. The ESP muscle has the following three muscle groups from medial to lateral, namely multifidus, longissimus thoracis, and Iliocostalis in the lumbar area. Dorsal rami divide into medial, lateral, and intermediate branches at the base of the multifidus and longissimus thoracis muscle. As the injection endpoint suggests, TLIP works on the dorsal rami, not the ventral.

Indications

Post-operative analgesia for all lumbar spine surgeries and spinal cord stimulator implant insertion procedures. TLIP is also indicated for chronic back pain (low back pain, post-spine surgery pain syndrome, etc.)

USG Procedure

The curvilinear probe is commonly used. Block is usually performed bilaterally. The patient is given a prone position. A transverse paramedian scan on either side of the spinous process in the lumbar area to identify erector spinae muscle morphology is the first step.

For the classic medial approach, LA (15–20 ml) is deposited between the plane between multifidus and longissimus thoracis closer to the superior articular process. LA spreads proximally to block all branches of the dorsal rami. Recently, its lateral approach was described as a safer option with similar analgesia where LA is deposited between the longissimus thoracis and iliocostalis muscles.

An additional second injection (5 ml) in the skin and subcutaneous tissue over ESP muscle ensures better coverage of subcutaneous nerve branches. The drug concentration used for this block is 0.2% ropivacaine or 0.125% bupivacaine or levobupivacaine.

Clinical Pearls

- Although its use is limited, the analgesia provided by TLIP in its described area is dense. Due to the anatomical structure of the lumbar vertebrae, the superior articular process is imaged in the same plane as the spinous process (spine), making the imaging easier. The transverse process lies a little cephalad to the spine. TLIP anatomy and deposition of LA (Fig. 41.4)

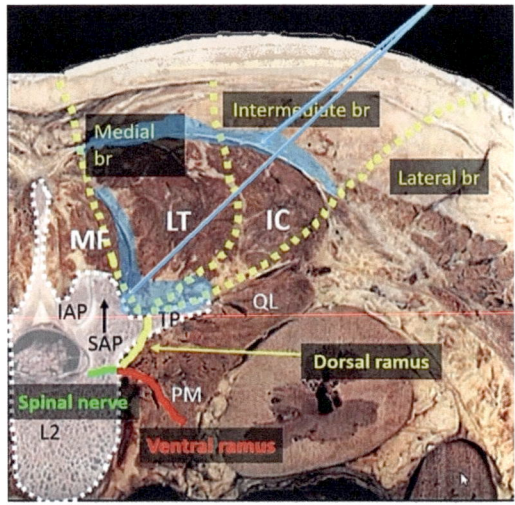

Fig. 41.4 TLIP anatomy and deposition of LA: Arrows represent needle trajectory, blue coloured area spread of LA, PM: psoas major, QL: quadratus lumborum, IC: iliocostalis, LT: longissimus thoracis, MF: multifidus muscle, L2: second lumbar vertebra, SAP: superior articular process, IAP: inferior articular process, TP: transverse process

- Arrows represent needle trajectory, blue coloured area spread of LA, PM- psoas major, QL- quadratus lumborum, IC- iliocostalis, LT- longissimus thoracis, MF- multifidus muscle, L2- second lumbar vertebra, SAP- superior articular process, IAP- inferior articular process, TP- transverse process A.

Questions

1. What are the indications of the Erector spinae plane block (ESPB)?
2. What is the target injection point and mechanism of action of ESPB?
3. What is the drug and dosage for ESPB for thoracotomies?
4. How do you perform ESPB?
5. Compare ESPB and paravertebral block (PVB) for breast surgeries.
6. How is the sacral approach to ESPB different from thoracic or lumbar ESPB?
7. What is the Thoracolumbar Interfascial Plane (TLIP) Block? What are the indications?
8. What is the difference between ESPB and TLIP block?

Suggested Reading

1. Chakraborty A. Blockmate: a practical guide for ultrasound guided regional anaesthesia.
2. Kaya C, Dost B, Tulgar S. Sacral erector spinae plane block provides surgical anesthesia in ambulatory anorectal surgery: two case reports. Cureus. 2021;13(1):e12598. https://doi.org/10.7759/cureus.12598. PMID: 33585088; PMCID: PMC7872479.
3. Krishnan S, et al. Erector spinae plane block [updated 2022 Feb 5]. In: StatPearls.
4. Adhikary SD, Liu WM, Fuller E, Cruz-Eng H, Chin KJ. The effect of erector spinae plane block on respiratory and analgesic outcomes in multiple rib fractures: a retrospective cohort study. Anaesthesia. 2019;74(5):585–93.
5. Kumar A, et al. Saudi J Anaesth. 2017;11(2):248–9.

Rectus Sheath Block

42

Arunangshu Chakraborty and Amit Dixit

Level of Difficulty Intermediate

Describe the Relevant Anatomy of the Block
The rectus sheath is a tendinous sheath (aponeurosis) which encloses the rectus abdominis (RAM) and the pyramidalis muscles. It is an extension of the tendons of the external oblique (EOM), internal oblique (IOM), and transversus abdominis muscles (TAM). It is formed of two layers- anterior and posterior rectus sheath. The layers fuse at the midline to form the linea alba.

The anterior rectus sheath covers all the rectus muscles anteriorly but differs in thickness. At the level above the costal margin, it is thin and formed by the aponeurosis of the external oblique muscle (Fig. 42.1). From the costal margin to midway between the umbilicus and the symphysis pubis (SP), the anterior rectus sheath becomes double layered, the two outer layers being contributed by the external oblique aponeurosis and the inner layer by the outer lamella of the internal oblique aponeurosis. Below this level, the anterior layer is at its thickest and is formed by fusion of the aponeurosis of the EOM, IOM, and TAM. The anterior rectus sheath is adherent to the rectus muscles along the three tendinous

intersections. As the tendinous intersections of the rectus muscle are not fused to the posterior rectus sheath, local anaesthetic from a single injection site can spread cephalocaudally within this compartment.

The posterior rectus sheath is deficient above the level of the costal margin, and the posterior surface of the rectus muscle lies directly on the 5th to 7th ribs. From the costal margin to one third of the distance between the umbilicus and the SP, the posterior rectus sheath is bilayered and is formed by the inner lamella of the aponeurosis of the IOM and the aponeurosis of the TAM (Fig. 42.1). Below this level, the posterior rectus sheath is deficient again. A crescent-shaped line called the arcuate line demarcates the end of the posterior rectus sheath. Below this level, the rectus muscle lies on the fascia transversalis as the aponeurosis formed by the three muscles of the anterior abdominal wall, namely the EOM, IOM, and TAM, passes above the rectus muscle to form a thick anterior rectus sheath.

The superior and inferior epigastric vessels run almost parallel to the midline at about the center of the rectus muscles and anastomose at about the midpoint between the umbilicus and the SP.

Which Nerves Are Blocked with the Rectus Sheath Block?
Terminal branches of the 7th–11th intercostal nerves, which run between IOM and TAM to penetrate the posterior wall of RAM and end in

A. Chakraborty (✉)
Sultan Qaboos Comprehensive Cancer Care and
Research Centre, Muscat, Oman

A. Dixit
Department of Anaesthesia, Ruby Hall Hospital,
Pune, India

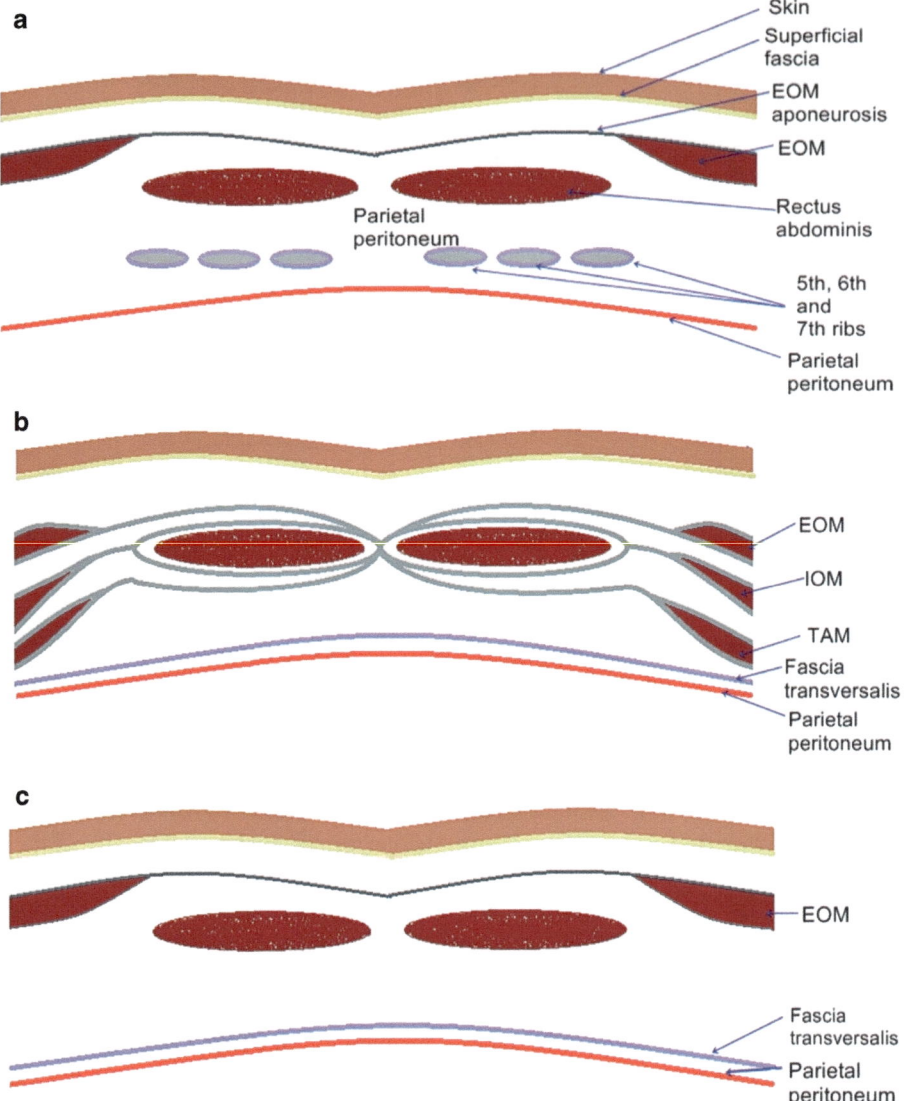

Fig. 42.1 Transverse sections through the anterior abdominal wall. (**a**) above the costal margin. (**b**) from the costal margin to the one-third between the umbilicus and SP, (**c**) below the arcuate line

an anterior cutaneous branch supplying the skin of the anterior abdominal wall near the midline. The anterior branches from the subcostal (T12) and the iliohypogastric nerves (L1) also travel in the plane below the RAM and enter the muscle close to the midline at the level below the arcuate line. The nerves from either side cross over at the midline, thus, the innervations of the midline come from both sides. Therefore, for surgical analgesia of a midline incision, bilateral rectus sheath block is to be employed.

Enlist the Indications of the Rectus Sheath Block

Rectus sheath block (RSB) can be employed for post-operative analgesia for abdominal surgeries involving a longitudinal midline/median incision as a single-shot injection or a continuous catheter.

What Are the Techniques of RSB?
Landmark-Based Technique

Landmarks: Costal cartilage, umbilicus, pubic symphysis

The RAM is palpated (difficult in obese patients) and pinched between opposing fingers and thumb. Blunt tipped block needle is inserted slowly in a perpendicular fashion along the midpoint of the muscle belly. After piercing the skin and subcutaneous fatty tissue, two distinct "pops" should be felt at the tip of the advancing needle when they pierce the superficial (anterior) and deep (posterior) surfaces of the RAM. After the second pop, upon a negative aspiration (for blood or peritoneal fluid), local anaesthetic (LA) is injected. A catheter can be placed after injection of LA or saline (thus creating space). Before injecting LA through the catheter, aspiration should be performed to rule out intravascular migration of the catheter tip.

Block Procedure

Position: Supine

Depth: 3–6 cm depending on body habitus

Needle size: 50–100 mm, 22 G short bevel needle

Needling technique: perpendicular to skin along the midpoint of the muscle belly

Drug choice: 0.25% or 0.5% ropivacaine, 0.25% bupivacaine

Drug volume: 10–20 ml of 0.25% ropivacaine, in children 0.1 ml/kg/side for single shot block; for continuous catheter dose would be 5–6 ml/h on each side in adults, 0.05 ml/kg/h in children, divided in equal volume for both the sides of 0.125% Bupivacaine or 0.2% Ropivacaine.

Clinical Pearls

- RSB is considered a learner's/beginner's block. The landmarks are easy to identify, and there is minimal risk of complications
- RSB, being a superficial block, can even be performed with a hypodermic needle. Blunting

the needle end helps in the appreciation of loss of resistance when the muscle is pierced

Complications

- Bleeding/hematoma,
- Wound infection
- Catheter migration to the intraperitoneal space.
- Bowel perforation and visceral solid organ injury

Ultrasound-Guided Block Technique
Scanning Technique

Medial to lateral approach:

A high-frequency linear array probe is placed in the midline, midway between the xiphisternum and the umbilicus, to identify the linea alba and the spindle-shaped rectus muscle. The anterior and posterior rectus sheath are identified as hyperechoic fascia surrounding the rectus muscle. The posterior rectus sheath and transversalis fascia together provide the "tramline" appearance; the peritoneum can be identified deep to the transversalis fascia (Fig. 42.2).

Lateral to medial approach:

A high-frequency linear array probe is placed between the costal margin and the iliac crest in the midclavicular line, the 3 layers of the abdominal wall (EOM, IOM and TAM) are identified, the probe is moved in a medial direction to identify the splitting of the layers of the IOM to enclose the spindle shaped RAM, the tramlines created by the posterior rectus sheath and transversalis fascia.

Colour Doppler should be used to identify the epigastric vessels.

A 22 G Tuohy needle is inserted into the plane along lateral to medial direction between RAM and the posterior rectus sheath (PRS) and 15–20 ml of LA is injected (Fig. 42.2). A catheter may be placed for a continuous block. For inserting the catheter, the probe is rotated by 90° and a plane is created between RAM and PRS by hydrodissection. The catheter is advanced 5–6 cm into space. Bilateral block/catheter is required for a midline surgery.

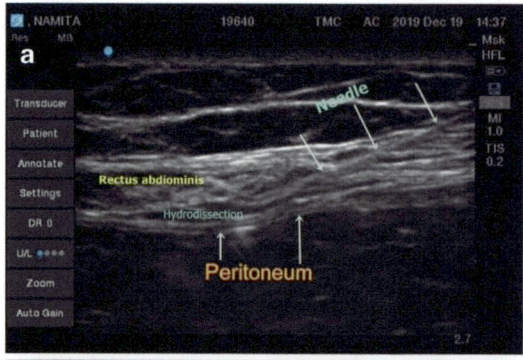
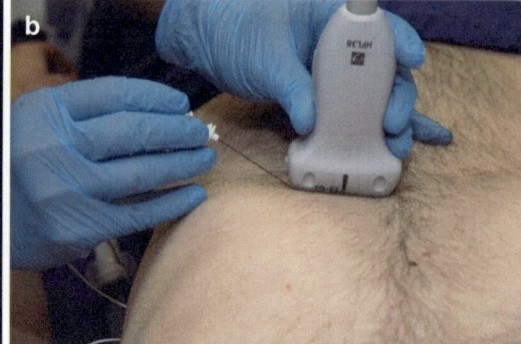
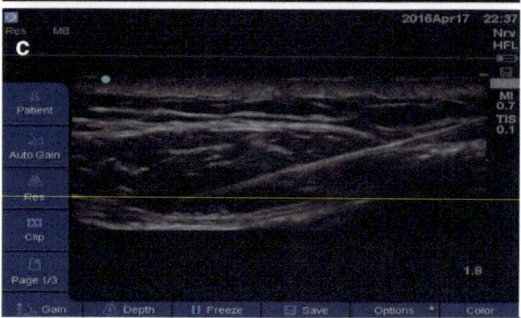

Fig. 42.2 Rectus sheath block. The structures visible in the USG-guided rectus sheath block. (**a**) Note the needle is inserted in-plane from lateral to medial direction, US transducer being held in a transverse orientation (**b, c**)

Structures to Identify

Rectus abdominis muscle, posterior rectus sheath, transversalis fascia, peritoneum, linea alba. If possible, epigastric vessels on colour doppler

Block Procedure

Position: Patient is positioned supine, arms by the side

Probe: linear probe (6–18 MHz), transverse or parasagittal on the abdomen, immediately superolateral to the umbilicus

Settings: Musculoskeletal resolution, compound imaging/multibeam

Depth: 3–6 cm depending on body habitus

Needle size: 50–100 mm, 22 G short bevel needle, 18 or 16 G Tuohy needle is used for catheter technique

Needling Technique

- Transverse approach: in-plane lateral to medial direction
- Parasagittal approach: in-plane cephalad to caudad direction

Needle Endpoint

The aim is to place the needle just posterior to the rectus muscle; hydrodissection with saline should produce a lentiform spread which separates the rectus muscle and lifts it off from the posterior rectus sheath.

Drug Choice

0.25% or 0.5% ropivacaine, 0.25% bupivacaine for single shot and 0.2% Ropivacaine or 0.125% Bupivacaine for infusions postoperatively.

Drug Volume

15–20 ml, in children 0.1 ml/kg/side for single shot block; for continuous catheter dose would be 10 ml/h on each side in adults, 0.05 ml/kg/h in children, divided in equal volume for both the sides.

Continuous Catheter Technique

Once the Tuohy needle is confirmed with the tip posterior to the rectus muscle, a catheter is inserted through the needle for a distance of 4–5 cm beyond the tip of the needle. The catheter is usually visible, resting on the posterior rectus sheath.

Clinical Pearls

- RSB is considered a learner's/beginner's block. The landmarks are easy to identify, and there is minimal risk of complications.
- Always use colour doppler to identify epigastric vessels in the trajectory of the needle.
- It is a very versatile block, and as with any fascial plane block, volume is the key to spread. The transducer can be held transversely or longitudinally. Accordingly, the needle is inserted from lateral to medial or from cephalad to caudal direction
- Bilateral blocks are needed for midline surgery. Sparing on T12 and L1 dermatomes often happens.
- Single-shot blocks can be performed with precision, but it is sensible to place catheters postoperatively due to the risk of catheters being entrapped or cut by surgical instruments.
- For catheter placement, hydrodissection can be performed with a single-shot B-bevel echogenic needle in the transverse-in-plane approach, and then the Tuohy needle can be inserted easily into the hydro-dissected space either in a transverse or parasagittal approach for catheter placement.
- When performed postoperatively, the ultrasound images may be distorted or suboptimal due to hematoma, oedema, air entrapment in tissues, sutures/mesh, and surgical dressings or drains.

- Complications: Bleeding/hematoma, wound infection, and catheter migration to intraperitoneal space, bowel perforation, and solid organ injury are known but rare complications of RSB.
- The ultrasound-guided technique is safer compared to the landmark-based technique as larger blood vessels such as the epigastric arteries (superior and inferior) can be easily identified and injury avoided with real-time ultrasound guidance.

Summary

RSB is effective in reducing pain and opioid requirements in children as well as adults. Use of ultrasound guidance makes the RSB and TAP blocks more reliable. Single-shot infiltration is useful for less extensive surgical procedures, while catheters are a useful alternative when thoracic epidural analgesia is contraindicated.

Rectus sheath block is a fascial plane block, and the volume required to be injected in a bilateral block is high, which can lead to higher than acceptable plasma levels of LA. Although it is relatively safe, adding adrenaline helps to mitigate this effect.

Suggested Reading

1. Gray H. Gray's anatomy. Elsevier; 2016. p. 1074–5.
2. Abrahams MS, Horn JL, Noles LM, Aziz MF. Evidence-based medicine: ultrasound guidance for truncal blocks. Reg Anaesth Pain Med. 2010;35:S36–42.
3. Snell R. Clinical anatomy. 8th ed. Baltimore: Lippincott Williams & Wilkins; 2008.
4. Cornish P, Deacon A. Rectus sheath catheters for continuous analgesia after upper abdominal surgery. ANZ J Surg. 2007;77:84.
5. Webster K. Ultrasound guided rectus sheath block – analgesia for abdominal surgery. Update Anaesth. 2010;26(12):17.
6. Hamill JK, Rahiri JL, Liley A, Hill AG. Rectus sheath and transversus abdominis plane blocks in children: a systematic review and meta-analysis of randomized trials. Paediatr Anaesth. 2016;26(4):363–71.
7. Uppal V, Sancheti S, Kalagara H. Transversus abdominis plane (TAP) and rectus sheath blocks: a technical description and evidence review. Curr Anesthesiol Rep. 2019;9:479–87. https://doi.org/10.1007/s40140-019-00351-y.
8. Rahiri J, Tuhoe J, Svirskis D, Lightfoot NJ, Lirk PB, Hill AG. Systematic review of the systemic concentrations of local anaesthetic after transversus abdominis plane block and rectus sheath block. Br J Anaesth. 2017;118:517–26. https://doi.org/10.1093/bja/aex005.

Spinal Anaesthesia

43

Namisha Goyal, Chang Chuan Melvin Lee, and Ashokka Balakrishnan

Introduction

Spinal anaesthesia is a commonly performed anaesthetic technique. It is generally regarded as a reliable regional anaesthetic technique (for appropriate surgical procedures), and its safe and competent conduct is a core skill in any anaesthetist's armamentarium. The method is straightforward: local anaesthetic is deposited intrathecally, directly into the cerebrospinal fluid surrounding the spinal cord and cauda equina within the subarachnoid space. Local anaesthetic produces inhibition of sodium channel-mediated impulse conduction and thus enables reversible pharmacologic denervation. The neural blockade is thought to follow a sequence starting with B fibres (preganglionic sympathetic), then C fibres (temperature sensation), Aδ (pinprick), Aβ (fine touch), and ending with Aα (motor) fibres. This produces differential blockade during a spinal anaesthetic—blockade of sympathetic outflow is two segments higher than sensory block, which

is, in turn, two segments higher than motor block; during emergence, the reverse occurs, starting with recovery of motor function. Additives to improve block quality or prolong analgesia are commonly used as part of the injectate.

The order of local anaesthetic differential blockade can be remembered by the mnemonic ATP—GTP—MTP

A: Autonomic preganglionic
T: Temperature (Ice)
P: Pin prick (pain)
G: Greater than pin prick (pain)
T: Touch
P: Pressure
M: Motor
T: Tactile localisation
P: Proprioception

Functional Anatomy to Consider During Spinal Anaesthesia

The spinal cord is enveloped in cerebrospinal fluid (CSF). A series of protective meninges encase the spinal cord, namely the pia mater, which covers the spinal cord, and the arachnoid mater, which is closely adherent to the outer fibrous dura mater. The subarachnoid, or intrathecal space, lies between the pia and the arachnoid mater and contains CSF, which cushions

N. Goyal (✉)
Department of Anaesthesia, Alexandra Hospital, National University Health System, Singapore, Singapore

C. C. M. Lee
Department of Anaesthesia, Toowoomba Base Hospital, Darling Downs Health, Toowoomba City, QLD, Australia

A. Balakrishnan
Department of Anaesthesia, National University Hospital, Singapore, Singapore

© The Author(s), under exclusive license to Springer Nature Switzerland AG 2026
S. Phillips et al. (eds.), *Regional Anaesthesia*, https://doi.org/10.1007/978-3-032-05165-3_43

and affords the spinal cord buoyancy, and surrounds it with a milieu of electrolytes and proteins.

Throughout its length, 31 pairs of spinal nerves emerge from the intervertebral foramina between each vertebra, and each is composed of anterior and posterior roots. The spinal cord then terminates as the conus medullaris, typically at the level of L1 in the average adult and approximately at L2–L3 in newborns and children up to the age of 12. Between the apex of the conus medullaris and the periosteum of the coccyx is the filum terminale, a non-functional fibrous band divided into intrathecal (cranial) and epidural (caudal) segments.

During spinal anaesthesia, a needle inserted via the midline approach transverses the following structures before entering the subarachnoid space: the skin, subcutaneous tissue, supraspinous ligament, interspinous ligament, ligamentum flavum, and the epidural space; it then pierces the dura and arachnoid mater (Fig. 43.1). In the paramedian approach, the needle passes through the paraspinal muscles before penetrating the ligamentum flavum and dura, thus bypassing the supraspinous and interspinous ligaments. The subarachnoid space ends at the level of S2. The subdural space lies between the dura and arachnoid and consists of a small volume of serous fluid and a neuroepithelial cell layer with connections between the two dural layers. Inadvertent injection into the subdural space can separate the neuroepithelial cell layer and its connections. This leads to an unpredictable spread of local anaesthetic within a limited space, and a consequent variable clinical presentation that can range from absent sensory loss to high, patchy sensory loss with intracranial extension of subdural local anaesthetic involving the cranial nerves.

Risks and Benefits of Spinal Anaesthesia

Absolute and relative contraindications to spinal anaesthesia are listed in Table 43.1. In addition, there is a "grey zone", mainly about surgical-related factors, where the use of spinal anaesthesia (especially a single-shot technique) might be controversial. Furthermore, there are other situations where a spinal anaesthetic may warrant careful consideration, such as immunocompromised patients. Patients with previous spinal surgery may present with technically challenging anatomy, with adhesions and scarring that might potentially limit the spread of local anaesthetic during central neuraxial blockade. Complications of spinal anaesthetics are listed in Table 43.2, and risk factors for hypotension are presented in Table 43.3.

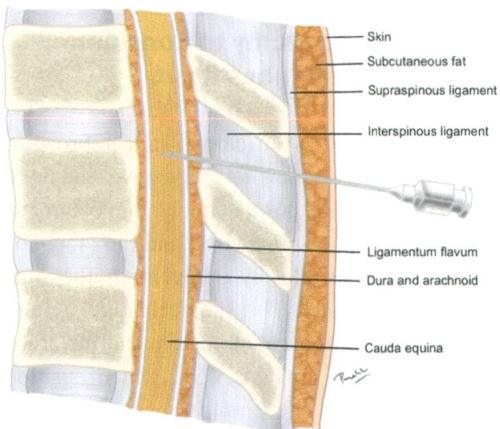

Fig. 43.1 Functional anatomy during spinal anaesthesia

Skin
Subcutaneous fat
Supraspinous ligament
Interspinous ligament
Ligamentum flavum
Dura and arachnoid
Cauda equina

Table 43.1 Contraindications of spinal anaesthesia

Absolute	Relative
Patient refusal	Neurological
Injection site infection	Myelopathy/peripheral neuropathy
Allergy to drugs used in spinal anesthesia	Spinal stenosis
Increased intracranial pressure (risk of brainstem herniation)	Previous spine surgery
	Spina bifida
	Cardiovascular instability: Aortic stenosis or fixed cardiac output state (eg, HOCM*), Hypovolemia (may present with exaggerated hypotensive response)
	Thromboprophylaxis
	Inherited coagulopathy
	Sepsis

Abbreviations: *HOCM* hypertrophic obstructive cardiomyopathy

Table 43.2 Complications of spinal anaesthesia

Due to Adverse/ exaggerated physiological responses	Due to needle/catheter insertion	Due to drug toxicity

Urinary retention	Misplacement
	  No effect/inadequate anaesthesia
	  Subdural block
	  Inadvertent intravascular injection
		Local Anaesthetic Systemic Toxicity (LAST)

High neural blockade, Total spinal anaesthesia	Dural puncture/leak
	  Postdural puncture headache
	  Diplopia
	  Tinnitus
		Transient Neurological Symptoms (TNS)

Cardiac arrest	Neural injury
	  Nerve root/spinal cord damage
	  Cauda equina syndrome	

Anterior spinal artery syndrome	Bleeding Intraspinal/epidural haematoma	

Horner syndrome	Inflammation/infection
	  Arachnoiditis
	  Meningitis
	  Epidural abscess	

Table 43.3 Risk factors for hypotension following a spinal anaesthetic

Patient factors	Anaesthetic factors	Surgical factors
Obesity (high body mass index)	Combined general and spinal anaesthetic	Emergency surgery
Pre-existing hypertension	High sensory blockade	
Hypovolaemia	Addition of vasoconstrictor to local anaesthetic solution	
Age >40 years		
Chronic alcohol consumption		

Subdural block Injection of local anaesthetic into the poorly distensible subdural space leads to an unpredictable spread with a variable clinical presentation that has been articulated earlier in this chapter. The extent of sensory loss can be disproportionate to the amount of local anaesthetic injected, and there is relative sparing of motor and sympathetic function. The subdural space extends intracranially, where it covers all neural structures in the distribution of the meninges, and thus accounts for potential cranial nerve involvement. This space extends laterally to cover the dorsal nerve roots. However, the dura and arachnoid mater are more adherent to the ventral nerve roots, and thus, the propensity for subdural spread is greater.

Indications and Benefits of Spinal Anaesthesia

Indications Central neuraxial anaesthesia is indicated in a patient when the surgical procedure can be performed with a sensory level of anaesthesia that does not cause adverse patient outcomes. Traditionally, this refers to surgeries involving the lower abdomen, pelvic girdle and perineum (such as urogenital or rectal procedures), and the lower extremities, with an injection performed in the lumbosacral region. However, spinal anaesthesia has also been described in lumbar vertebral surgeries and laparoscopic cholecystectomy, and thoracic spinal anaesthesia has been described in several studies. Furthermore, neuraxial blockade can be performed to provide analgesia, such as the addition of spinal opioids such as diamorphine or morphine for prolonged postoperative analgesia.

Benefits By the provision of adequate intraoperative and postoperative anaesthesia/analgesia, spinal anaesthesia avoids the risks related to a general anaesthetic, such as the need for airway instrumentation and positive pressure ventilation; particularly in patients at risk of pulmonary aspiration, those with significant respiratory compromise, or those with features of a difficult airway. However, one has to be mindful of the inherent risk of failure and that emergent conversion to a general anaesthetic can be worse than one that is carefully planned and conducted. Spinal anaesthesia also attenuates the surgical stress response and can reduce the risk of venous thromboembolism and surgical blood loss.

Although it is commonplace for elderly patients to undergo lower-body surgical procedures under a spinal anaesthetic, several studies have failed to demonstrate a benefit in postoperative cognitive dysfunction or delirium with central neuraxial blockade over a general anaesthetic in elderly patients across different clinical settings. Lastly, whether a spinal anaesthetic confers mortality and/or morbidity benefits over a general anaesthetic is a subject of ongoing debate, and heterogeneity in available data makes it difficult to draw meaningful conclusions.

Pharmacology

The primary target of local anaesthetics is the voltage-gated sodium channel, a complex molecule comprising a large α-subunit and one to two β subunits. Each α-subunit shall consist of 4 domains and 6 transmembrane segments. Following deposition into the cerebrospinal fluid surrounding the spinal cord and nerve roots, local anaesthetics bind to the α-subunit of voltage-gated sodium channels (amongst other proteins), in a complex interaction that culminates conformational changes which block sodium permeability across the cell membrane and thus inhibit axonal electrical impulse propagation. However, the exact mechanisms of local anaesthetic binding to voltage-gated sodium channels and gating modifications are beyond the scope of this chapter.

Pharmacokinetics

Following administration into the intrathecal space, local anesthetic distribution is determined by multiple factors. The dose of local anaesthetic is proportional to the local anesthetic concentration achieved by which diffusion occurs, while the spread of the injectate is also affected by patient positioning and the baricity of the local anesthetic solution.

Hyperbaric solutions are manufactured by adding glucose, which increases the specific gravity of the local anesthetic solution relative to the cerebrospinal fluid. Conversely, the addition of sterile water to a local anesthetic generates a hypobaric solution. Although hyperbaric solutions demonstrate a greater mean spread, the final height of sensory blockade achieved is influenced by patient positioning. When a patient is in a seated position, the perineum is in the dependent position, and a saddle block can be achieved by the use of hyperbaric solutions and maintaining the patient in the upright position for 3–10 min. In the lateral decubitus position, hyperbaric solutions preferentially distribute to the dependent side, while hypobaric solutions spread to the nondependent side, and can thus produce unilateral blockade if the patient is left in the lateral position following the spinal anaesthetic. The spread of isobaric solutions is not significantly affected by patient positioning. Caution should be used if hypobaric solutions are used, due to the osmotic stress they place on neural tissues. Of note, most glucose-free local anesthetic solutions are slightly hypobaric at core body temperature, although they are somewhat hyperbaric at lower (room) temperatures (23 °C).

Factors affecting the distribution, or spread of local anaesthetic in the subarachnoid space are listed in Table 43.4. The effect of some of these variables have been described using pharmacokinetic models, such as in a two compartment open pharmacokinetic model comprising of a spinal compartment, a systemic compartment, and an effect-site, which interestingly showed a negative effect of age and body weight on sensory block duration, and unsurprisingly, an increase in block intensity and duration with increasing dose.

Anatomical variations can alter the spread of a spinal anaesthetic. Dural ectasia is when the dural sac widens in the lumbosacral region with an associated increase in CSF volume. This can result in variable or inadequate spread of local anaesthetic within the dural sac, leading to a higher failure rate of spinal anaesthesia.

Concentration is not thought to affect the spread of local anaesthetic, as it mixes with the surrounding cerebrospinal fluid, resulting in a new concentration. Administration of Phenylephrine may be associated with decreased cephalic spread of subarachnoid local anaes-

thetic, and its use has been associated with a lower block height or increased requirement; the mechanism by which this is mediated is unclear, although hypotheses relating to cerebrospinal fluid shifts or changes in epidural space pressure (and hence subarachnoid and intracranial space pressure) have been proposed. The dose of local anaesthetic required in a spinal is a function of the factors listed above in Table 43.4, as well as the choice of local anaesthetic type, surgical procedure, and surgical time. For caesarean delivery, the clinically relevant 95% effective dose (ED95%) of various intrathecal local anaesthetics is shown in Table 43.5.

The pharmacokinetics of intrathecally-administered opioids differs from local anaesthetics, and is influenced by the lipophilicity of the molecule. This is discussed below in the intrathecal additives section.

Table 43.4 Possible Factors that may affect the spread of spinal local anaesthetic

	Anaesthetic factors	
Patient factors	Drug factors	Technique
Raised intra-abdominal pressure (pregnancy, obesity, ascites, etc.)	Baricity	Direction of needle bevel
Spinal column anatomy	Volume	Rate of injection
Patient position (e.g., supine)	Specific gravity	Barbotage
Duration patient remains in (sitting/lateral) position after injection	Viscosity	Site of injection
Patient height	Dose	Epidural volume extension
	Vasoconstrictor use	

Pharmacodynamics

The onset, duration, and potency of local anaesthetic-induced sensorimotor blockade is dependent on the pKa, protein binding, and lipid solubility of the local anaesthetic molecule respectively. The choice of local anesthetic is influenced by expected surgical procedure duration as well as local availability. Bupivacaine is highly protein-bound (approximately 95%) compared to prilocaine (approximately 55%). Chloroprocaine is an ester local anaesthetic which has one of the lowest protein binding capacity of all local anesthetics in clinical use.

Table 43.5 Estimates of the 95% effective dose of local anaesthetic for caesarean delivery

Drugs	ED95	Confidence interval of ED95 (mg)
Bupivacaine, isobaric (with Fentanyl 10 mcg and Morphine 200 mcg)	13.0 mg	9.1–16.2
Bupivacaine, hyperbaric	11.7 mg	9.9–22.8
Ropivacaine, hyperbaric (with Sufentanil 5 mcg)	15.2 mg	13.5–18.8
Levobupivacaine (with Sufentanil 2.5 mcg and Morphine 100 mcg)	12.9 mg	11.1–17.9
Prilocaine, hyperbaric (with Sufentanil 2.5 mcg and Morphine 100 mcg)		45–50

Shorter surgical procedures of less than 60 min may be performed with chloroprocaine, while prilocaine may produce sensorimotor blockade up to 90 min to facilitate ambulatory surgery.

Intrathecal Additives

Various agents have been used intrathecally to provide anaesthesia and/or analgesia, either as a single agent or a combination.

Opioids Typically administered as adjuvants to local anaesthetics, intrathecally-administered opioids produce a significant analgesic effect by binding to pre- and post-synaptic opioid receptors located in the spinal cord as well as cranially in the brainstem. The pharmacokinetics of intrathecal opioids are influenced by the lipophilicity of the molecule. The spinal cord is composed of grey and white matter. The latter is lipid-rich due to the presence of myelinated neurons; lipophilic (or hydrophobic) opioids, such as fentanyl, thus preferentially bind to elements within the white matter, while hydrophilic opiates, such as morphine, tend to distribute into the grey matter. The grey matter contains a high density of G-protein coupled opioid receptors. Lipophilic agents such as fentanyl and sufentanil typically have a short onset of action due to rapid diffusion into surrounding neuronal tissues; but also uptake into non-neuronal elements (eg. epidural fat). Binding of intrathecal opioids to spinal opioid receptors exert and analgesic effect by a decrease in pre-synaptic release of excitatory neurotransmitters (eg. substance P and glutamate) as well as indirect post-synaptic activation of descending pain modulation pathways. Lipophilic opioids, except for diamorphine, are quickly cleared from the CSF. Although highly lipophilic, diamorphine is metabolised in the spinal cord into active but less lipophilic metabolites and thus has a longer duration of action than fentanyl and sufentanil. The addition of spinal fentanyl to intrathecal bupivacaine (with or without morphine) can reduce the need for intraoperative rescue analgesia and pro-

long the time to the first analgesia request in the postoperative period. Intrathecal fentanyl also reduces postoperative nausea and vomiting but is associated with a higher incidence of intraoperative pruritus with a recommended safe maximum dose of less than 25 µg. Lipophilic opioids thus have a short duration of action with limited rostral spread, and are used to augment the sensory block of intrathecally-administered local anaesthetics.

In contrast, hydrophilic opioids have a slower onset of effect. Hydrophilic opioids spread into the grey matter, including the dorsal horn, which contains a high concentration of opioid receptors. High solubility within the CSF results in decreased spread to surrounding tissues and reuptake into spinal capillaries. These molecules thus have a longer half-life in the CSF, and migrate beyond the level of injection, rostrally to act on receptors in the brainstem; producing a wider covered area and longer-lasting analgesia. However, late respiratory depression can occur. Additionally, intrathecal opiates can be associated with other undesirable adverse effects such as postoperative urinary retention and pruritus.

Additionally, phenylpiperidines, such as pethidine, exhibit close structural similarities to local anaesthetics, and may demonstrate local anaesthetic-like effects on sensory C afferent nerve fibres.

Beyond the addition of µ-receptor agonists, the intrathecal use of nalbuphine, a synthetic opioid with mixed agonist-antagonist activity, has been described. Nalbuphine is a µ-receptor antagonist and κ-receptor agonist, which can prolong the sensory regression time and the average duration of analgesia of spinal anaesthesia without increasing the incidence of adverse reactions and reducing the occurrence of hypotension, shivering, and pruritus as compared to other potent opioids. The use of remifentanil as intrathecal opioid is contraindicated, owing to the inhibitory effect on spinal conduction.

Clonidine Clonidine is an α_2 adrenoceptor agonist with supraspinal, spinal, and peripheral activity. The spinal cord binds to presynaptic receptors within the substantia gelatinosa following subarachnoid administration. Clonidine has a high specificity for α_2 receptors compared to α_1 (220:1). When administered intrathecally as an adjuvant to bupivacaine, clonidine prolongs sensory and motor blockade. However, it also increases the incidence of hypotension and sedation. In combination with intrathecal opiates, neuraxial clonidine increases the duration of analgesia and postoperative opioid requirement.

Dexmedetomidine A highly selective α_2 adrenoceptor agonist with approximately 8 times higher specificity for α_2 receptors compared to clonidine (1620:1, α_2:α_1). Given intravenously, dexmedetomidine may prolong the duration of spinal anaesthesia. However, the mechanism by which this occurs is unclear. Neuraxial dexmedetomidine shortens the onset time of spinal or epidural block, prolongs postoperative analgesia and block duration, and reduces postoperative shivering; although there is no recommended dose at present, doses of between 2.5 and 15 μg have been studied. A meta-analysis has suggested that hypotension and bradycardia are not statistically significant, although further studies on the safety of dexmedetomidine as a spinal adjuvant are required.

Other agents Other pharmacological agents can be administered intrathecally for analgesia in situations beyond the typical provision of perioperative anaesthesia and/or analgesia, such as in chronic cancer and non-cancer pain. Drugs include baclofen, a centrally-acting muscle relaxant with gamma-aminobutyric acid B receptor activity used in conditions associated with painful muscle spasms and clonus; and ziconotide, a N-type voltage-gated channel antagonist which reduces neurotransmitter release and nociceptive signals. A discussion of these drugs is beyond the scope of this chapter.

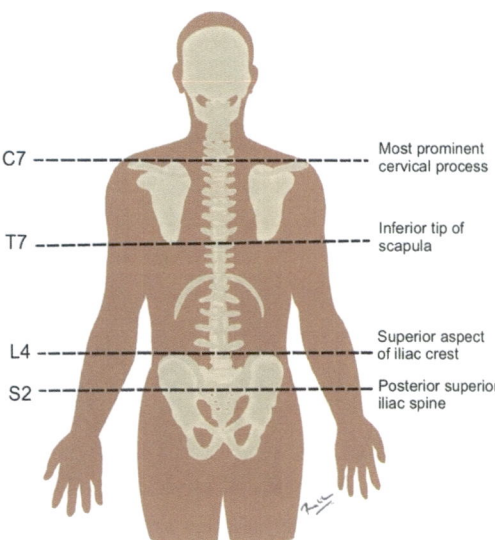

Fig. 43.2 Surface Anatomy and dermatomal landmarks

Surface Anatomy

The midline is identified by palpating the spinous processes. C7 is the most prominent cervical spinous process (vertebra prominens). The medial end of the spine of the scapula is usually located at the level of T3. At the same time, its inferior angle (with the arms by the side) typically corresponds to the T7 vertebra. An imaginary line between the highest points of both iliac crests usually crosses the L4 body or L4–5 interspace (Tuffier's line) (Fig. 43.2).

Ultrasound can be used to define landmarks when spinous processes are not palpable to identify anatomy, such as midline, identity of the intervertebral space, and estimated depth to the posterior complex, which may improve the success rate of subsequent needle insertion. Preprocedural static transverse and parasagittal scans are typically obtained. In addition, real-time ultrasound-guided spinal anaesthesia can be performed using either a paramedian-sagittal-oblique or paramedian transverse scan; both in-plane and out-of-plane approaches have been described (Fig. 43.3).

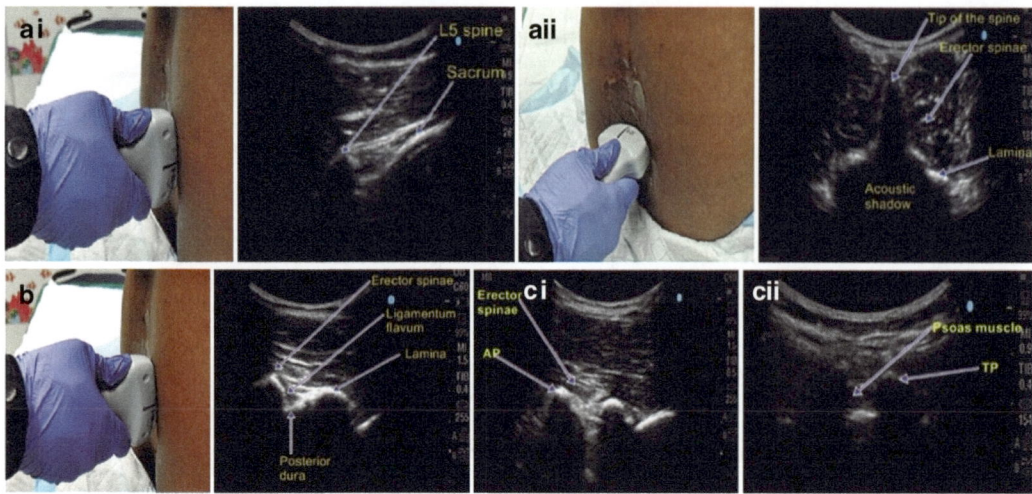

a i) Identifying the lumbar spine with the help of the L5-S1 interspace
a ii) Transverse scan at spinous process
b) Sagittal scan at lamina
c i) Paramedian sagittal scan at the level of the Articular Process (AP)
c ii) Paramedian sagittal scan at the level of the Transverse Process (TP)

Fig. 43.3 Sonoanatomy of the lumbar spine. (Blockmate: A practical guide for Ultrasound Guided Regional Anaesthesia. 133–136. Springer Nature)

Technique

Spinal needles can be broadly divided into 2 types: (1) sharp, cutting needle designs, such as the Quincke, which has the orifice located at the tip; and (2) blunt, pencil-point (rounded) tipped needles with a lateral orifice for injection (Whitacre) (Fig. 43.4). In the latter, the needle is closed-ended, and the orifice is located 2 mm from the tapering tip. The Sprotte needle is a pencil-point needle with a more extended opening than the Whitacre design. The incidence and severity of post-dural puncture headache are reduced with the use of pencil-point needles and lower-gauge needles. In a pencil-point, or non-cutting needle design, the tip is postulated to separate the longitudinal fibres of the dura atraumatically, thus reducing CSF leakage following needle withdrawal as the fibres return to a state of closed apposition. Furthermore, pencil-point needles might produce better tissue feedback with a more appreciable "give" or "click" when penetrating the dura.

Patient Positioning

The sitting position is commonly adopted when performing a central neuraxial block as it "opens" up the intervertebral space by reducing lumbar lordosis (Fig. 43.5). In addition, the sitting position pushes the dural sac more superficially. Commercial devices that facilitate positioning for central neuraxial anaesthesia are available, such as the EpiHug® pillow (Deep Creek Medical Products, Springville, UT). In certain situations, the sitting position may not be feasible, such as patients with pain from a lower limb or hip fracture, or those who require sedation, and the conduct of a spinal anaesthetic in the lateral position is required. Either way, appropriate flexion of the whole spine, hips, and knees places the patient in a foetal position, maximising the interspinous and interlaminar distances between the lumbosacral vertebrae. Avoidance of rotation or lateral flexion of the spine is important, as is assistance in maintaining this position during the spinal

Fig. 43.4 Types of
spinal needles

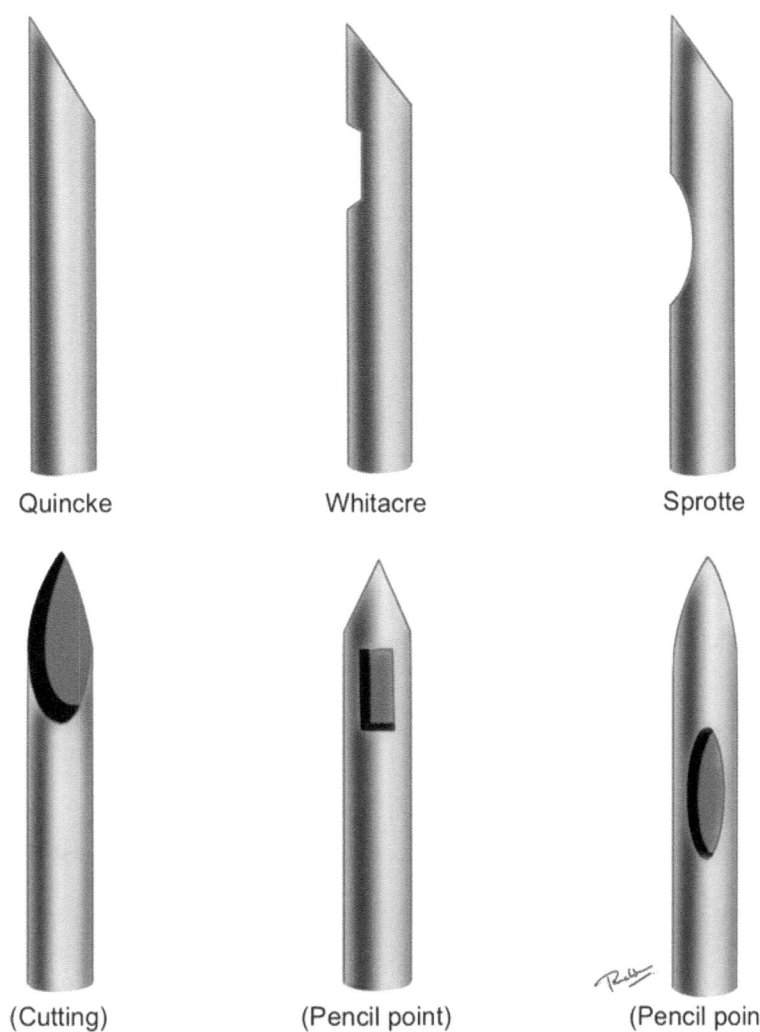

Quincke   Whitacre   Sprotte

(Cutting)   (Pencil point)   (Pencil point)

anaesthetic. The Oxford position is a modification of the lateral position in which the patient is
placed slightly head down, with 3 pillows supporting the head, and a support placed under the
left shoulder, such as an air-inflated bag.

Depending upon the anatomic approach, the
technique for spinal anaesthesia can be either (1)
midline or (2) paramedian. The traditional midline approach is commonly used as the spinous
processes are easily palpable and the technique
requires less 3-dimensional perception. The paramedian approach may be performed with an
entry site 1 cm lateral and 1 cm caudal to the spinous process, with the needle directed approximately 45° cephalad and medially—although

some variations in the description exist. The
paramedian approach may confer some advantage in technically difficult patients, such as in
the elderly, where there might be calcification of
the interspinous ligaments, or when the lumbar
interspace is narrow, as it bypasses most of the
bony structures that hinder advancement of the
needle. Furthermore, the angled approach might
facilitate catheter insertion. Taylor's approach is
a paramedian approach at the level of L5/S1,
which (1) has been thought to be the widest interspace, and (2) might be less likely affected by
degenerative processes, thus potentially offering
an advantage in a patient with a difficult spinal
(Fig. 43.6). The insertion point is 1 cm inferior

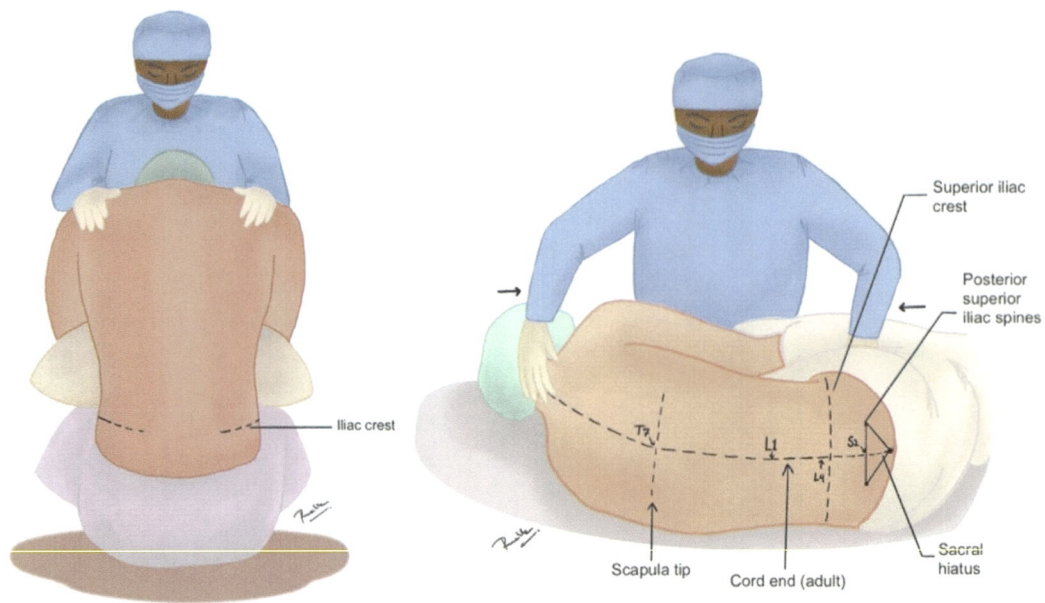

Fig. 43.5 Patient positioning (sitting and lateral decubitus); with assistant helping to provide maximal flexion

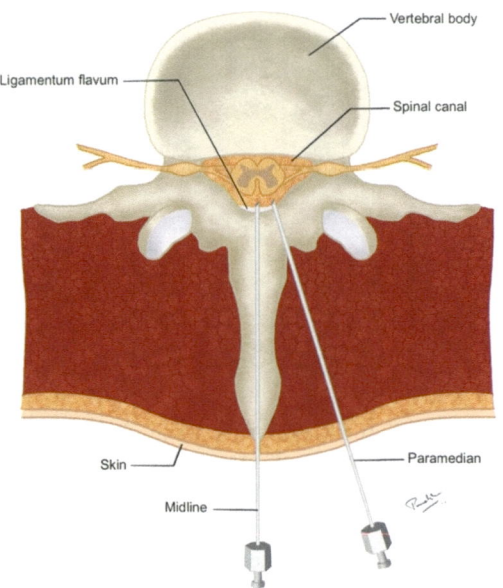

Fig. 43.6 Paramedian approach for spinal anaesthesia

and 1 cm medial to the posterior superior iliac spine, and the needle is directed cephalad and medially around 45°–50°, approximating the angle formed by the dorsal aspect of the sacrum and the skin. Lastly, the paramedian approach may be performed under real-time ultrasound-guidance with the probe placed in a paramedian sagittal oblique position.

Continuous Spinal Anaesthesia

Somewhat under-utilised, placement of an intrathecal catheter for continuous spinal anaesthesia allows small titrated local anesthetic doses to be administered. This can minimize cardiovascular instability as it will enable careful titration of local anaesthetic after the patient has been positioned, and incremental intrathecal injection can be titrated against vasoactive drugs to counteract the sympatholysis caused by central neuraxial blockade. Injection directly into the cerebrospinal fluid allows a desired block height with the rapid onset and density of a spinal anaesthetic to be achieved— one that can (theoretically) be prolonged indefinitely. Unlike a combined spinal epidural, much smaller volumes (10–15 times) of local anaesthetic are used, which can alleviate concerns of local anaesthetic systemic toxicity. Short-acting local anaesthetics can be used to facilitate early recovery from anaesthesia, or subarachnoid opiates such as Diamorphine or Morphine can be administered for post-operative analgesia.

However, compared to single-shot spinal anaesthesia, continuous spinal anaesthesia can be technically challenging, particularly regarding the threading of microcatheters, which can easily kink. Post-dural puncture headache from leakage of cerebrospinal fluid is another concern, as might be the safety of the technique in institutions with limited expertise. Furthermore, microcatheter use has been associated with reports of cauda equina syndrome, which prompted the withdrawal of microcatheters by the United States Food and Drug Administration. Such reports were largely associated with hyperbaric Lignocaine, and one postulated mechanism is displacement of cerebrospinal fluid and exposure of the cauda equina to maldistribution of local anaesthetic, which can be neurotoxic at high concentrations with repeated dosing and long exposure time.

Troubleshooting Difficulties with the Administration of Spinal Anaesthetic

A functional, effective spinal anaesthetic with surgical blockade is a necessity for safe conduct of anaesthesia and adequate patient comfort. Understanding how to troubleshoot the difficulties while advancing a spinal needle and having a structured approach is paramount. While pencil-point needles are associated with a reduced incidence of post-dural puncture headache, the orifice is located proximal to the tip, and maintaining its position within the intrathecal space requires expertise to prevent misplacement or displacement.

Questions
1. What anatomical structures does the spinal needle pass through when performing spinal anaesthesia?
2. What is the approximate clinically effective dose of Bupivacaine in a spinal anaesthetic in the context of a caesarean delivery?
3. Name the essential surface landmarks while performing spinal anaesthesia.

4. What are the absolute contraindications for spinal anaesthesia?
5. What are some of the factors that affect the spread of local anaesthetic in spinal anaesthesia?
6. What is the difference between high spinal and total spinal?
7. A patient is made to lie supine after a spinal anaesthetic in the sitting position. She feels a sudden onset of breathlessness and voice change. Explain the pathophysiology.
8. What are your thoughts on the prevention of hypotension with spinal anaesthetics?
9. What is your preferred regimen for spinal anaesthesia for a caesarean section and knee arthroplasty?

Acknowledgement for Figures Dr. Parisha Malik (MBBS, MSc), Digital Illustrator, UK. Email: parisha@theartisticscroll.com.

Suggested Reading

1. Cousins MJ, Bridenbaugh PO, Carr DB, et al. Cousins and Bridenbaugh's neural blockade in clinical anesthesia and pain medicine. 4th ed. Philadelphia: Lippincott Williams & Wilkins; 2008. p. 219.
2. Brouwers E, van de Meent H, Curt A, et al. Definitions of traumatic conus medullaris and cauda equina syndrome: a systematic literature review. Spinal Cord. 2017;55:886–90.
3. Agarwal D, Mohta M, Tyagi A, Sethi AK. Subdural block and the anaesthetist. Anaesth Intensive Care. 2010;38:20–6.
4. Xu C, Liu S, Huang Y, Guo X, Xiao H, Qi D. Phenylephrine vs ephedrine in cesarean delivery under spinal anesthesia: a systematic literature review and meta-analysis. Int J Surg. 2018;60:48–59.
5. Chooi C, Cox JJ, Lumb RS, Middleton P, Chemali M, Emmett RS, Simmons SW, Cyna AM. Techniques for preventing hypotension during spinal anaesthesia for caesarean section. Cochrane Database Syst Rev. 2020;7(7):CD002251.
6. Brull R, Macfarlane AJR, Chan VWS. Spinal, epidural, and caudal anaesthesia. In: Miller's anaesthesia, vol. 1. 9th ed; 2020. p. 1413–49.
7. le Roux JJ, Wakabayashi K, Jooma Z. Defining the role of thoracic spinal anaesthesia in the 21st century: a narrative review. Br J Anaesth. 2022:S0007-0912(22)00131-3.
8. Lacassie HJ, Millar S, Leithe LG, Muir HA, Montaña R, Poblete A, Habib AS. Dural ectasia: a likely cause of

inadequate spinal anaesthesia in two parturients with Marfan's syndrome. Br J Anaesth. 2005;94:500–4.

9. Yang HJ, Baek IC, Park SM, Chun DH. Inadequate spinal anesthesia in a parturient with Marfan's syndrome due to dural ectasia. Korean J Anesthesiol. 2014;67(Suppl):S104–5.

10. Ginosar Y, Mirikatani E, Drover DR, Cohen SE, Riley ET. ED50 and ED95 of intrathecal hyperbaric bupivacaine coadministered with opioids for cesarean delivery. Anesthesiology. 2004;100(3):676–82.

11. Bouvet L, Da-Col X, Chassard D, Daléry F, Ruynat L, Allaouchiche B, Dantony E, Boselli E. ED_{50} and ED_{95} of intrathecal levobupivacaine with opioids for Caesarean delivery. Br J Anaesth. 2011;106:215–20.

12. Goffard P, Vercruysse Y, Leloup R, Fils JF, Chevret S, Kapessidou Y. Determination of the ED95 of intrathecal hyperbaric prilocaine with sufentanil for scheduled cesarean delivery: a dose-finding study based on the continual reassessment method. BMC Anesthesiol. 2020;26(20):293.

13. Ramaswamy S, Wilson JA, Colvin L. Non-opioid-based adjuvant analgesia in perioperative care. Contin Educ Anaesth Crit Care Pain. 2013;13:152–7.

14. Engelman E, Marsala C. Efficacy of adding clonidine to intrathecal morphine in acute postoperative pain: meta-analysis. Br J Anaesth. 2013;110:21–7.

15. Shen QH, Li HF, Zhou XY, Yuan XZ, Lu YP. Dexmedetomidine as an adjuvant for single spinal anesthesia in patients undergoing cesarean section: a system review and meta-analysis. J Int Med Res. 2020;48:300060520913423.

16. Conroy PH, Luyet C, McCartney CJ, McHardy PG. Real-time ultrasound-guided spinal anaesthesia: a prospective observational study of a new approach. Anesthesiol Res Pract. 2013;2013:525818.

17. Chen L, Huang J, Zhang Y, Qu B, Wu X, Ma W, Li Y. Real-time ultrasound-guided versus ultrasound-assisted spinal anesthesia in elderly patients with hip fractures: a randomized controlled trial. Anesth Analg. 2022;134:400–9.

18. Arevalo-Rodriguez I, Muñoz L, Godoy-Casasbuenas N, et al. Needle gauge and tip designs for preventing post-dural puncture headache (PDPH). Cochrane Database Syst Rev. 2017;4:CD010807.

19. Soltani Mohammadi S, Piri M, Khajehnasiri A. Comparing three different modified sitting positions for ease of spinal needle insertion in patients undergoing spinal anesthesia. Anesth Pain Med. 2017;7:e55932.

20. Rucklidge MW, Paech MJ, Yentis SM. A comparison of the lateral, oxford and sitting positions for performing combined spinal-epidural anaesthesia for elective caesarean section. Anaesthesia. 2005;60:535–40.

21. Zeng W, Shi Y, Zheng Q, Du S. Ultrasound-assisted modified paramedian technique for spinal anesthesia in the elderly. BMC Anesthesiol. 2022;30(22):242.

22. Gupta K, Rastogi B, Gupta PK, Rastogi A, Jain M, Singh VP. Subarachnoid block with Taylor's approach for surgery of lower half of the body and lower limbs: a clinical teaching study. Anesth Essays Res. 2012;6(1):38–41.

23. Chong SE, Mohd Nikman A, Saedah A, Wan Mohd Nazaruddin WH, Kueh YC, Lim JA, Shamsul Kamalrujan H. Real-time ultrasound-guided paramedian spinal anaesthesia: evaluation of the efficacy and the success rate of single needle pass. Br J Anaesth. 2017;118:799–801.

24. Farquhar-Smith P, Chapman S. Neuraxial (epidural and intrathecal) opioids for intractable pain. Br J Pain. 2012;6(1):25–35.

25. Hocking G, Wildsmith JA. Intrathecal drug spread. Br J Anaesth. 2004;93(4):568–78.

26. Grape S, El-Boghdadly K, Albrecht E. Management of adverse effects of intrathecal opioids in acute pain. Best Pract Res Clin Anaesthesiol. 2023;37(2):199–207.

Lumbar and Thoracic Epidural

44

Ashokka Balakrishnan, Kai Yin Hwang, Chen Hui Ng, and Geraldine Pei Chin Cheong

Level of difficulty Intermediate

Anatomy

The Spine

The vertebral column comprises seven cervical, 12 thoracic, five lumbar, five fused sacral, and four coccygeal vertebrae. It has a normal cervical and lumbar lordosis, and thoracic and sacral kyphosis. The general structure of each vertebra consists of an anterior body and a posterior bony arch. The arch is made of the pedicles extending from the posterolateral margins of the vertebral body, laminae on each side, and the spinous process at the fusion of the laminae at midline. In addition, paired transverse processes, superior and inferior articular processes, emerge from the junction of the pedicles and laminae. The vertebral canal is formed within the vertebral arches of adjacent vertebrae (Fig. 44.1).

The Vertebrae

Cervical vertebrae have small vertebral bodies and a wide vertebral canal. C3–C6 vertebrae have short bifurcated spinous processes, while C7 has a long horizontal spinous process that protrudes at the base of the neck. Thoracic vertebral bodies are larger than cervical vertebral bodies and wider posteriorly than anteriorly. Spinous processes of thoracic vertebrae are long and thin, and angled caudally at steep angles. The steepest-angled spinous process is between T4 and T9, thus complicating the midline approach of epidural insertion in the midthoracic area. The vertebrae beyond T10 gradually resemble lumbar vertebrae, so a helpful feature to distinguish them is that each thoracic vertebra articulates with the ribs laterally (Fig. 44.1). Lumbar vertebrae bodies are thicker anteriorly than posteriorly, and their spinous processes are large, wide, and point posteriorly. It is common to have anatomical variations such as sacralization of the last lumbar vertebrae or lumbarization of S1 and S2 (fusion incomplete).

The Spinal Cord

The spinal cord lies within the vertebral canal and is covered by protective layers of pia, arachnoid, and dura. The spinal cord ends in the conus medullaris, most commonly at T12 in adults. Anterior and posterior nerve roots exit from the

A. Balakrishnan · K. Y. Hwang (✉) · C. H. Ng
Department of Anaesthesia, National University Hospital, Singapore, Singapore

G. P. C. Cheong
Department of Anaesthesia, Khoo Teck Puat Hospital, Singapore, Singapore

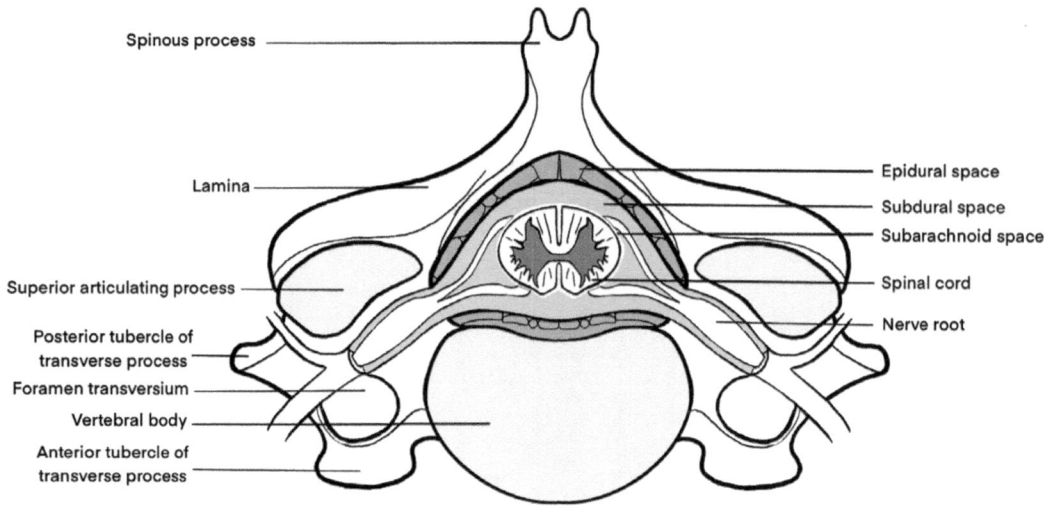

Fig. 44.1 Cross section of vertebra and spinal cord

spinal cord dorsally and ventrally at specific vertebral levels, and travel out via the intervertebral foraminae. The dorsal roots carry afferent sensory axons while the ventral roots carry efferent motor axons. Together, they form the spinal nerve, which splits into the dorsal and ventral rami. The dorsal ramus innervates the dorsal trunk (skin and epi-axial muscles of the back) and transmits visceral motor, somatic motor, and sensory information. The ventral ramus innervates the ventral trunk (ventrolateral body surface, body wall), upper and lower limbs (hypaxial muscles), and transmits visceral motor, somatic motor, and sensory information. Meningeal branches of the spinal nerve reenter the intervertebral foramen to innervate the ligaments, dura, blood vessels, intervertebral discs, facet joints, and periosteum of the vertebrae. Autonomic nervous information is added to spinal nerves via the rami communicantes, where visceral motor and sensory input is supplied and received to and from visceral organs.

Thoracic

Thoracic spinal nerves enter the paravertebral autonomic ganglia to transmit and receive sympathetic nervous information to the organs and glands in the body. The anterior rami of T1–T12 form the intercostal nerves that run between the ribs (except the T12 intercostal nerve that runs

below the 12th rib. The posterior rami of T1–T12 supply the skin and back muscles such as the semispinalis dorsi, multifidus, and longissimus dorsi.

Lumbar

Lumbar nerves are split into anterior and posterior divisions. The posterior division is further divided into medial and lateral branches, which supply the multifidus and erector spinae muscles. Anterior divisions of the lumbar nerves accompany the lumbar arteries along the sides of the vertebrae, running beneath the psoas major. They are also connected to the lumbar part of the sympathetic trunk by the white ramus communicans. L1–L3 supply the quadratus lumborum and form the lumbar plexus, while L4–L5 contribute to the lumbosacral trunk.

Blood Vessels of Clinical Significance

Vertebral and segmental arteries supply the spinal cord. Vertebral arteries give rise to a single anterior and two posterior spinal arteries to supply the anterior two-thirds and posterior one-third of the spinal cord, respectively. The artery of Adamkiewicz is the largest segmental artery, commonly unilateral, arising between T8 and L1. Anterior and posterior spinal veins anastomose with the internal vertebral plexus in the epidural space. Intervertebral venous plexus is formed by two anterior and two posterior longitudinal vessels. The veins drain into the azygos and hemiazygos veins in the thoracic and abdominal levels and the internal iliac veins in the pelvis. Because the veins are valveless, blood flow can be bidirectional, and intra-abdominal/ intrathoracic pressure can cause engorgement of epidural vessels, leading to enhanced absorption of epidural drugs and more rapid onset of action. Pregnant mothers in active labour with venacaval compression in supine position can result in further engorgement of the venous plexus, resulting in a higher propensity for high spinal blockade, or additionally the risk of intravenous placement of epidural catheters (Fig. 44.2).

Ligaments of Clinical Significance

The anterior and posterior longitudinal ligaments support the vertebral column and the intervertebral discs between them. The Posterior Longitudinal Ligaments (PLL) form the anterior wall of the vertebral canal. Intervertebral disc hernia occurs commonly in the paramedian area of the PLL, but this region is the anterior epidural space, which is away from the epidural needle placement in the posterior epidural space. The ligamentum flavum is a dense connective tissue connecting the adjacent vertebrae's lamina. The supraspinous ligament connects the tips of the spinous processes, and the interspinous ligament is a thinner membranous ligament along the length of adjacent spinous processes.

The Epidural Space

The epidural space is a potential space that lies superficial to the dura mater circumferentially. It extends cranially from the foramen magnum to the sacrococcygeal ligament caudally. It contains passing nerve roots, dural sac, epidural arteries, valveless venous plexi, and fatty tissue. It is bounded anteriorly by the posterior longitudinal ligament, laterally by the vertebral pedicles and intervertebral foramina, and posteriorly by the ligamentum flavum. Midline septae, which are membranes connecting dura to the ligamentum flavum, can sometimes be found in the epidural

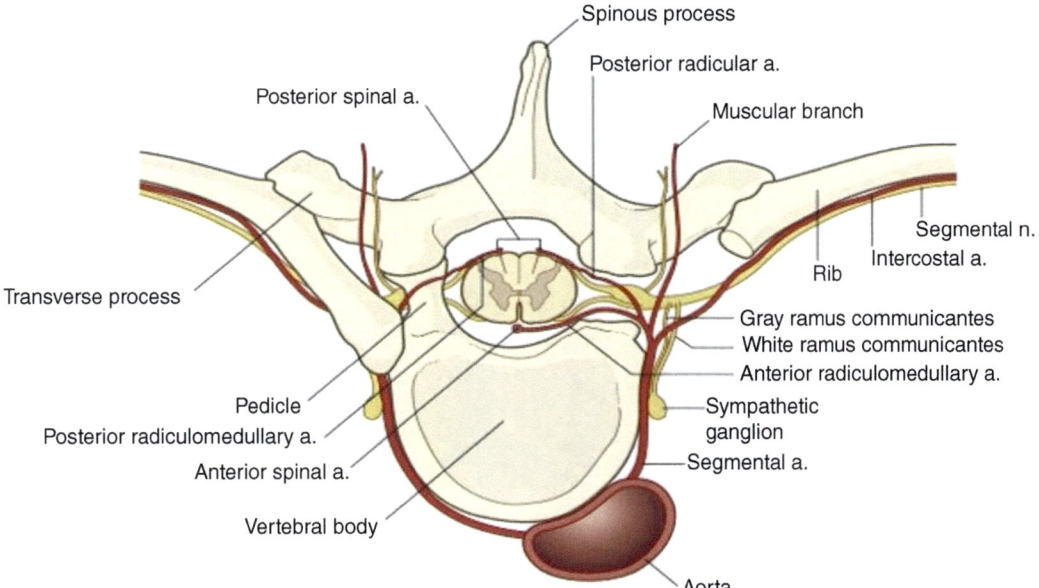

Fig. 44.2 Cross section of spinal cord with its blood supply. (Image obtained with permission from Parmar and Ashokka [1])

space, but are not found to be clinically significant to affect bilateral LA spread or onset of regional anaesthesia, to obstruct catheter movement, or to result in accidental dural punctures.

Surface Anatomy (Fig. 44.3)

Caveats:

- Variation in vertebral levels of the landmarks occurs
- Palpation of landmarks in obese patients (especially the scapula and 12th rib) is difficult
- Intercristal line (between the superior border of bilateral iliac crests can appear to be higher in pregnant, elderly, and obese patients (by 1–2 levels)

Sonographic Anatomy

Curved array transducers and low frequency ultrasound (2–5 MHz) can be used to image the spine and epidural space. This helps identify the midline, estimate depth to epidural space, and determine the required needle approach and angle. It is often used just immediately before the epidural procedure to locate and mark out the site of injection (Figs. 44.4 and 44.5).

Lumbar Level

With a transverse scan, the spine can be imaged at the spinous process level or the interspinous level. A scan at the spinous process level will show a hyperechoic spinous process at the apex nearest the ultrasound probe, and lamina extending out on both sides. Dark acoustic shadows obscure deeper structures. Nevertheless, this helps the procedurist to identify the midline when the spinous process is not easily palpable (e.g., obese patients or patients with scoliosis).

Next, a scan at the interspinous level (through tilting or sliding the transducer) will reveal the interspinous space, the spinal canal in midline, and laterally on both sides, as well as the articular and transverse processes. In the midline, from posterior to anterior, lie the epidural space, posterior dura (first horizontal hyperechoic structure), intrathecal sac, anterior complex (second horizontal hyperechoic structure), and vertebral body.

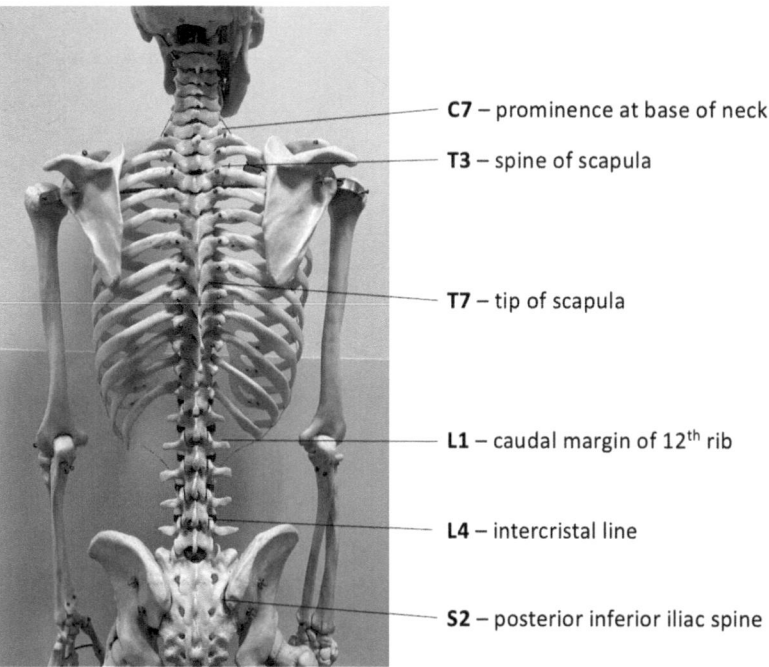

Fig. 44.3 Picture of a skeleton denoting important surface landmarks of the spine

C7 – prominence at base of neck

T3 – spine of scapula

T7 – tip of scapula

L1 – caudal margin of 12th rib

L4 – intercristal line

S2 – posterior inferior iliac spine

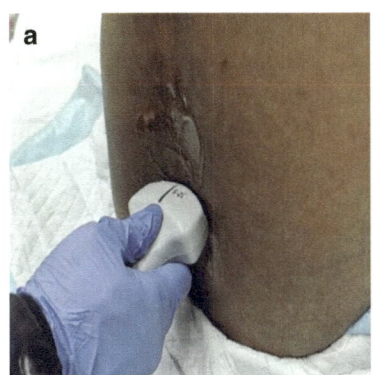
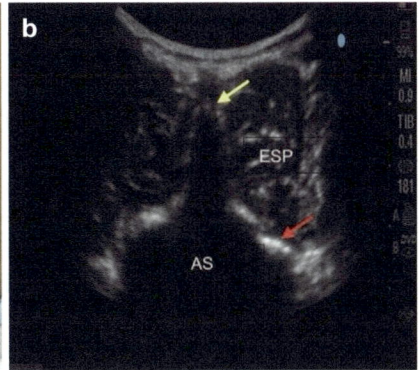

Fig. 44.4 Transverse Scan of the lumbar vertebra using the low-frequency ultrasound probe at the spinous process level. The image obtained shows the spinous process (yel- low arrow), lamina (red arrow), erector spinae muscle (ESP), and acoustic shadow (AS). (Image obtained with permission from Parmar and Ashokka [1])

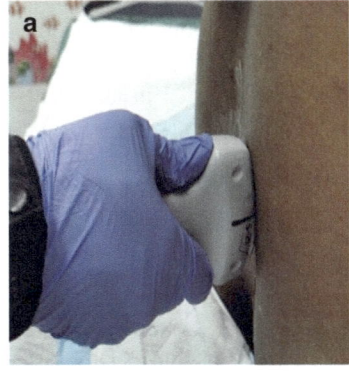
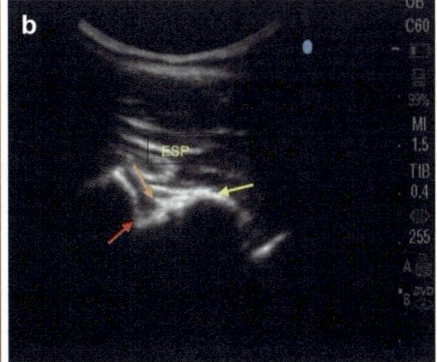

Fig. 44.5 Sagittal scan of the lumbar vertebra at the lamina using the low-frequency ultrasound probe. The image obtained shows the erector spinae muscle (ESP), lamina (yellow arrow), ligamentum flavum (orange arrow), and posterior dura (red arrow). (Image obtained with permission from Parmar and Ashokka [1])

Thoracic Level

Ultrasound imaging of the thoracic spine is more challenging due to the steep angle of the spinous processes of the upper to mid thoracic vertebrae. The image of the interspinous level is almost impossible to achieve. Epidural space is best visualized in the paramedian sagittal scan. The lamina is a flat hyperechoic structure with posterior acoustic shadows, and the ligamentum flavum connects the laminae on either side in the interspinous spaces. The posterior dura is seen as a hyperechoic structure, before the dark hypoechoic intrathecal space. The anterior complex lies deepest to it and is a bright horizontal hyperechoic structure.

Physiological Effects of Epidural Blockade

Differential blockade may be observed at the onset and regression of epidural anaesthesia. The sympathetic nervous system is blocked first, and can be two to six dermatomes higher than a sensory block. Sensory blockade happens sequentially in the order of temperature, pain, and then touch. Motor nerves are one of the last to be blocked, followed by proprioception, and often at a lower level than the sensory dermatomes.

The central nervous system appears to be depressed by epidural anaesthesia, more so for midthoracic block rather than lower lumbar blocks. Sedative effects of epidural anaesthesia have been found to reduce hypnotic requirements for both intravenous and volatiles.

Cardiovascular changes caused by epidural anaesthesia are mainly due to sympathetic blockade, inhibiting sympathetic outflow to blood vessels and heart (T1–T4 cardiac accelerator sympathetic fibers), and a decrease in endogenous catecholamine release from adrenal glands. There is a resultant venous and arterial vasodilation, reduced systemic vascular resistance, and changes in chronotropy and inotropy, thus decreasing cardiac output and hypotension. The vasodilatory effect is more markedly seen in the T6–L1 block because sympathetic outflow to the splanchnic beds is blocked, resulting in extensive vasodilation. However, the degree of hypotension is not as severe as when compared to that caused by spinal anesthesia, as the onset of epidural anaesthesia can be slowed with controlled LA infusion into the epidural catheter. Spinal anaesthesia, in addition, results in profound venodilation of extremities and reduced preload. Thoracic epidural anaesthesia has been found to improve myocardial blood flow and oxygen balance, have antianginal effects, and improve recovery from reversible myocardial ischaemia.

Respiratory function can be affected in high epidural blocks. While tidal volume remains unchanged, vital capacity can be reduced due to blocked accessory muscles involved in expiration, reducing expiratory reserve volume. However, inspiratory muscles are unaffected and ventilation is often adequate. When a thoracic epidural is used postoperatively for thoracic operations, the analgesic effect has the added advantage of preventing hypoventilation from pain. Respiratory arrest from high epidural block is due to hypoperfusion of the brainstem respiratory center rather than direct LA effects on the phrenic nerve or CNS.

The gastrointestinal system also receives sympathetic outflow from T5 to T12. Sympathectomy results in unopposed parasympathetic vagal tone, resulting in increased peristalsis, relaxed sphincters, and increased secretions. This aids in rapid restoration of GI function and prevents postoperative ileus.

Epidural anesthesia minimally affects renal function because of the presence of native renal blood flow autoregulation in healthy patients. Blockade of S2–S4 affects sympathetic and parasympathetic outflow to the bladder, leading to temporary urinary retention.

Indications and Contraindications

What are the indications for epidural anaesthesia? (Table 44.1)

Specific indications for epidural anaestheia for Obstetric caesarean section include [2]

- Maternal cardiovascular disease (e.g., peripartum cardiomyopathy, congenital heart disease). Patient is at an elevated risk of haemodynamic instability with spinal

Table 44.1 Indications for lumbar epidural anaesthesia/analgesia

Category	Procedures	Sensory level required
Lower limb major orthopaedic surgery	Pelvic and hip surgeries (e.g., Hip arthroplasty, acetabular, and femur surgeries)	T10
	Knee surgeries (e.g., Total knee replacement, knee arthroscopy)	T12
	Ankle and foot	T12
Vascular surgery	Lower limb vascular surgeries (e.g., embolectomy, thrombectomy, vein excision)	T8
	Abdominal aortic aneurysm repair	T6
Genitourinary & gynaecological	Nephrectomy	T4
	Prostatectomy and urethral stone extraction	T8
	Hysterectomy, dilatation and curettage	T10
Obstetric	Labour analgesia	T10
	Caesarean section	T4

Table 44.2 Indications for thoracic epidural anaesthesia/analgesia

Category	Procedures	Sensory level required
Thoracic surgery	Cardiac surgery with cardiopulmonary bypass	T1–T5
	Thoracotomy, video-assisted thoracic surgery	T1–T10
	Thoracic aortic aneurysm repair, thymectomy	T1–T10
Upper abdomen	Esophagectomy, gastrectomy, pancreatectomy, cholecystectomy	T5–T8 (T4–T8 if laparoscopic)
Lower abdomen	Colectomy, bowel resection, sigmoidectomy	T7–T9
	Abdominal perineal resection	T9–T11
Urogenital/gynaecologic	Extracorporeal shock wave lithotripsy	T6–T12
Breast procedures	Modified radical mastectomy	C5–T7 (placement at T2–T4)
	Mastectomy with transverse rectus abdominus myocutaneous flap reconstruction	C5–L1 (placement at T8–T10)
	Partial mastectomy, breast augmentation	T1–T7
Suprainguinal vascular procedures	Aortofemoral bypass	T6–T12 if extensive abdominal incision
	Renal artery bypass	
	Abdominal aortic aneurysm repair	T4–T12 if visceral denervation is required

anaesthesia, and a slow onset of surgical anaesthesia is desired
- Maternal characteristics of a potentially difficult spinal technique (that would be challenging if an urgent caesarean is required)
  - Severe scoliosis
  - Ankylosing spondylosis
  - High body mass index
- High risk of conversion from vaginal delivery to emergency caesarean section
  - Preeclampsia
  - High risk for assisted delivery (e.g., breech/multiple gestation)
  - Trial of labour after caesarean section
  - Anticipated difficult airway/risk factors for general anaesthesia

Contraindications to an epidural
Absolute

- Patient refusal
- Severe coagulation abnormalities (e.g., disseminated intravascular coagulation)

Relative

- Sepsis
  - Epidural anaesthesia risks causing relative hypovolemia, refractory hypotension, and introduction of possible infection into the epidural/subarachnoid space

- Elevated intracranial pressure
  - In patients with elevated intracranial pressure from obstructed cerebrospinal fluid flow due to mass effect, any accidental dural puncture can lead to cerebral herniation.
- Anticoagulant or antiplatelet medications
  - Patients are at increased risk of epidural hematoma. Timing for block initiation, catheter removal, anticoagulant drug omission, and restarting needs to be deliberated. See Chap. 34
- Thrombocytopaenia
  - There is no universally accepted platelet count, but a platelet count of 70 k is acceptable in the absence of bleeding for inserting and removing an epidural catheter. A trend of rapid fall is more significant than an absolute number.
  - Besides platelet count, platelet function should be considered as well. Preeclampsia and thrombotic thrombocytopenic purpura may affect this in pregnant patients
  - If platelet number or function deteriorates after the catheter is placed, the catheter should not be removed until coagulopathy is reversed
- Other bleeding diatheses: hemophilia, von Willebrand disease, and disorders related to lupus anticoagulant and anticardiolipin antibodies

- Preexisting central nervous system disorders (e.g., multiple sclerosis, post-polio syndrome)
  - Possible association with disease recurrence (e.g., Multiple sclerosis relapse)
- Fever/infection (e.g., varicella zoster virus)
  - Risk of infectious spread to epidural/subarachnoid space
- Preload dependent states (e.g., aortic stenosis)
  - Epidural-induced decrease in SVR would lead to acute decompensation. This leads to decreased coronary perfusion and contractility, further reducing cardiac output and worsening hypotension.
- Previous back surgery, preexisting neurologic injury, back pain
  - Technical difficulties may complicate epidural catheter placement and risk PDPH
  - Subsequent epidural blood patch to manage PDPH, if indicated, would be equally technically challenging
  - Spread of LA in the epidural space may be irregular, limited, or excessive
  - No established causal relationship between epidural and back pain
- Placement in anaesthetized adults
  - Increased risk of spinal cord injuries as patients cannot respond to the pain of intraneural injection and provide early feedback
- Needle placement through tattoo
  - Theoretical risk of introducing potentially toxic or carcinogenic pigment into epidural

Advantages of epidural anaesthesia

In obstetric and most non-obstetric procedures, effective epidural analgesia is advantageous in controlling postoperative pain, avoiding opioid-related side effects, and hence improving functional outcomes and patient satisfaction. In patients undergoing abdominal, thoracic, suprainguinal vascular and major lower limb surgery, the risk of cardiac, pulmonary and thromboembolic complications is reduced, due to earlier resolution of ileus in abdominal surgery, and for the rest, facilitation of mobilization and reduced

hospital stay. When done for thoracic surgery, lumbar and sacral nerves are spared, which reduces the incidence of postoperative urinary retention and lower limb motor block. The coronary blood supply is enhanced for cardiac surgery, improving left ventricular function and reducing perioperative arrhythmia [3]. In patients with chronic spinal cord injury and autonomic dysreflexia, attenuation of hypertensive crises and reflex bradycardia from surgical stimulus helps avoid life-threatening complications perioperatively. Central neuraxial techniques are also helpful in this group of patients to avoid repeated General Anaesthesia (GA) for recurrent simple procedures such as cystoscopy and lithotripsy.

Some procedures may be done safely with a lumbar epidural as the sole modality of anaesthesia, which helps to avoid GA and its complications. Patients who may benefit from this include those at the extremes of age, those with neurological conditions, and those at risk of pulmonary complications. In the elderly, avoidance of general anaesthesia reduces the risk of postoperative delirium and cognitive dysfunction, provided that intraoperative hypotension is minimized. Paediatric patients may still require a concomitant general anaesthetic technique, but doses required will be less, resulting in earlier awakening and discharge. If general anaesthesia is avoided entirely in infants less than 60 weeks postmenstrual age, the risk of postoperative apnoea and need for continuous monitoring is significantly reduced. Patients with neurological diseases such as myasthenia gravis and myotonia are at risk of postoperative hypoventilation and infection. By avoiding GA in these patients, muscle relaxants and opioids, respiratory function and cough are preserved, and the risk of prolonged mechanical ventilation is reduced. Patients with malignant hyperthermia may also benefit from regional techniques, as triggers such as volatile agents and succinylcholine are easily avoided.

Surgeries which are amenable to pure epidural technique include caesarean sections, major lower limb, suprainguinal vascular, and urogenital surgeries. In particular, epidural is especially beneficial in transurethral prostate resection for early detection of TURP syndrome and bladder/capsular perforation, and in enabling patient cooperation with the cough test for urinary incontinence surgery.

Compared to other regional techniques, epidurals are advantageous over spinals as they have a slower onset with less haemodynamic compromise. This is essential in high-risk patients with fixed cardiac output states such as critical aortic stenosis or reduced ejection fraction from cardiomyopathy. Compared with spinal, epidural block height and duration can be titrated if a catheter is left in situ, allowing for anaesthesia that can adapt to the surgical requirements. Additionally, epidurals also result in dense sympathetic blockade, which is superior for visceral analgesia in extensive abdominal surgery, compared with truncal plane or nerve blocks (e.g., TAP block, ESP). This sympathetic blockade results in vasodilation, which may improve graft patency in vascular surgery, mucosal perfusion in bowel anastomosis, and blunts sympathetic responses to surgical stimulus, which helps reduce blood loss in major limb surgery.

Disadvantages of epidural anaesthesia

The main disadvantages of epidural anaesthesia stem from its interindividual variability in clinical effectiveness, as well as the potential serious complications during placement. In some patients, the block may be incomplete over particular segments, leading to sparing and pain. In autonomic dysreflexia, this can lead to life-threatening hypertensive crises; in lower limb surgery, the tourniquet pain may not be adequately covered, which can lead to breakthrough pain. Additionally, the vasodilation from epidural anaesthesia may lead to intraoperative hypotension, which can complicate the haemodynamics in major open vascular surgery during clamping and unclamping of vessels. There may also be profound postoperative postural hypotension, hampering mobilization and necessitating excessive fluid resuscitation, which results in pulmonary and interstitial edema from third spacing.

Due to the size of the needle bore used, the risk of epidural haematoma after needle insertion or catheter placement is higher after full heparin-ization for cardiac and major vascular surgery. Large-bore dural puncture may also pose a significant concern for post-dural puncture headache and intracranial hypotension, which may be debilitating in postpartum mothers, who are also at highest risk for these complications. In parturients, the second stage of labour may also be prolonged, with a higher risk of instrumental delivery.

Overzealous motor blockade may delay discharge for ambulatory surgery and complicate postoperative lower limb assessment after thoracic aortic stenting. Residual sacral parasympathetic block can also lead to prolonged urine retention, requiring longer duration of urinary catheterization and its associated complications, including increased length of stay.

Block Performance

Equipment (Fig. 44.6)

Positioning

- Sitting, upright with shoulders relaxed and spine in flexion, OR
- Lateral decubitus position, knees drawn towards the chest and spine in flexion

Technique [4]
1. Aseptic technique with cleansing solution and sterile drapes
2. Identification of the level of insertion using the landmark and palpation technique or using ultrasound pre-scanning
    (a) Midline approach: between 2 spinous processes
    (b) Paramedian approach: 1–2 cm lateral to the spinous process
3. Skin infiltration with 1% Lidocaine 3–5 ml using a 25G hypodermic needle
4. A Touhy needle (16G or 18G) is inserted about 2 cm, the stylet is then removed, and a low resistance Loss-of-resistance (LOR) syringe is connected to the Touhy needle. Depending on preference, the syringe may be filled with air or saline.

Fig. 44.6 Equipment necessary for the performance of epidural anaesthesia with catheter insertion. Labels A—cleansing solution, B—Gauze, C—5-ml syringe with 25G hypodermic needle with 1% Lidocaine, D—Touhy needle, E—Loss of Resistance syringe, F—Catheter-securing clip, G—Filter, H—Epidural catheter, J—water-resistant and transparent dressing. (Equipment appearance may differ between different institutions and packaging)

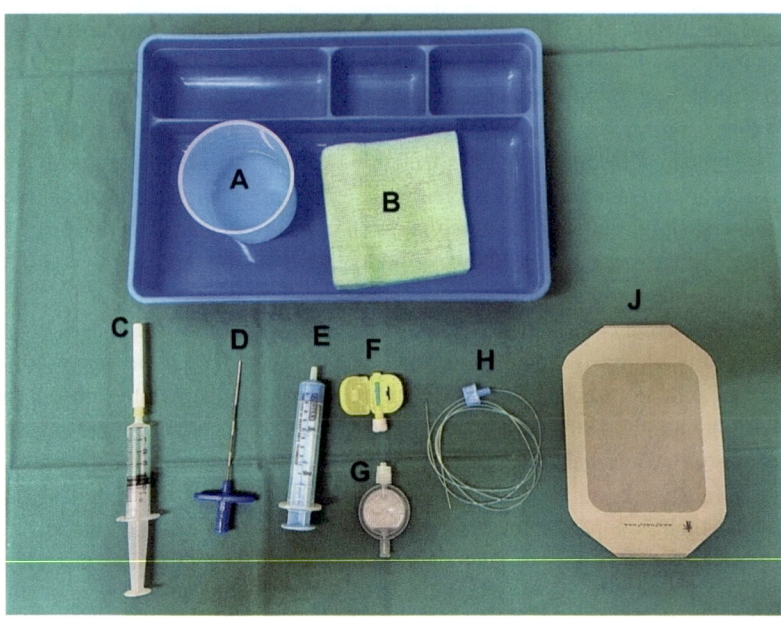

5. The Touhy needle is advanced until the ligamentum flavum is passed, and the LOR syringe empties efficiently. If bone is encountered, the needle trajectory is redirected cephalad (technique commonly termed as "walking off" the lamina).
6. The catheter is inserted through the Touhy needle, which is removed once a sufficient length has been inserted.
7. Withdraw the catheter to the desired length (usually 4–5 cm in epidural space) and connect to the clip and filter.
8. Carefully aspirate, verifying there is no CSF or blood, and inject a test dose of 3 ml of 1% Lidocaine with 1:200,000 adrenaline. Monitor for rapid increase in heart rate, blood pressure, or profound weakness, which may suggest intravascular or intrathecal insertion respectively.
9. Secure the catheter with a sterile dressing.

Controversies in technique

The above summarizes the steps to one of the possible techniques in epidural insertion. Several debates exist in the literature as different techniques and approaches are used worldwide,

partly due to variations and preferences in practice, training, and other patient profiles.

Midline Versus Paramedian

The midline approach is favoured for lumbar epidural placement due to the less steep angulation of spinous processes and accessibility of the midline for needle insertion. The paramedian approach may be more suitable for thoracic epidural placement due to the overlap of spinous processes, steeper needle angulation, and longer distance to space via midline approach. However, the midline approach may occasionally lack the characteristic tactile pop due to gaps left by incomplete fusion of ligamentum flavum, which may result in excessive needle advancement and inadvertent dural puncture. The midline approach in non-parturients may also result in more paraesthesia and bleeding. The paramedian approach is less dependent on spinal flexion, [5] resulting in faster catheter placement and more reliable cephalad passage [6]. However, preprocedure local anaesthetic infiltration should be generous as the large bore needle passes through the erector spinae muscles rather than less sensitive connective tissue of the midline approach.

Tactile Sensation During Either Approach

Both supra and interspinous ligaments are made of collagenous fibers that make a distinct "crunching" sensation as the Tuohy needle advances. The ligamentum flavum comprises thick elastic fibers arranged longitudinally in a tight network, and is thickest in the lumbar area. A characteristic "pop" sensation is felt when penetrating the ligamentum flavum. Midline gaps in the ligamentum flavum from incomplete fusion between left and right ligamentum flava may affect the identification of the epidural space by the procedurist [7].

Paramedian approach penetrates paraspinous tissues and not the supraspinous and interspinous ligaments. As a result, there is less resistance before the ligamentum flavum is reached. However, the bony landmark of the vertebral lamina is contacted before 'walking off' superomedially into the intervertebral space, which also presents as a 'give' using the LOR syringe.

LOR to Saline or Air

Loss of resistance is tested by depressing the plunger of a low-resistance syringe, connected to a Touhy needle and either filled with saline or air. If using saline, a constant pressure is applied to the plunger during needle advancement. If using air, intermittent rapid pressure is applied instead. Loss of resistance to air has been reported to put the patient at risk for pneumocephalus, retroperitoneal air, subcutaneous emphysema, venous air embolism, and neurological compression. However, in a Cochrane review, low-level evidence showed no difference in the identification of epidural space nor complications encountered for LOR to both saline and air [8].

What is the expected distance from the skin to the epidural space?
Different levels of the vertebra have varying depths from skin to epidural space. Parturients have an average depth from skin to space of 4–6 cm, but some patients have a shallow depth of 2–4 cm. These patients are at an elevated risk of accidental dural puncture because this shallow depth can also be reached with the LA infiltration needle.

How much catheter should be left in the epidural space?
The epidural catheter should be left approximately 4–5 cm within the epidural space. Insufficient length within the epidural space risks migration of the epidural catheter superficially out of the epidural space, with higher chances of that occurring in a multi-orifice catheter where the proximal hole can be 1.5 cm from the tip of the catheter. Excessive length within the epidural space risks a unilateral block because of the laterality of the catheter tip. In previous studies, epidural catheters were found to be rarely in the posterior midline, with about half of them deviating towards intervertebral foramina.

What is the purpose of the test dose?
The purpose of the test dose is to detect intrathecal or intravascular catheter placement, as a secondary check after negative aspiration of blood or CSF from the epidural catheter. The test dose should only be performed after the epidural catheter is withdrawn to the desired length within the epidural space. Typically, 3 ml of 1.5% lignocaine is administered. If intrathecal, dense lower limb motor block would be apparent within 5 minutes on assessment of the Bromage score. If intravascular, the patient may not experience central nervous system symptoms such as tinnitus or perioral numbness. If 1:200,000 epinephrine is administered in the test dose, an increase in heart rate by >20% would also be noted within a minute. In patients with preexisting beta-blockade, an increase in systolic blood pressure by >20 mmHg may be observed instead.

Troubleshooting

How would you manage paraesthesia on needle insertion/movement?
Patients may report paraesthesia during epidural needle or catheter placement. This signifies that

the needle is too near a nerve. The needle should be withdrawn and reinserted at a different angle or level. Before inserting an epidural catheter, it may be helpful to inject normal saline into the Touhy needle to displace spinal nerves and dura away from the needle tip (Fig. 44.7).

If there is resistance to catheter insertion, how do you manage this?

It should not be forced if difficulty is encountered in threading the catheter into the epidural space. A catheter inserted past the Touhy needle should not be withdrawn from the needle for the risk of shearing the catheter tip. The Touhy needle and catheter assembly should first be removed from the patient as one unit. Repeat epidural needle insertion with LOR should be done, and normal saline injected to displace the spinal nerves/spinal cord before reinserting the catheter (Fig. 44.7).

You aspirate blood from the epidural catheter. What do you do now?

Blood aspirated from the epidural catheter or needle likely means there is epidural vein cannulation. This could mean the needle placement is too lateral and should be redirected midline, or the catheter was inserted during a contraction while in labour. The epidural catheter should be flushed with saline to prevent blood from clotting within and blocking the catheter. The catheter should then be withdrawn by 1–2 cm, and re-aspirated for blood. If blood is still aspirated, remove the catheter and repeat the procedure.

How do you manage a unilateral block?

Unilateral block reflects the epidural catheter tip being too lateral, entering the intervertebral foramen, or too close to a nerve. Withdraw the catheter by 1–2 cm and recheck the sensory block

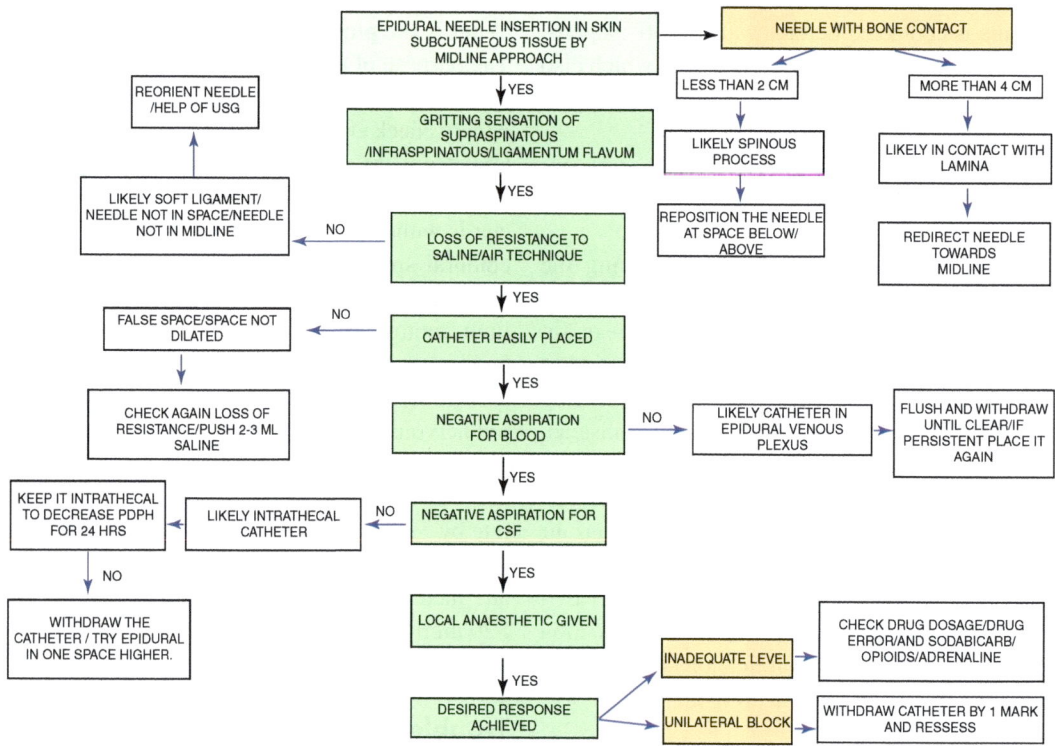

Fig. 44.7 Structured approach for troubleshooting needle placement in epidural anaesthesia. (Produced with permission from Parmar and Ashokka [1])

level. The patient can also be placed in the lateral position with the unblocked side on the dependent side, and several milliliters of dilute LA can be administered. If unresolved, the procedure should be repeated.

Why do some epidurals lead to a patchy block?

A patchy block can manifest as persistent pain despite adequate block height. It can result from epidural air injected during LOR to air technique, catheter migration, or anatomical variation. Top-ups of additional LA, with or without opioids, are reasonable. The catheter can also be withdrawn by 1–2 cm, and the patient positioned dependent on the less blocked side. If unresolved, replace the catheter.

Drug Choice

Drugs commonly given in an epidural catheter or single-shot bolus include local anaesthetics, opioids, and additives. After deposition in the epidural space, they are postulated to diffuse across the dura into the cerebrospinal fluid in the subarachnoid space to act on the spinal cord and nerve roots.

Factors affecting the use of local anaesthetic

2-chloroprocaine has the shortest onset (5–15 minutes) and duration of action (30–90 minutes), and can provide surgical analgesia with expedited postoperative recovery [9]. The fast onset is due to its high concentration when administered, because it has fast metabolism and thus low risk for systemic toxicity despite high doses. The duration of action is short due to low protein binding, and it is hence quickly eliminated. However, as it is an ester local anaesthetic, its metabolite para-aminobenzoic acid (PABA) may be associated with allergic reactions. It was also previously manufactured with preservatives such as ethylenediaminetetraacetic (EDTA) acid and bisulfites, and hence adverse effects such as back pain and adhesive arachnoiditis were reported when accidentally injected into the subarachnoid space [10].

2% lidocaine is often used to top up a preexisting epidural catheter to allow for rapid ascent of the epidural level and density for surgery, with an onset time of 10–20 minutes and duration of action of 1–2 hours. However, it has been associated with the adverse effects of intense shivering and transient neurological symptoms, including pain radiating from the buttock to both lower limbs after recovery of the central neuraxial blockade [11].

Ropivacaine and bupivacaine both have an onset time of 15–20 minutes, and can last almost 4 hours after each bolus. If given in a dilute form (0.1–0.25%), it is sufficient for analgesia (e.g., labour contractions). However, surgical anesthesia requires a higher concentration (e.g., 0.5%). Ropivacaine is slightly less long acting than bupivacaine, and may produce a less-dense motor block at equivalent doses. Bupivacaine has a low CC/CNS ratio of 2 (compared to the 7 of lidocaine), and hence runs a higher risk of severe refractory cardiotoxic adverse reactions such as hypotension, heart block, and ventricular fibrillation if given intravascularly at therapeutic epidural doses. Levobupivacaine has fewer of these toxic effects; however, it has a slower onset but similar duration of motor block compared to ropivacaine and bupivacaine [12].

For pre-cesarean epidural top-ups, 2% lidocaine with epinephrine and fentanyl gives the fastest onset, whilst ropivacaine 0.75% gives the best quality sensory blockade. Bupivacaine 0.5% was the least effective solution [13].

Mixing of local anaesthetics before administration via an epidural

Mixing local anaesthetics is not practical for hastening onset or prolonging duration. Mixing likely dilutes local anaesthetics below their effective concentration for potency of onset, and a continuous infusion of a single drug is sufficient. The dilution of local anaesthetics in normal saline has been found to achieve a lower level of sensory block and a less potent epidural blockade. For a top up for surgical anaesthesia, 15 ml of lidocaine 2% (with fentanyl and sodium bicarbonate) took the same time to establish a block to sensation at T4 level when compared to 0.5%

levobupivacaine and 0.75% ropivacaine [14]. However, the duration of action was significantly longer with levobupivacaine compared with ropivacaine, and again when compared with lidocaine.

The density of the motor block depends on the concentration of local anaesthetic injected—a lower concentration bolus produces a sensory band with motor sparing. Using a lower concentration local anaesthetic also helps decrease the total dose required for clinical labour anaesthesia. To maintain adequate analgesia, a third to half of the initial epidural bolus can be repeated after the initial sensory block has receded by two dermatomal levels. Alternatively, local anaesthetic can be run as an infusion, and a higher concentration of local anaesthetic provides better analgesia but a longer lasting motor block and a dilute anaesthetic at the same rate. However, if a high concentration solution is run at a slower infusion rate, the motor blockade and haemodynamic instability are reduced when compared to a high infusion rate of a low concentration solution.

Regimes for a labour epidural

Programmed Intermittent Epidural bolus (PIB) achieves the same degree of labour analgesia as continuous epidural infusion, reducing the total local anaesthetic consumption and degree of motor block. Using slower PIB injection rates (125 ml/h/h vs 250 ml/h) does not affect the maximum sensory level, but may reduce the incidence of hypotension [15]. The optimal interval between boluses for a dilute solution containing plain bupivacaine (0.0625%) and fentanyl (2 mcg/ml) has been found to average 40 minutes during the first stage of labour [16].

Instituting patient-controlled top-ups results in an equivalent analgesic effect compared to a continuous infusion rate, but it also reduces the overall local anaesthetic consumption and motor blockade.

Use of opioids in an epidural

Fentanyl, sufentanil, and morphine have been added to epidural bolus and infusions. They help increase the density of the epidural blockade and

reduce the absolute volume of local anaesthetic bolus and infusion required to achieve the same clinical effect, hence reducing the risk of local anaesthetic toxicity [17].

Problems with epidural morphine

The use of a morphine infusion may slightly decrease the overall morphine-equivalent opioid usage when compared to fentanyl or sufentanil (by 1.2 mg morphine). However, it also results in more pruritus and postoperative nausea or vomiting. Morphine is more hydrophilic than fentanyl and sufentanil. It may tend to migrate further cephalad in the intrathecal space, resulting in nausea and vomiting and a risk of delayed respiratory depression. In addition to the activation of opioid receptors, its additional mechanism of histamine release may also intensify its pruritic side effect. It is also less lipophilic, which reduces its diffusion into the epidural fat. It promotes its persistence in the epidural depot, prolonging its effect in the intrathecal space and reducing the dose required.

Extended release morphine (DepoFoam) consists of microscopic lipid membrane-coated vesicles containing morphine, which slowly release the drug over 48 hours. Longer clinical analgesic effect and fewer side effects compared to intrathecal morphine have been demonstrated, and these include less nausea, pruritus, drowsiness, and respiratory depression [18].

Other additives for epidural anaesthesia

Adding 1:200,000 epinephrine to an epidural lidocaine, 2-chloroprocaine, or mepivacaine prolongs their duration of action. It is less effective for ropivacaine and bupivacaine. This acts via vasoconstriction of the surrounding epidural vessels, reducing diffusion of local anaesthetic into the blood and prolonging the effect of local anaesthetic around the epidural nerve roots. Other vasoconstrictors, such as phenylephrine, have not shown similar effectiveness.

Adding sodium bicarbonate 8.4% mixed with or just before lidocaine, 2-chloroprocaine or mepivacaine, converts more of the local anaesthetic to the lipid soluble nonionised form (the extent of which depends on their pKa), which facilitates transmembrane diffusion of local anaesthetic molecules and hastens the onset of clinical analgesia. Ropivacaine and bupivacaine will precipitate when mixed with sodium bicarbonate.

Similar to opioids, clonidine increases the density of analgesic block and reduces the dose of local anaesthetic used to maintain the level of block. The latter thus results in fewer motor blocks and less arterial hypotension. Clonidine may also prolong the block duration due to its effect on the hyperpolarization-activated current in neuronal cells, rather than its action on alpha 2 receptors. Additionally, it also has a synergistic effect with epidural opioids and modulates the stress response after thoracic surgery. However, dependent side effects include sedation, brady-cardia, hypotension, and dry mouth [19].

Dexamethasone in the form of a 2 ml 8 mg bolus has been shown to hasten the sensory onset and increase the duration of lumbar epidural anaesthesia, as well as reduce the incidence of postoperative nausea and vomiting, in patients undergoing unilateral inguinal herniorraphy [20, 21]. It has also shown similar results in a 1 ml 4 mg bolus in thoracic epidurals. This may be related to the direct suppression of pain and sensory transmission in unmyelinated nociceptive C fibres by steroids, as well as the suppression of spinal cord phospholipase A2 and cyclo-oxygenase 2, with resultant reduced prostaglandin synthesis.

Factors affecting the spread and duration of epidural drugs

When delivered into the epidural space, drugs distribute into three compartments, namely the epidural fat, CSF, and blood in epidural vessels. The analgesic effect results from its diffusion in the CSF and subsequent direct action on the spinal cord and nerve roots. Individual variation in CSF volume affects the pharmacokinetics of drugs. Drugs distributed into the blood are cleared from the epidural space and metabolised by the body. The epidural fat acts as a lipid sink which traps lipophilic drugs and reduces their bioavailability, with the most excellent affinity for bupivacaine, then ropivacaine, followed by

lidocaine (in the order of 2 each time). Consequently, a higher amount of epidural adiposity results in a lower degree of motor blockade and faster block regression to S3. Conversely, a reduction in epidural fat with age leads to higher levels and quicker onset of anaesthesia in older people.

Epidural drugs spread freely within the epidural space. However, several factors affect the spread of epidural medications and the extent of action along the spinal cord [22]. A higher dose or volume of local anaesthetic results in a greater spread along the spinal cord. Thoracic epidural injections tend to spread cranially, whilst more extensive nerve roots limit caudal spread to the lumbosacral region. Additionally, the direction of the bevel of the Tuohy needle affects the predominant spread of local anaesthetic cephalad or caudally, when rotated towards the respective directions. This effect is significant in those >40 years old, possibly due to connective tissue fibrosis and dural thickening with age. Higher dural surface area may lower the peak block level achieved and delay the onset of peak epidural block.

The epidural volume required for spread per spinal segment in young patients is 1.7–1.8 ml [23]. Less volume per spinal segment is required with advancing age, shorter patient height, supine position (compared to sitting), and when using a higher concentration solution. Pregnancy has been shown to reduce the dose required by a third, possibly due to raised intra-abdominal pressure causing epidural vein engorgement and reduction of epidural space. Speed of injection does not affect the extent of spread. However, a higher speed correlates with higher epidural pressure, which may be hazardous in patients with pre-existing spinal stenosis or at risk for intracranial hypertension. Increasing the block height via the 'epidural volume effect' has also been described. This involves administering a volume of saline into the epidural space within 20 minutes of drug delivery or diffusion into the intrathecal space, or before the block level has receded by two or more segments, and is based on the mechanism of dural sac compression with reduction of CSF volume. The latter correlates with a higher peak block height, shorter onset time, and longer action duration. A decrease in CSF volume may be achieved through abdominal compression and/or hyperventilation, both of which cause epidural vein plexus enlargement that compresses the dural sac.

Potential complications of epidural

Complications of epidural anaesthesia can be drug or procedure-related. For clinical relevance, complications are listed in order of severity and frequency of occurrence (Table 44.3).

Clinical Pearls

- Some clinical tips include:
  - In the sitting position, a squared pelvis, relaxation of both shoulders, forward flexion of the spine and neck, and legs supported with a stool is the optimal position during block performance.
  - Ultrasound used to identify bony landmarks and depth of epidural space is invaluable in difficult surface landmarks such as obesity and pregnancy.

Table 44.3 Complications of epidural block

Severity	Complication	Risk
Minor, common	Nausea	1:10
	Shivering	1:10
	Pruritus	1:10
	Motor block	1:10
	Transient hypotension	1:1000
Major, common	Partial/incomplete block requiring resiting/ adjustment	1:10–20
	PDPH	1:100
Major, uncommon	LA toxicity [24]	1:10,000
	High block	1:10,000
	Transient neurological weakness due to nerve injury	1:15,000
	Meningitis	1:100,000
	Epidural abscess	1:100,000
	Epidural haematoma	1:100,000
	Spinal cord injury and paralysis	1:1,000,000

- The appropriate level of catheter insertion is important for adequate dermatomal coverage—e.g., T7–T8 or T8–T9 for midline laparotomy incisions and T9–T10 or T10–T11 for subumbilical incisions. Placing at the wrong level may require larger volumes or higher rates of infusion to achieve adequate analgesia, resulting in more hypotension.
  - Lowering the concentration of local anaesthetics and opioids helps to reduce the side effects in elderly patients—0.1% Ropivacaine with 1 mcg/ml Fentanyl instead of 0.2% Ropivacaine with 2 mcg/ml Fentanyl.
- In addition to meticulous execution of the block, system factors, such as well-established management protocols, adequate post-insertion monitoring by trained nursing personnel, and an acute pain service team, contribute to the success of epidural analgesia.

Questions

1. Outline the relevant anatomy encountered whilst doing an epidural
2. Describe the physiological impact after epidural anaesthesia is achieved for a thoracotomy.
3. How would you perform a safe thoracic epidural for Ivor Lewis Oesophagectomy?
4. What are the advantages of a plain epidural over a CSE or spinal?
5. Discuss the differences between the midline and paramedian approaches
6. Discuss the local anaesthetics commonly given in an epidural
7. What are the adjunct drugs that can be administered via an epidural catheter
8. Discuss the techniques that can be utilized to decrease the overall epidural local anesthetic usage whilst achieving the same clinical analgesic effect
9. Eight hours after the removal of an epidural catheter, a postpartum parturient has persistent right foot drop and paraesthesia over the lateral leg and right dorsum foot. What are

the possible causes and the appropriate management?

10. Six hours after a labour epidural catheter has been placed, the patient complains of breakthrough labour pain. A sensory check suggests the level is at T10 on the right and T12 on the left. The Bromage score is zero. Discuss the possible causes and your management.

References

1. Parmar S, Ashokka B. Central neuraxial blockade. In: Chakraborty A, editor. Blockmate: a practical guide for ultrasound guided regional anaesthesia. Singapore. ISBN 978-981-15-9201-0, ISBN 978-981-15-9202-7 (eBook): Springer; 2021. p. 121–46. https://doi.org/10.1007/978-981-15-9202.

2. Hawkins JL. Epidural analgesia for labor and delivery. N Engl J Med. 2010;362(16):1503–10.

3. Nygård E, Kofoed KF, Freiberg J, Holm S, Aldershvile J, Eliasen K, et al. Effects of high thoracic epidural analgesia on myocardial blood flow in patients with ischemic heart disease. Circulation. 2005;111(17):2165–70.

4. Toledano RD. Epidural anesthesia and Analgesia [Internet]. NYSORA. 2022 [cited 2022 Jul 12]. Available from: https://www.nysora.com/topics/regional-anesthesia-for-specific-surgical-procedures/abdomen/epidural-anesthesia-analgesia/.

5. Podder S, Kumar N, Yaddanapudi LN, Chari P. Paramedian lumbar epidural catheter insertion with patients in the sitting position is equally successful in the flexed and unflexed spine. Anesth Analg. 2004;99:1829–32.

6. Blomberg RG. Technical advantages of the paramedian approach for lumbar epidural puncture and catheter introduction. A study using epiduroscopy in autopsy subjects. Anaesthesia. 1988;43(10):837–43.

7. Igarashi T, Hirabayashi Y, Shimizu R, Saitoh K, Fukuda H, Mitsuhata H. The lumbar extradural structure changes with increasing age. Br J Anaesth. 1997;78(2):149–52.

8. Pedro L, Paulo NG, Leandro GB, João VPD, Norma SPM, Regina ED. Air versus saline in the loss of resistance technique for identification of the epidural space. Cochrane Database Syst Rev. 2014;2014(7):CD008938.

9. Datta S, Corke BC, Alper MH, Brown WU, Ostheimer GW, Weiss JB. Epidural anesthesia for cesarean section: a comparison of bupivacaine, chloroprocaine, and etidocaine. Anesthesiology. 1980;52(1):48–51.

10. Mims SC, Zanolli NC, Fuller M, Habib AS. Intrathecal bupivacaine versus chloroprocaine for transvaginal cervical cerclage placement: a retrospective cohort study. Int J Obstet Anesth. 2022;50:103276.

11. Forget P, Borovac JA, Thackeray EM, Pace NL. Transient neurological symptoms (TNS) following spinal anaesthesia with lidocaine versus other local anaesthetics in adult surgical patients: a network meta-analysis. Cochrane Database Syst Rev. 2019;(12):CD003006.

12. Kopacz DJ, Allen HW, Thompson GE. A comparison of epidural levobupivacaine 0.75% with racemic bupivacaine for lower abdominal surgery. Anesth Analg. 2000;90(3):642–8.

13. Hillyard SG, Bate TE, Corcoran TB, Paech MJ, O'Sullivan G. Extending epidural analgesia for emergency caesarean section: a meta-analysis. Br J Anaesth. 2011;107(5):668–78.

14. Peduto VA, Baroncini S, Montanini S, Proietti R, Rosignoli L, Tufano R, Casati A. A prospective, randomized, double-blind comparison of epidural levobupivacaine 0.5% with epidural ropivacaine 0.75% for lower limb procedures. Eur J Anaesthesiol. 2003;20(12):979–83.

15. Mazda Y, Arzola C, Downey K, Ye XY, Carvalho JCA. Programmed intermittent epidural bolus for labour analgesia: a randomized controlled trial comparing bolus delivery speeds of 125 mL·hr-1 versus 250 mL·hr-1. Can J Anaesth. 2022;69(1):86–96.

16. Kanczuk ME, Barrett NM, Arzola C, Downey K, Ye XY, Carvalho JCA. Programmed intermittent epidural bolus for labor analgesia during first stage of labor: a biased-coin up-and-down sequential allocation trial to determine the optimum interval time between boluses of a fixed volume of 10 mL of bupivacaine 0.0625% with fentanyl 2 μg/mL. Anesth Analg. 2017;124(2):537–41.

17. Youssef N, Orlov D, Alie T, Chong M, Cheng J, Thabane L, et al. What epidural opioid results in the best analgesia outcomes and fewest side effects after surgery? A meta-analysis of randomized controlled trials. Anesth Analg. 2014;119(4):965–77.

18. Cohen M, Zuk J, McKay N, Erickson M, Pan Z, Galinkin J. Intrathecal morphine versus extended release epidural morphine for postoperative pain control in pediatric patients undergoing posterior spinal fusion. Anesth Analg. 2017;124(6):2030–7.

19. Kroin JS, Buvanendran A, Beck DR, Topic JE, Watts DE, Tuman KJ. Clonidine prolongation of lidocaine analgesia after sciatic nerve block in rats is mediated via the hyperpolarization-activated cation current, not by alpha-adrenoreceptors. Anesthesiology. 2004;101(2):488–94.

20. Razavizadeh MR, Fazel MR, Heydarian N, Atoof F. Epidural dexamethasone for postoperative analgesia in patients undergoing unilateral inguinal herniorrhaphy: a comparative study. Pain Res Manag. 2017;2017:7649458–5.

21. Naghipour B, Aghamohamadi D, Azarfarin R, Mirinazhad M, Bilehjani E, Abbasali D, et al. Dexamethasone added to bupivacaine prolongs dura-

tion of epidural analgesia. Middle East J Anaesthesiol. 2013;22(1):53–7.

22. Higuchi H, Adachi Y, Kazama T. Factors affecting the spread and duration of epidural anesthesia with ropivacaine. Anesthesiology. 2004;101(2):451–60.

23. Lee I, Soehartono RH, Yamagishi N, Taguchi K, Yamada H. Distribution of new methylene blue injected into the dorsolumbar epidural space in cows. Vet Anaesth Analg. 2001;28(3):140–5.

24. Christie LE, Picard J, Weinberg GL. Local anaesthetic systemic toxicity. Continuing education in anaesthesia. Crit Care Pain. 2015;15:136–42.

Combined Spinal Epidural Block

45

Roche John Alexis Martin, Ashokka Balakrishnan, Premi Cynthia, and Jessie Paul

Introduction

Regional anaesthesia techniques have gained widespread use in surgical, obstetric, and postoperative pain management settings. In the combined spinal–epidural (CSE) technique, an initial dose of medication is administered into the subarachnoid space, followed by the placement of an epidural catheter through which subsequent doses can be delivered. Although now a common practice, the CSE remains a technically demanding procedure. This approach provides rapid onset of analgesia or anaesthesia from the spinal component, while the epidural catheter allows for continued maintenance of anaesthesia and effective postoperative pain control.

Functional Anatomy to Consider During CSE

Understanding the skin-to-epidural space distance (SED) and the width of the posterior epidural space (PED) is essential when performing a combined spinal–epidural (CSE) technique. These measurements help reduce the risk of inadvertent dural penetration or injury to neural structures. An inaccurate estimate of the PED may lead to the spinal needle protruding beyond the

epidural needle tip, particularly in the needle-through-needle configuration, thereby increasing the risk of neural trauma. Measures of these distances have been obtained using techniques such as MRI, CT, and ultrasound, as well as by recording the tip-to-tip distance between the epidural (Tuohy) needle and the spinal needle in CSE set-ups. For example, one study in parturients found a mean SED of approximately 5.6 cm (±1.6) at the L3–4 level. The width of the PED varies by spinal level: it is widest in the mid-lumbar region (about 5–6 mm) and becomes narrower in the mid-thoracic (approximately 3–5 mm) and lower cervical regions (about 1.5–2 mm). These anatomic findings have informed the design of spinal needles that project approximately 10–15 mm beyond the epidural needle tip. Additionally, other important anatomic considerations include the thickness of the ligamentum flavum and the distance from the dorsal dura—both of which change at different vertebral levels (Table 45.1).

The ligamenta flava do fuse variably in the midline, and this fusion or lack of fusion of ligamentum flavum occurs at different levels of the vertebral column. Various studies found the highest incidence of absent midline fusion at the

R. J. A. Martin (✉)
North Hampshire Hospital Trust, HHFT, Basingstoke, UK

A. Balakrishnan · P. Cynthia · J. Paul
St. Michael's Hospital, Toronto, ON, Canada

Table 45.1 Distance from skin to ligamentum flavum and thickness of ligament at various levels

Site	Skin to Ligament (cm)	Thickness of ligament (mm)
Cervical	–	1.5–3.0
Thoracic	–	3.0–5.0
Lumbar	3.0–8.0	5.0–6.0
Caudal	Variable	2.0–6.0

lower thoracic level (T10–11, 35.5%) and the weakest at the mid-thoracic level (T7–8, 2.1%). This midline fusion loss decreases the ability to appreciate the loss of resistance when using a midline approach.

Applications of the CSE

Various advantages that have stood out for CSE's popularity are faster onset, decreased failure rate, more pronounced motor block in non-obstetric cases, and minimal risk of toxicity in obstetric cases.

Obstetrics

The use of combined spinal–epidural (CSE) anaesthesia has grown significantly over the past decade, both for providing analgesia during labour and for anaesthesia in caesarean section procedures. The advantages of CSE in labour include a faster onset of pain relief compared with the conventional epidural technique—particularly in the later stages of labour—while allowing the mother to remain ambulant. A Cochrane review of 14 randomised controlled trials comparing CSE with standard epidural analgesia confirmed

that CSE offers quicker and more effective pain relief, along with greater maternal satisfaction. However, no significant differences were found between the two techniques in terms of maternal mobility, incidence of post-dural puncture headache, or the rates of instrumental or caesarean deliveries. CSE has also been shown to provide more reliable analgesia and muscle relaxation than conventional epidural anaesthesia, with a lower total dose of local anaesthetic required for caesarean section. Although demonstrating advantages over single-shot spinal anaesthesia can be more challenging, CSE offers the important benefit of prolonged anaesthesia when surgery is expected to extend beyond the duration of a single spinal injection. Performing neuraxial techniques in obstetric patients requires special consideration due to anatomical and physiological changes during pregnancy. These include exaggerated lumbar lordosis, increased adiposity around the paraspinal area, difficulty palpating bony landmarks, subcutaneous oedema, and engorgement of the epidural venous plexus, which can fluctuate with intra-abdominal pressure during labour. Additionally, positioning may be suboptimal due to the gravid uterus and frequent movement in advanced labour, necessitating careful adjustment of anaesthetic technique and dosing (Fig. 45.1).

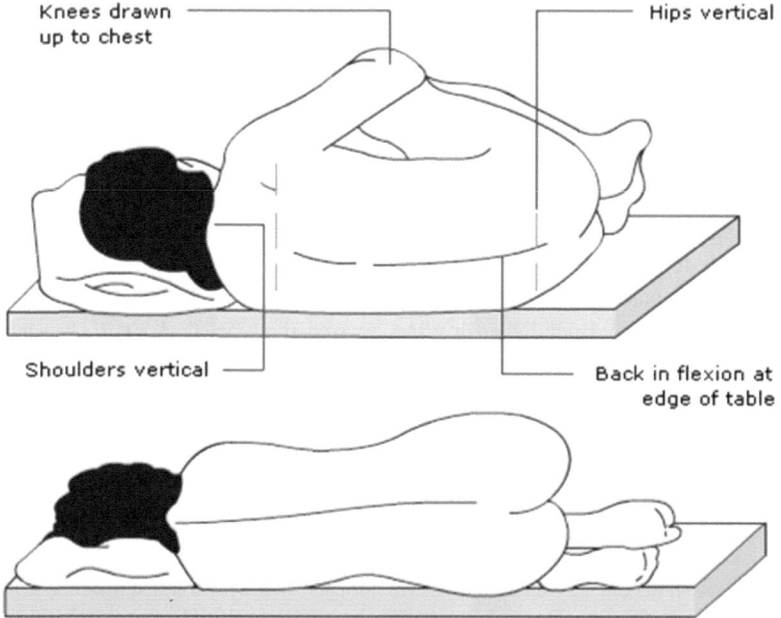

Fig. 45.1 Positioning for combined spinal epidural (**a**: With full back flexion; **b**: Without back flexion)

Knees drawn up to chest

Hips vertical

Shoulders vertical

Back in flexion at edge of table

Non-obstetric

CSE has been used for various non-obstetric surgery in adults, including orthopaedic, urological, vascular, gynaecological, and general surgical procedures. The technique has also been used for inguinal hernia repair in neonates.

Technical Consideration of CSE

Combined Spinal Epidurals can be placed using two primary techniques

1. The needle-through-needle technique (NTN) and
2. The separate-needle technique (SN).

Both midline and paramedian approaches can be used for each of the techniques described below:

The Needle-Through-Needle Technique (NTN)

The needle-through-needle technique is the most widely used CSE technique. This technique has led to the design of epidural needles with 'black-eyes or holes' in the greater curvature of the needles, which allow the epidural catheter to be inserted away from the dural puncture site, thereby reducing the inadvertent placement of epidural catheter in the subarachnoid space (Fig. 45.2).

Other developments include the design of spinal needles which lock onto the epidural needle after dural puncture, thus reducing the risk of spinal needle displacement during intrathecal injection and failure of spinal anaesthesia.

The epidural catheter can be inserted into the epidural space before the spinal block. However, it holds the disadvantage of misplacement of the

catheter or epidural needle and risks damage to the epidural catheter as the spinal needle is inserted.

With this technique, the epidural catheter location is not tested before spinal anaesthetic administration and is quicker to perform and better tolerated by patients.

Separate Needle (SN)

This technique uses two separate needles to perform the spinal and epidural components of the CSE. Both needles can be inserted at the same vertebral interspace or two separate interspaces. Again, the spinal and epidural components of the CSE can be performed in either order. The advantages and risks of performing the epidural component first are the same as those described for the needle-through-needle technique above. The advantage of performing the spinal component first is that the almost instantaneous onset of analgesia reduces the risk of the patient moving during the subsequent epidural needle insertion. The SN technique allows for testing the epidural catheter before administering the spinal anaesthetic.

Studies comparing the needle-through-needle technique with the separate needle technique have found a higher failure rate of the spinal component with the needle-through-needle technique. Failure rates of 5–20% have been reported for the NTN technique (although in experienced hands this is as low as 1–5%), compared with 0.5% for the separate needle technique.

With the NTN technique, the epidural catheter location is not tested before spinal anaesthetic administration. Success with the SN and NTN techniques differs. Casati et al. found that SN and NTN had similar failure rates. A dual-lumen CSE needle was recently introduced in Europe (Fig. 45.3).

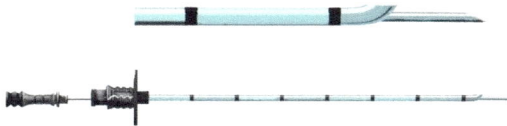

Fig. 45.2 Needle through needle technique

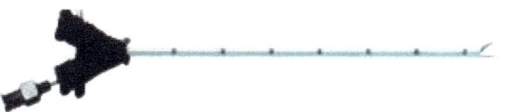

Fig. 45.3 Dual-lumen technique

Applied Anatomy of Standard Approaches to Epidural Space

Midline/Interlaminar Approach

The needle is inserted at the midline between the spinous processes. In the lumbar region, the needle is advanced with a relatively flat trajectory, whereas in the thoracic region, a slight cranial angulation is required. The needle passes sequentially through the following tissue layers: skin, subcutaneous tissue, supraspinous ligament, interspinous ligament, and ligamentum flavum.

Paramedian Approach

In this approach, the needle is inserted slightly caudal and lateral to the lower border of the spinous process at the selected interspace. The needle is then advanced and "walked off" the lamina until it engages the ligamentum flavum. The epidural needle traverses the following structures: skin, subcutaneous tissue, connective tissue, and ligamentum flavum. This technique is particularly useful for patients with limited positioning ability or altered spinal anatomy, such as those with kyphoscoliosis.

Taylor's Approach

This technique serves as an alternative paramedian approach at the L5–S1 interspace for patients with difficult anatomy where a midline approach is not feasible. The L5–S1 level provides the largest interlaminar space and is typically the least affected by arthritic or degenerative changes. The needle is inserted approximately 1 cm medial and 1 cm caudal to the posterior superior iliac spine, directed in a medio-cranial trajectory. If bone is encountered, the needle should be walked off the sacrum until the ligamentum flavum is engaged. Other possible approaches include the transforaminal technique (targeting the anterior epidural space under fluoroscopic guidance) and the transsacral or caudal approach.

Different Drugs Used and Their Duration of Action

The most commonly used local anaesthetic agents in combined spinal–epidural (CSE) anaesthesia are bupivacaine, levobupivacaine, and ropivacaine. Among these, bupivacaine produces the most pronounced motor blockade. Intrathecal administration of bupivacaine allows for a reduced dose of intrathecal fentanyl, thereby minimising opioid-related side effects such as pruritus and respiratory depression. The table below summarises the commonly used agents and their median effective intrathecal doses required to achieve motor blockade in parturients, as assessed by the Bromage Scale (Grades 1–3: feet/knees) (Table 45.2).

Sufentanil and fentanyl, either alone or in combination with local anaesthetics, are the agents most commonly administered intrathecally to provide analgesia for labouring women undergoing combined spinal–epidural (CSE) anaesthesia (Table 45.3).

In combined spinal–epidural (CSE) anaesthesia, a lower dose of local anaesthetic is administered intrathecally since the anaesthesiologist has the option to maintain or extend the block through the epidural component. A more recent advancement is the practice of administering a 10 ml saline "top-up" into the epidural space, which can significantly extend the level of a low sub-

Table 45.2 Common drugs used and their median effective local anaesthetic intrathecal doses for motor blockade in parturients

Drugs	ED50 (mg)	Confidence interval of ED50 (mg)
Ropivacaine	5.79	4.62–6.96
Levobupivacaine	4.83	4.35–5.32
Bupivacaine	3.44	2.55–4.34

Table 45.3 Standard intrathecal opioid doses for labour analgesia

	Fentanyl (mcg)	Sufentanil (mcg)
Dose Range	10–25	2.5–10
ED50	5.5	2.5
ED95	17.4	8.9

arachnoid block in a cephalad direction—a phenomenon known as epidural volume extension (EVE). This effect is thought to occur due to compression of the subarachnoid space, promoting the upward spread of the intrathecal drug. To achieve a noticeable increase in sensory block height, 5–10 ml of saline is typically required, with minimal effect seen at 5 ml. The extent of epidural volume extension is influenced by several factors, including the timing of saline injection, the injected volume, the baricity of the intrathecal solution (hyperbaric vs. hypobaric), patient positioning during or after spinal anaesthesia, and whether the procedure is performed in obstetric or non-obstetric settings.

Complications of the CSE Technique

1. Failure of spinal component-this is relatively common, especially with the needle-through-needle technique.
   - The spinal needle may be too short to extend sufficiently beyond the epidural tip or may only tent the dura without penetrating it.
   - Failure to enter the dura can occur when substantial resistance is encountered and inadequate force is applied.
   - Deviation from the midline may occur even after correct identification of the epidural space.
2. Failure of epidural component
   - Delayed placement of the epidural catheter may alter the level of the established block.
   - Rarely, the catheter may migrate through the dural puncture site into the subarachnoid space, leading to an unintended spinal block.
3. Failure of the needle component
   - A long, fine-gauge spinal needle may advance excessively through the dura if cerebrospinal fluid (CSF) reflux is delayed.
   - A long pencil-point spinal needle that is poorly anchored in the epidural needle or

tissue can move during injection, causing partial administration of the drug into the subarachnoid space.
4. Subarachnoid placement or migration of the epidural catheter: The likelihood of this complication depends on the size of the needle and the number of dural punctures.
5. Damage to the spinal needle or epidural catheter.
6. Subarachnoid spread of epidurally administered drugs.
7. Neurological injury: The incidence has been estimated at approximately 1.14 per 1,000 CSE cases in retrospective analyses.
8. Drug-related complications.
9. Post-dural puncture headache (PDPH): The reported incidence ranges from 0.8% to 2.5%, comparable to that of conventional epidural anaesthesia. Since lower doses of local anaesthetic are typically used in CSE, the overall incidence and severity of drug-related side effects are generally lower than with standard epidurals.
10. Maternal hypotension in obstetric patients: CSE may cause a rapid and profound sympathetic blockade, resulting in a sudden drop in blood pressure. Continuous maternal and fetal monitoring is essential, particularly in patients with compromised uteroplacental perfusion, non-reassuring fetal status, fixed cardiac output states (e.g., stenotic valves), or reduced intravascular volume (e.g., pregnancy-induced hypertension).

- Other potential complications are similar to those observed with standard spinal or epidural anaesthesia and include: Hypotension Needle-induced trauma Tissue coning Infection, including meningitis Cauda equina syndrome.

Contraindications in CSE

The contraindications are similar to those for spinal or epidural anaesthesia.

Absolute Contraindications
1. Patient refusal
2. Sepsis
3. Hypovolemia
4. Coagulopathy or therapeutic anticoagulation
5. Increased Intracranial pressure
6. Infection at the procedure site

Relative Contraindications
1. Current neurologic pathology
2. Severe psychiatric disease
3. Dementia
4. Aortic Stenosis
5. Left ventricular outflow tract obstruction
6. Alteration of the vertebral column secondary to prior surgery

Questions
1. What are the advantages of CSE over plain epidural vs dural puncture epidurals in obstetric patients?
2. Describe your technique for performing a CSE.
3. Choice and dose of local anaesthetics?
4. What are your thoughts on the test dose in CSE?
5. What would be your preferred positioning of patients for performing a CSE-sitting or lateral?
6. What is your opinion about epidural volume extension (EVE)?
7. A patient is breathless and uncomfortable 15 min after starting an epidural infusion in the CSE technique. What are your chief differentials?
8. Upon performing the loss of resistance to saline, disconnecting the syringe requires a continuous flow of large volume clear fluid through the Touhey. What would be your first step in management?
9. After the baby is delivered, the midwife is attempting to remove the epidural catheter, but feels there is resistance upon pulling it. What is your following line of management?
10. You have been called to attend to a break-through pain in a labouring patient after 1 h of epidural infusion on flow, 1 h after CSE. Upon giving a top-up to a patient, she feels lightheaded and has ringing in her ears. How do you manage further?.

Suggested Reading

1. NYSORA-regional-anesthesia-for-specific-surgical-procedures/abdomen/combined-spinal-epidural-anaesthesia/.
2. Ong K-B, Sashidharan R. Combined spinal–epidural techniques. Contin Educ Anaesth Crit Care Pain. 2007;7(2):38–41.
3. Hughes D, Simmons SW, Brown J, Cyna AM. Combined spinal-epidural versus epidural analgesia in labour. Cochrane Database Syst Rev. 2003;(4):Art. No: CD003401. https://doi.org/10.1002/14651858.CD003401.
4. Ekeoduru RA, Rahangdale R. Combined spinal epidural (CSE). 2019.

Superior Trunk Block

Franklin Wou

Level of Difficulty Difficult

Anatomy and Surface Anatomy

The superior trunk block (STB) was first described in 2014 as a refinement of the interscalene block. The superior trunk is formed by joining the ventral rami of the C5 and C6 nerve roots as they travel through the interscalene groove between the anterior and middle scalene muscles. The trunk bifurcates into the anterior and posterior divisions posterior to the clavicle to form the plexus cords.

Important Anatomical Structures

Subclavian Artery
Anterior and middle scalene muscles

Surface Landmark

Interscalene groove, subclavian artery pulsations

Indications

As per interscalene nerve block
Arthroscopic shoulder surgery

Contraindications
Relative

Unclear sonoanatomy
Severe pulmonary disease

Absolute

Patient refusal
Allergy to local anaesthetic

Advantages Over Other Techniques

The STB is performed distal to the interscalene block. This has the advantage of less spread of local anaesthetic to the phrenic nerve, leading to less hemidiaphragmatic paralysis and dyspnoea, but the rates are not zero. However, the degree of phrenic nerve involvement may be volume or injection site-dependent.

Under ultrasound imaging, the superior trunk is visible as a connective tissue sheath surrounds it. This may provide a degree of protection against needle injury compared to the nerve roots, as seen in the interscalene block, which has relatively little connective tissue.

Nerves Blocked

Superior trunk
Suprascapular nerve
Lateral pectoral nerve

Positioning

Supine, semi-recumbent, head turned to contralateral side of block

F. Wou (✉)
Queen Victoria Hospital NHS Foundation Trust,
East Grinstead, UK
e-mail: franklin.wou@nhs.net

© The Author(s), under exclusive license to Springer Nature Switzerland AG 2026
S. Phillips et al. (eds.), *Regional Anaesthesia*, https://doi.org/10.1007/978-3-032-05165-3_46

Anatomical Block Techniques

There have been no described landmark anatomical block approaches

Ultrasound Techniques

Scanning Protocol

Identification of the C5 and C6 nerve roots is performed as per the interscalene nerve block. Once seen in the interscalene groove, the roots are traced distally to where they coalesce to form the superior trunk (Fig. 46.1). It is important to identify the take-off of the suprascapular nerve from the lateral aspect of the superior trunk before it dives under the omohyoid muscle, as this is a key nerve in the innervation to the shoulder joint (Fig. 46.2).

No studies have examined the optimal injection point for local anaesthetic. Still, it is important to ensure adequate spread around the trunk to guarantee maximal success of the block.

Structures to Identify

Scalenus medius
Scalenus anterior
Suprascapular nerve
Middle trunk
Subclavian artery

The transverse cervical and dorsal scapular arteries can overlie the superior trunk
Omohyoid muscle

Block Performance

Position/Ergonomics: The patient is in the semi-recumbent position with their head turned to the contra-lateral side to the block side. The ultrasound machine is placed on the opposite side of the block to ensure needling is performed in line with the visualisation of the ultrasound (Fig. 46.3).

Probe: High frequency linear probe 8–14 mHz
Settings: Multi-beam resolution
Depth: 2–3 cm
Needle size: 22 g short bevel, 50 mm insulated stimulating needle

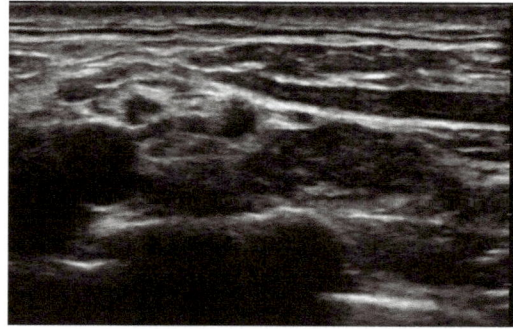

Fig. 46.2 Suprascapular nerve branching off from the superior trunk under the omohyoid muscle

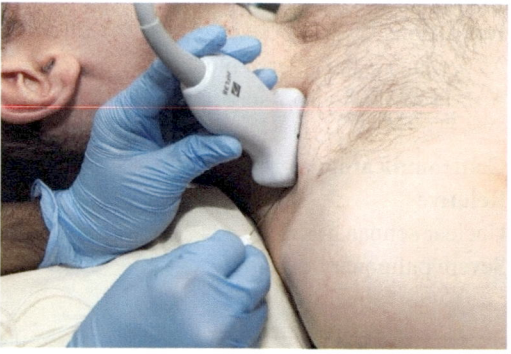

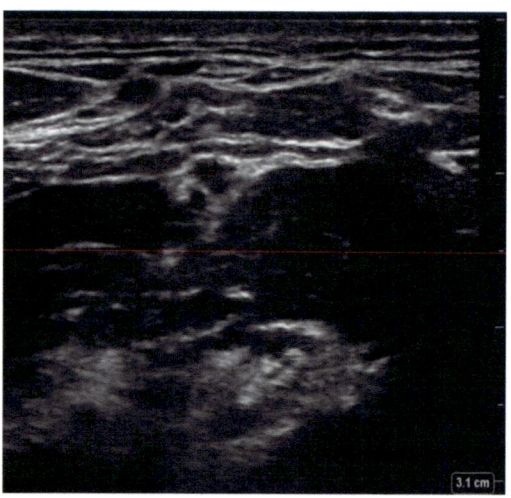

Fig. 46.1 Superior trunk sandwiched between anterior and middle scalene muscles

Fig. 46.3 Transverse in-plane, lateral to medial needling for STB

Needling Technique
In-plane, posterior lateral to anterior medial, passing under the deep cervical fascia and superficial to the scalenus medius muscle, aiming lateral to the superior trunk before the take-off of the suprascapular nerve.

Optimal Needle Tip Position
Close to the superior trunk to ensure adequate peri-truncal spread. The needle tip can be placed posterior/laterally and then moved anteriorly.

Drug Choice and Volume
Surgical anaesthesia: 10–15 ml 0.5% (levo)bupivacaine or 0.75% ropivacaine
Analgesia: 10–15 ml of 0.25% (levo)bupivacaine or 0.375% ropivacaine
Optimal current if nerve stimulation is used: 0.2–0.5 mA
   Muscle responses acceptable: Biceps/deltoid (C5/C6)

Testing Block Success
Inability to perform shoulder abduction
Inability to perform elbow flexion
Loss of sensation to cold over C5–C6 dermatomes

Clinical Pearls
Ensure that the suprascapular nerve is blocked before it branches off from the superior trunk. To identify this nerve, scan from proximal to distal until you see the nerve (hypoechoic) branch off the trunk's lateral side (Fig. 46.2). Aim to block proximal to the branching off of the nerve.

Side Effects
Phrenic nerve blockade
Hoarseness (recurrent laryngeal nerve blockade)

Complications Specific to the Block
- Infection.
- Bleeding/Hematoma.
- Puncture of vascular structure.
- Epidural or subarachnoid injection.
- Local anaesthetic toxicity.
- Permanent nerve injury.
- Total spinal anaesthesia.

- Horner syndrome
- Pneumothorax
- Diaphragm paresis and respiratory compromise
- Recurrent laryngeal nerve block

Continuous Regional Anaesthesia Techniques
Indications
As per the interscalene catheter insertion

Catheter
Multiorifice catheter

Regime
2 ml/h 0.125% (levo)bupivacaine +/− bolus 5 ml

Questions
1. Why choose a superior trunk block over an interscalene block?
2. What additional blocks are needed for shoulder cover when a low-volume superior trunk block is performed?
3. What is the incidence of diaphragm paresis after the superior trunk block?
4. What vascular structure could be seen crossing the superior trunk?

Suggested Reading

1. Amaral S, Arsky Lombardi R, Medeiros H, Nogueira A, Gadsden J. Superior trunk block is an effective phrenic-sparing alternative to interscalene block for shoulder arthroscopy: a systematic review and meta-analysis. Cureus. 2023;15(11):e48217. https://doi.org/10.7759/cureus.48217. PMID: 38050517; PMCID: PMC10693833.
2. Robles C, Berardone N, Orebaugh S. Effect of superior trunk block on diaphragm function and respiratory parameters after shoulder surgery. Reg Anesth Pain Med. 2022;47(3):167–70. https://doi.org/10.1136/rapm-2021-102962. Epub 2022 Jan 10.
3. Kim DH, Lin Y, Beathe JC, Liu J, Oxendine JA, Haskins SC, Ho MC, Wetmore DS, Allen AA, Wilson L, Garnett C, Memtsoudis SG. Superior trunk block: a phrenic-sparing alternative to the interscalene block: a randomized controlled trial. Anesthesiology. 2019;131(3):521–33. https://doi.org/10.1097/ALN.0000000000002841.
4. Sinha C, Kumari P, Kumar A, Kumar A, Kumar A, Bhar D, Arun SK, Vamshi C. Superior trunk versus

interscalene brachial plexus block in humerus surgery: a randomised controlled trial. Anaesthesiol Intensive Ther. 2024;56(3):194–8. https://doi.org/10.5114/ait.2024.142772. PMID: 39451166; PMCID: PMC11484482.

5. Lee MG, Shin YJ, You HS, Lim CH, Chang YJ, Shin HJ. A comparison of anesthetic quality between interscalene block and superior trunk block for arthroscopic shoulder surgery: a randomized controlled trial. Pain Physician. 2021;24(3):235–42.

6. Vijayakumar V, Ganesamoorthi A, Subramaniyan N, Kasirajan P. Ultrasound-guided superior and middle trunk brachial plexus block with superficial cervical plexus block for shoulder surgeries in high-risk patients: case series. J Med Ultrasound. 2020;28(3):185–7. https://doi.org/10.4103/JMU.JMU_73_19. PMID: 33282665; PMCID: PMC7709537.

Combined Axillary and Suprascapular Block

47

Roche John Alexis Martin, Ashokka Balakrishnan, Premi Cynthia, Jessie Paul, and Louise Frost

Level of Difficulty Expert

Anatomy and Surface Anatomy

Price first described the combined suprascapular and axillary nerve block ("The Shoulder Block") in 2007 as a technique for blocking the significant nerves supplying the shoulder joint.

The suprascapular nerve (SSN) supplies 60–70% of the sensation to the shoulder joint. It originates from C5 and C6 nerve roots and branches off the superior trunk before running deep to the omohyoid muscle in the supraclavicular region towards the posterior triangle of the neck. It then runs through the suprascapular notch under the superior transverse scapular ligament into the supraspinous fossa where it gives off branches to supraspinatous muscle. It travels obliquely and exits through the spinoglenoid notch into the infraspinous fossa, where it provides terminal branches to the infraspinatous muscle. After passing through the suprascapular notch, it divides into several branches.

It provides sensation to the posterior shoulder capsule, acromioclavicular joint, subacromial bursa, coracoclavicular ligament, and motor branches to the supraspinatus and infraspinatus muscles.

The axillary nerve arises from the C5 and C6 nerve roots, the terminal branch of the posterior cord of the brachial plexus. It provides 25–30% shoulder joint innervation. From its origin at the lateral border of the subscapularis, it winds around the surgical neck of the humerus beneath the shoulder joint. It passes through the quadrilateral space alongside the posterior humeral circumflex artery. The quadrilateral space is a small opening bordered by the teres minor above, the Teres Major below, the long head of the biceps medially, and the proximal humerus laterally (Fig. 47.1). After the nerve passes through this space, it branches into its anterior and posterior divisions

Suprascapular Nerve Approaches

Two approaches have been described: the posterior and anterior approaches.

The posterior approach targets the SSN close to the suprascapular notch or within the supraspinous fossa. The nerve course is related to bony landmarks, which provide identifiable structures for landmark and ultrasound techniques. The anterior approach aims to block the SSN immediately after branching from the superior trunk. This is a relatively new ultrasound-located peripheral nerve block. It courses laterally under the omohyoid muscle, where it can be targeted.

R. J. A. Martin
North Hampshire Hospital Trust, HHFT,
Basingstoke, UK

A. Balakrishnan · P. Cynthia · J. Paul
St. Michael's Hospital, Toronto, ON, Canada

L. Frost (✉)
Department of Anaesthesia, Waikato Hospital,
Hamilton, New Zealand
e-mail: louise.frost@doctors.net.uk

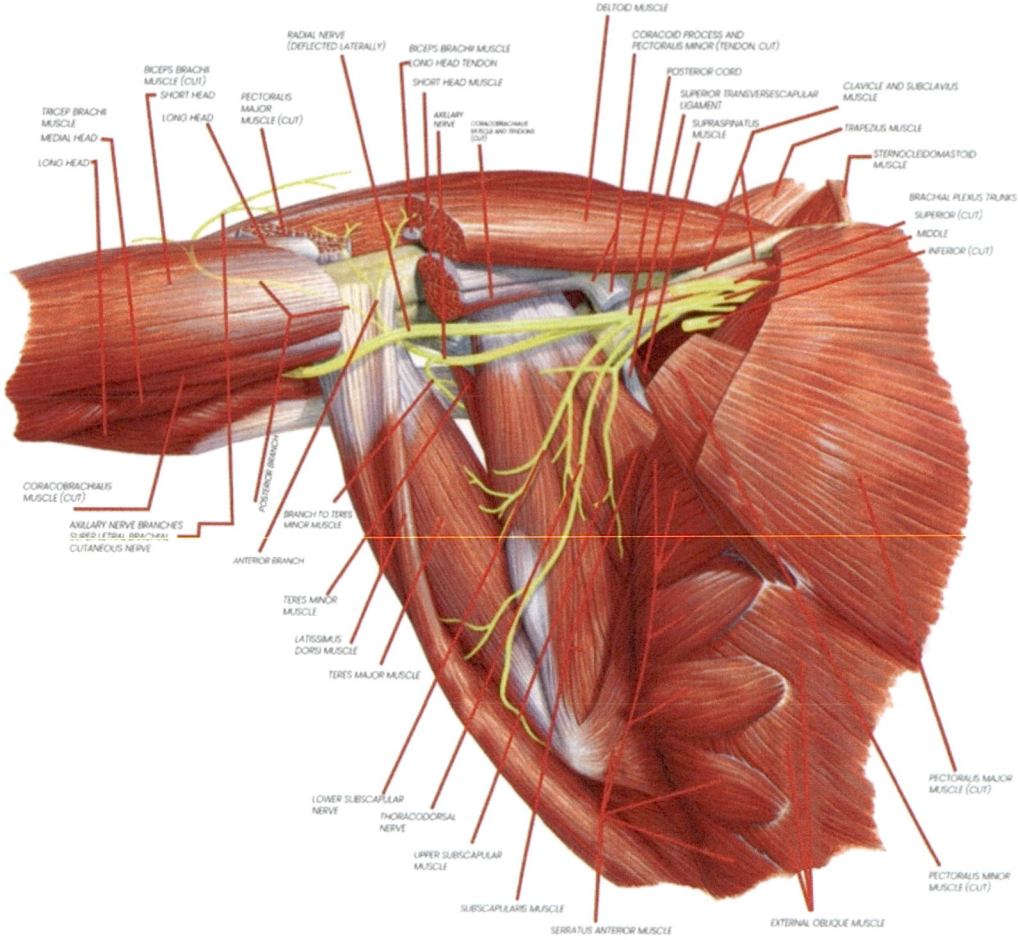

Fig. 47.1 Anatomy for axillary nerve block

Important Anatomical Structures
Axillary Nerve

The posterior humeral circumflex artery runs together with the axillary nerve. US Colour Doppler can be used to identify the structure before needling.

Suprascapular Nerve (posterior)

The suprascapular artery travels close to the suprascapular nerve (above the superior transverse scapular ligament) as it transversus through the notch. This can be identified using US color Doppler. Pleura can be damaged as the needle trajectory in some approaches is towards the thoracic cavity when targeting the suprascapular notch. This can be minimised by elevating the scapula from the posterior chest wall with the ipsilateral hand on the opposite shoulder. This manoeuvre will increase the distance of the skin from the chest wall.

Surface Landmark
Axillary Nerve

Acromion

Inferior angle of the scapula

Posterior humeral shaft

Suprascapular Nerve (posterior)

Acromion

Spine of the scapula

Indications

Shoulder block: Analgesia for shoulder operations (Minor)

Anterior suprascapular nerve block: Analgesia for shoulder operations (major and minor)

Contraindications

Axillary Nerve block

Relative

Coagulopathy

Absolute

Patient refusal

Allergy to local anaesthetic

Infection at the block site

Suprascapular Nerve block

Relative

Severe respiratory disease (anterior approach)

Absolute

Patient refusal

Allergy to local anaesthetic

Advantages Over Other Techniques

The main advantage of the shoulder block (combined axillary and suprascapular nerve) in shoulder surgery is that it does not lead to any diaphragmatic paralysis/phrenic nerve involvement due to the distal nature of the injections. It can provide surgical analgesia, albeit inferior to the interscalene block (ISB), for major shoulder surgery in the first 24 h. Caution must be made if surgical anesthesia is sought, as it does not block the other nerves innervating the shoulder (lateral pectoral nerve and subscapular nerve)

Studies comparing the anterior suprascapular nerve block to the ISB have demonstrated non-inferiority to the interscalene block for providing analgesia post-shoulder surgery, most likely due to its spread to the superior trunk. The study group used volumes of 10–15 ml. As the block is performed more distal and lateral to the ISB, there is a lower risk of phrenic nerve involvement, mainly if smaller volumes are used.

Nerve Blocked

Suprascapular nerve

Axillary Nerve

Landmark Techniques

Posterior Axillary Nerve

Price first described this technique as part of his 'Shoulder block'. The patient is seated with the arm in full adduction. Two planes are visualized to identify the passage of the nerve through the quadrilateral space.

1. Horizontal plane between the anterior aspect of the acromion and the inferior angle of the scapula. A horizontal line is drawn from the midpoint of this plane.
2. The vertical plane from the posterior-lateral aspect of the acromion down directly behind the humerus

A line is drawn midway from the horizontal plane, and the point at which this intersects with the vertical plane is the point of injection. The needle is inserted perpendicular at this point (100 mm), looking for the twitched posterior deltoid at a 6–8 cm depth. 10–15 ml of LA is injected

Suprascapular Landmark

Since Wetheim et al. first described SSN (posterior) approaches in 1941, several landmark approaches have been described in the literature.

Ideally, the nerve should be blocked proximally (in the suprascapular notch) to ensure the proximal acromial and subacromial branches are covered, but this is associated with a risk of pneumothorax.

The technique described by Meier al and adopted by Price blocks the nerve in the supraspinous fossa, minimizing the risk of pneumothorax. With the patient sitting and shoulder in full adduction, a line is drawn connecting the lateral part of the acromion with the medial end of the spine of the scapula. The needle insertion point is 2 cm medial and 2 cm cephalad to the midpoint of this line. The needle is directed with a 45° inclination in the corneal plane and 30° inclination in the ventral plane to a depth of 4–6 cm along the bony surface of the supraspinous groove. 15 ml of LA is injected after stimulation of the infraspinatus is noted.

An alternative approach described by Checcuci in their 'shoulder block' identified the needle entry point as 2 cm medial to the medial border of the acromion and 2 cm cranial to the superior margin of the scapular spine. The needle is inserted perpendicular to the skin in a cranial-caudal direction, again looking for stimulation of the supraspinatus and infraspinatus muscles. This is performed with the patient in the lateral decubitus position. 15 ml of LA is injected

Ultrasound Techniques
Axillary Nerve

A high-frequency linear probe, HFL, is placed 2 cm postero-lateral to the acromion, parallel to the long axis of the humerus. A view is obtained of the teres minor (oval shaped) lying immediately above the humeral shaft, the axillary nerve in the triangular shaped neurovascular bundle inferior (confirmed using Doppler US), the deltoid muscle overlying superficially, and the triceps muscle causally. The image can be optimised by moving the probe medially until the humeral shaft is lost, then back slightly laterally until the shaft reappears. An in-plane cephalad to caudal approach aims to inject below the deltoid.

LAX Axillary Nerve View

Price proposes an alternative approach using a short-axis view of the humerus, with the neurovascular bundle viewed longitudinally. In his opinion, this provides a more stable view as small probe movements using Rothes' approach will lead to loss of image. The end injection point is the same, below the posterior deltoid.

SAX Axillary Nerve View

For both techniques, 5–15 ml of LA is injected through an 80–100 mm needle, which is adequate to provide analgesia. Higher volumes may result in radial nerve blockage due to spread to the posterior cord.

Suprascapular Nerve

The suprascapular nerve can be anaesthetized using two approaches (anterior or posterior). The anterior approach may provide better analgesia compared to the posterior approach due to the take-off of the cutaneous and articular branches proximal to the superior transverse scapular ligament and spread towards the superior trunk.

Anterior Suprascapular Nerve

The nerve is found deep in the inferior belly of the omohyoid muscle and superficial to the prevertebral fascia in the supraclavicular region. Using an HFL probe, C5 and C6 nerve roots are identified in the interscalene groove. Following the nerves distally, they coalesce to form the superior trunk. The suprascapular nerve is recognized as a branch off the superior trunk and can be traced travelling below the omohyoid muscle (thin, hypoechoic appearance) away from the brachial plexus.

Posterior Suprascapular Nerve (Fig. 47.2)

A HFL probe is placed in the transverse orientation parallel to the spine of the scapula. The probe is then translated cranially to identify the supraspinous fossa. Layers seen on ultrasound are the trapezius, supraspinatus, and the bony outline of the supraspinous fossa.

The probe is moved laterally towards the acromion to locate the suprascapular notch, and the suprascapular nerve can be seen as a round, hyperechoic structure beneath the transverse scapular ligament. Note that the pleura is anterior to the suprascapular notch.

The nerve is seen in the supraspinous fossa by tilting the probe into the chest before transversing

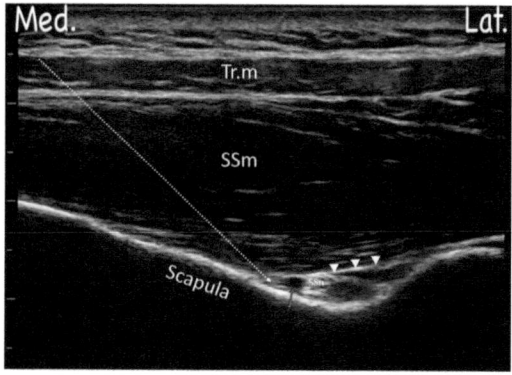

Fig. 47.2 Ultrasound-guided anatomy of the suprascapular nerve (posterior approach). This ultrasound image demonstrates the posterior approach to the suprascapular nerve (SSn) at the suprascapular notch, visualizing key structures such as the trapezius muscle (Tr.m), supraspinatus muscle (SSm), scapula, and adjacent fascial planes. The suprascapular nerve is identified as it courses near the scapular notch

the spinoglenoid notch. The nerve is always between the supraspinous fossa's floor and the supraspinatus muscle's deep fascia. Colour Doppler can identify the suprascapular artery that runs near the nerve and help determine the nerve.

Needling (100 mm) is performed in-plane onto the fossa floor when the nerve is between the suprascapular and spinoglenoid notch. 10–15 ml of local anaesthetic is injected to block the nerve.

Structures to Identify
Axillary Nerve
- Humeral shaft
- Teres minor muscle
- Deltoid muscle
- Posterior circumflex humeral artery

Suprascapular Nerve (Posterior)
- Trapezius
- Supraspinatus
- Supraspinous fossa
- Suprascapular artery

Suprascapular Nerve (Anterior)
- Subclavian artery
- Superior trunk/brachial plexus
- Omohyoid muscle
- The superficial cervical artery can sometimes be seen as superficial to the nerve.

Block Performance
Position/ergonomics: The block is performed with the patient sitting for the axillary and posterior suprascapular nerve. The ultrasound machine is placed inline in front of the patient.

For the anterior suprascapular nerve, the block is performed with the patient semi-recumbent with their head turned to the contralateral side.

The ultrasound machine is placed inline on the opposite side of the block.

Probe: High-frequency linear probe for both axillary and suprascapular nerve blocks.

Settings
Depth
Axillary Nerve 3–4 cm
Suprascapular nerve (posterior) 4–5 cm
Suprascapular nerve (anterior) 1–2 cm

Needle size: 22 g Short bevel, 50–100 mm insulated block needle

Needling Technique
Axillary Nerve—In-plane cranio-caudally
Suprascapular nerve (posterior)—In-plane medial to lateral. Imagining the needle may be difficult due to the steep insertion angle.
Suprascapular nerve (anterior)—In-plane lateral to medial

Optimal Needle Tip Position
Axillary Nerve—close to the axillary nerve, below the deltoid muscle, caudal to the fascia of the teres minor, and just cranial to the posterior circumflex humeral artery (Fig. 47.3).

Suprascapular nerve (posterior)—The needle tip is placed near the suprascapular nerve in the suprascapular notch under the transverse scapular ligament, initially described by Harmon and Hearty. There is a pneumothorax risk due to the pleura anterior proximity to this notch and its spread towards the brachial plexus. Instead, a safer approach is to block the nerve halfway between the suprascapular notch and the spinoglenoid notch, which can be achieved by tilting the probe posteriorly into the chest.

It is important to note that the neurovascular bundle is not always visible, so that the needle tip can be placed on the floor of the supraspinous fossa below the supraspinatus. The aim is to lift the supraspinatus off the floor of the fossa.

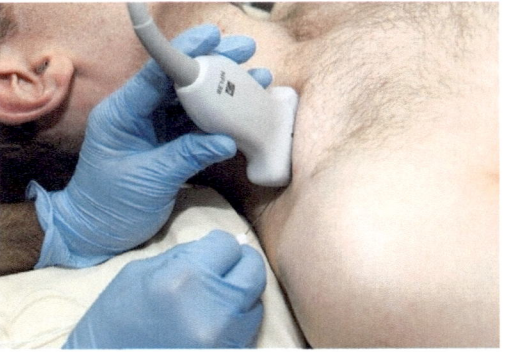

Fig. 47.3 Needle insertion for anterior suprascapular block

Suprascapular nerve (anterior)—The needle tip targets the suprascapular nerve under the omohyoid muscle.

Drug Choice

Axillary Nerve 5–15 ml of local anesthetic (high volumes may lead to radial nerve blockade)

Suprascapular nerve (posterior) 10–15 ml of local anesthetic

Suprascapular nerve (anterior) 10–15 ml of local anesthetic. Lower volumes may be used if adequate spread is seen.

Optimal current if nerve stimulation used: 0.5 mA

Muscle Responses Acceptable
Suprascapular Nerve

Contraction of the supraspinatus and infraspinatus

Axillary Nerve

Anterior Deltoid muscle contraction. The posterior deltoid may occur at 2–3 cm due to direct stimulation as the needle passes through.

Testing Block Success
Suprascapular Nerve

Sensory block to the scapula

Axillary Nerve

Sensory block to the deltoid.

Inability to abduct and externally rotate the shoulder

Side Effects

Axillary Nerve

Radial nerve blockade

Suprascapular nerve (posterior)

High volumes may spread toward the brachial plexus.

Complications Specific to the Block

- Axillary Nerve
- Nerve injury
- Intravascular injection (posterior humeral circumflex artery)
- Suprascapular nerve (posterior)
- Pneumothorax (1%)
- Intravascular injection (suprascapular artery and vein)
- Suprascapular nerve (anterior)
- Phrenic nerve blockade
- Brachial plexus (upper and middle trunk) blockade
- Proximity to the pleura and pneumothorax

Continuous Regional Anesthesia Techniques
Indications

Suprascapular (posterior) catheters have been described for severe posterior pain after major shoulder surgery.

Catheter

Multiorifice catheter; 6 ml/h low-dose local anesthetic

Suggested Reading

1. Price DJ. The shoulder block: a new alternative to interscalene brachial plexus blockade for the control of postoperative shoulder pain. Anaesth Intensive Care. 2007;35(4):575–81. https://doi.org/10.1177/0310057X0703500418. PMID: 18020078.
2. Chan VW, Perlas A, McCartney CJ, Brull R, Xu D, Abbas S. Ultrasound guidance improves success rate of axillary brachial plexus block. Can J Anaesth. 2007;54(3):176–82. https://doi.org/10.1007/BF03022637. Erratum in: Can J Anaesth. 2007 Jul;54(7):594. PMID: 17331928.

3. Brull R, Lupu M, Perlas A, Chan VW, McCartney CJ. Compared with dual nerve stimulation, ultrasound guidance shortens the time for infraclavicular block performance. Can J Anaesth. 2009;56(11):812–8. https://doi.org/10.1007/s12630-009-9170-2. PMID: 19728002.

4. Zhou Y, Zhao Y, Lin HH, Wang TL. Comparison of blockage effect of axillary brachial plexus block between ultrasound guidance alone and ultrasound guidance plus neurostimulation. Zhonghua Yi Xue Za Zhi. 2013;93(21):1649–52. Chinese. PMID: 24125675.

5. Vermeylen K, Engelen S, Sermeus L, Soetens F, Van de Velde M. Supraclavicular brachial plexus blocks: review and current practice. Acta Anaesthesiol Belg. 2012;63(1):15–21. PMID: 22783706.

6. Sehmbi H, Johnson M, Dhir S. Ultrasound-guided subomohyoid suprascapular nerve block and phrenic nerve involvement: a cadaveric dye study. Reg Anesth Pain Med. 2019;44(5):561–4. https://doi.org/10.1136/rapm-2018-100075. Epub 2019 Mar 13. PMID: 30867276.

7. Tran J, Peng PWH, Agur AMR. Anatomical study of the innervation of glenohumeral and acromioclavicular joint capsules: implications for image-guided intervention. Reg Anesth Pain Med. 2019:rapm-2018-100152. https://doi.org/10.1136/rapm-2018-100152. Epub ahead of print. PMID: 30635516.

8. Wiegel M, Moriggl B, Schwarzkopf P, Petroff D, Reske AW. Anterior suprascapular nerve block versus interscalene brachial plexus block for shoulder surgery in the outpatient setting: a randomized controlled patient- and assessor-blinded trial. Reg Anesth Pain Med. 2017;42(3):310–8. https://doi.org/10.1097/AAP.0000000000000573. PMID: 28257388.

9. Checcucci G, Allegra A, Bigazzi P, Gianesello L, Ceruso M, Gritti G. A new technique for regional anesthesia for arthroscopic shoulder surgery based on a suprascapular nerve block and an axillary nerve block: an evaluation of the first results. Arthroscopy. 2008;24(6):689–96. https://doi.org/10.1016/j.arthro.2008.01.019. Epub 2008 Mar 21. PMID: 18514113.

Infraclavicular Block

Anju Gupta and Louise Frost

Level of Difficulty Intermediate

Anatomy & Surface Anatomy

The cords of the brachial plexus emerge from under the clavicle, where they lie deep to the pectoral muscles and lateral about the axillary artery. As the artery descends laterally towards the axilla, the cords rotate around the artery into their respective lateral, medial, and posterior positions. Considerable anatomical variation exists in their position relative to the artery.

The anatomical arrangement of the three cords at the paracoracoid level is as follows:

Lateral Cord
Typically found at a 7–9 o'clock position. Gives rise to:
Musculocutaneous nerve
Part of the **median** nerve
Lateral Pectoral nerve

Posterior Cord
Often at a 6 o'clock" position. Gives rise to:
Axillary nerve

A. Gupta
Anesthesiology Pain and Critical Care, All India Institute of Medical Sciences, New Delhi, India

L. Frost (✉)
Department of Anaesthesia, Waikato Hospital, Hamilton, New Zealand
e-mail: louise.frost@doctors.net.uk

Radial nerve
Upper and lower subscapular nerves
Thoracodorsal nerve

Medial Cord
Located at approximately 3 o'clock. Gives rise to:
Ulnar nerve
Part of the **median** nerve
Medial pectoral nerve
Medial brachial cutaneous nerve
Medial antebrachial cutaneous nerve

Important Anatomical Structures

Surface Landmarks
Clavicle, pectoralis muscles, and deltopectoral groove.

Indications
Anaesthesia and analgesia for arm, elbow, forearm, and hand surgery.

Contraindications

Absolute
Patient refusal

Relative
Coagulopathy, as the plexus is less compressible at this point.

Severe respiratory disease, as there is a small-risk phrenic nerve blockade or pneumothorax, may worsen respiratory function.

The subcoracoid infraclavicular view may be more challenging in patients with a thick chest wall.

Advantages Over Other Techniques

- Infraclavicular blocks do not necessitate arm abduction, so this is an option where this is not possible. However, arm abduction may improve the ultrasonographic appearance of the plexus by moving it superficially.
- It provides reliable coverage of the radial nerve, the most challenging nerve to visualise when performing an axillary brachial plexus block.
- The infraclavicular approach can be helpful when siting a nerve catheter, as the comparatively deep site may be less prone to movement and accidental dislodgement.
- There is a lower risk of phrenic nerve blockade than supraclavicular block, though it is still possible with high volumes.
- Spread of local anaesthetic may block the intercostobrachial nerve (T2, occasionally T1), resulting in less tourniquet discomfort.

Nerves Blocked

Brachial plexus at the level of the cords.

Technique

Ultrasound Techniques

The plexus can be viewed using costoclavicular (medial) or subcoracoid (lateral) approaches. (Fig. 48.1).

Structures to Identify

Pectoralis Major.
Pectoralis Minor (sub-coracoid).
Subclavius (costoclavicular).
Axillary Artery.
Axillary vein.
Brachial plexus.

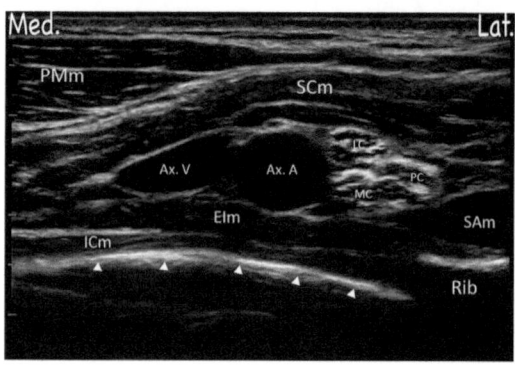

Fig. 48.1 USG image of an Costoclavicular approach to Infraclavicular brachial plexus block. Pectoralis major muscle (PMm), Subclavius muscle (SCm), Axillary artery (Ax.A), Axillary Vein (Ax.V), Lateral cord (LC), Posterior cord (PC), Medial cord (MC), Serratus anterior muscle (SAm), External intercostal muscle (EIm), Internal intercostal muscle (ICm). Arrowheads- Pleura

Serratus anterior (sub-coracoid).
Pleura.

Scanning Protocol

Costoclavicular block

Place the probe underneath and parallel to the midpoint of the clavicle. Identify the overlying pectoralis major and subclavius muscles and the axillary artery with the axillary vein lying medial to it. The cords and divisions are found lateral to the artery, with a "bunch of grapes" appearing on ultrasound, reminiscent of the supraclavicular view of the plexus. Note the pleura's position, which lies close to the plexus, and can be confirmed with the "sliding lung sign." The cords can be traced laterally to view them in their medial, lateral, and posterior positions (Fig. 48.1).

Subcoracoid block

For the subcoracoid view, place the transducer in a parasagittal plane in the deltopectoral groove, medial to the coracoid process. Scan laterally in the parasagittal plane until the vessels come into view. Identify the overlying pectoral major and minor muscles and the axillary artery, with the vein lying caudad to the artery. The chest wall and pleura may be visible deep in the artery. Continue to trace the artery laterally; you may note the appearance

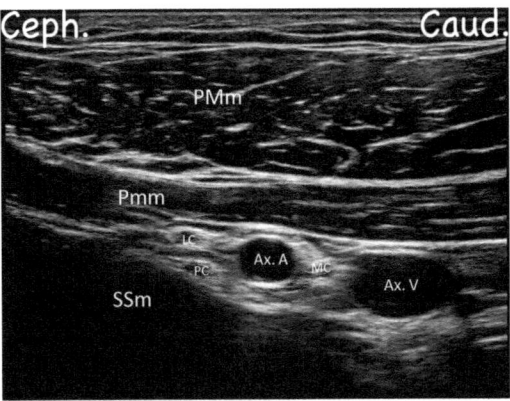

Fig. 48.2 USG image of the Subcoracoid Infraclavicular brachial plexus block. The Axillary artery (AA) is visualised with surrounding brachial plexus cords- lateral (LC), medial (MC), posterior (PC), deep to the pectoralis major (PMm) and pectoralis minor muscle (Pmm). Axillary vein (Ax.V), Subscapularis muscle (SSm)

of the serratus anterior between the vessels and the chest wall. More laterally, the subscapularis muscle lies deep in the vessels. Inserting the block needle with the probe positioned lateral to the pleura is optimal to maximise safety.

It can be challenging to note the exact positioning of the cords in this view. The lateral cord is cephalad, at about 7–9 "o'clock" relative to the artery. The medial cord is usually found at around 3 o'clock and may be difficult to identify, whilst the posterior cord lies at six o'clock, and is often the most challenging to approach, note the cords have attained their final positions in relation to the artery and vein (Fig. 48.2).

Block Performance

Position/Ergonomics

The patient should be positioned supine with their head turned away from the side of the block. A pillow behind the head and opposite shoulder may optimise conditions. The ipsilateral arm can be positioned at the patient's side. However, abducting the arm to 90 degrees can improve the ultrasound view by raising the clavicle and bringing plexus to a more superficial position.

Probe
Linear transducer 8–14 mHz
Consider a curvilinear probe if the artery depth is >5 cm.

Settings
Multibeam resolution

Depth
1–3 cm- costoclavicular.
3–5 cm- subcoracoid.

Needle Size
22 g short bevel insulated, 50 mm needle-costoclavicular.
22 g 80 mm or 100 mm short bevel, insulated-sub coracoid.

Needling Technique
Costoclavicular
Needling lateral to medial, just below the clavicle, advance the needle in-plane to enter the plexus (Fig. 48.3a). Inject 1–2 mls and observe spread. Once a satisfactory spread is observed within the sheath, inject 15–20 mls, aspirating regularly. The needle may need repositioning to ensure that the spread is visualised throughout the whole sheath. Up to 30mls may be used.
Sub-coracoid
The injection technique here has been described as a two-compartment technique. The first compartment contains the lateral cord; the second includes both the posterior and medial cords. Note in particular the location of the lateral cord. Needling cephalad-caudad, insert the needle just below the clavicle (Fig. 48.3b), aiming to enter the lateral compartment by passing close to the cord on an overall trajectory towards a 6 "o'clock" position in relation to the artery. A "pop" may be felt upon entering the compartment. Deposit 0.5–2 ml here to confirm the position and move the lateral cord out of the needle's path. Advance the needle towards 6 "o clock" aiming to "pop" into the second compartment. Position in the second compartment can be confirmed by visualising the artery moving slightly upwards and the local anaesthetic pushing down and around the artery. The posterior cord may also be witnessed

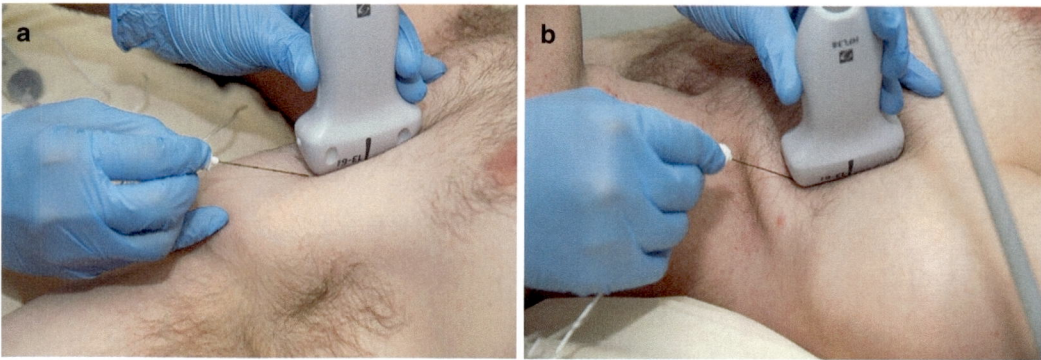

Fig. 48.3 Ergonomics, probe position and needling direction for (**a**) Costoclavicular approach (**b**) Subcoracoid infraclavicular approach

to move downwards with the flow of local anaesthetic ("double bubble sign.") Around 20 mls of local anaesthetic should be injected here. Next, slightly withdraw the needle to inject 5–10 mls in the lateral compartment. The anaesthetic should now form a U shape around the artery. If there is concern that the medial cord is not covered, consider withdrawing the needle and repositioning the tip above the artery at a 1 o'clock position, with a further injection of approximately 5mls at this point.

Nerve Stimulator Technique

Vertical Infraclavicular Block
Position: Supine, Head turned to the contralateral side. Forearm positioned on abdomen or chest.

Landmarks
The midpoint of a line from the middle of the jugular notch and the ventral process of the acromion is just below the clavicle. For reference, note the position of the subclavian artery above the clavicle- the plexus must be lateral to this point after the artery passes under the clavicle.

Direction Absolute vertical. NO MEDIAL ANGULATION. Inject once the distal stimulus is achieved at 0.5 mA or less. Do not insert more than 6 cm. If there is no response, redirect caudad or cephalad only.

Increased risk of pneumothorax if:
Needle insertion depth > 6 cm
Medial insertion point
The medial direction of the needle

Subcoracoid Technique
With the patient in the supine position, mark a needle insertion point 2 cm caudad and 1–2 cm medial to the coracoid process.

Direction-absolute vertical, depth 3–8 cm.

NO MEDIAL ANGULATION, cephalad-caudad only if redirection is required.

Drug Choice
20–40 ml local anaesthetic.
Optimal current if nerve stimulation is used
  ≤ 0.5 mA.
Muscle responses acceptable
  Wrist/finger extension (posterior cord)

Unacceptable Muscle Responses
- Pectoral muscle twitch, needle too superficial.
- Posterior scapular movements, needle too deep
- Elbow flexion (lateral cord), needle to cephalad or superficial.

- Wrist flexion and thumb adduction (medial cord) are acceptable if surgery is performed in the ulnar distribution.
- No twitch; the needle may be too lateral; careful re-evaluation is required

Testing Block Success
Inability to flex the elbow (musculocutaneous)
Failure to extend the elbow and wrist (radial)
Inability to flex wrist and fingers (median)
Failure to oppose the thumb and little finger (ulnar)

Side Effects & Complications Specific to the Block
Pneumothorax
Haemothorax
Very rare phrenic nerve block

Continuous Regional Anaesthesia Techniques

The same needling technique may be used when inserting a catheter. Once the correct position is confirmed at 6 o'clock, advance the catheter 2–4 cm into the space and secure it.

Indication
For extended analgesia following complex/elbow, forearm or hand surgery.

Catheter
Multi-orifice catheter.

Regime
5 mls/h 0.125% bupivacaine

+/– bolus's of 8mls

Questions
1. What are the anatomical positions of the three brachial plexus cords in relation of axillary artery in the costoclavicular and lateral infraclavicular approaches?
2. What are the nerves which branch off from the cords at infraclavicular level?
3. What are the two compartments which separate the cords in the infraclavicular approach and what precautions are needed to cover all the three cords during injection?
4. What is the advantage of infraclacular approach over supraclavicular and axillary blocks?

Suggested Reading

1. Ellis L. Anatomy for anaesthetists. 9th ed. Wiley Blackwell publishing; 2014.
2. Hazdic A. Hazdic's textbook of regional anaesthesia and pain management. 2nd ed. McGraw-Hill Education; 2017.
3. Hu Z, Hu J, Ai Z, Xu S, Li H, Guo R, Wang Y. Effect of ultrasound-guided extra-prevertebral fascial suprascapular nerve and infraclavicular brachial plexus block on postoperative analgesia and phrenic nerve function in shoulder arthroscopy: a pilot study. J Pain Res. 2024;17:4453–62. https://doi.org/10.2147/JPR.S487562. PMID: 39720322; PMCID: PMC11668314.
4. Zhang G, Hou X, Wang H, Han C, Fan D. Infraclavicular versus supraclavicular nerve block for upper limb surgeries: a meta-analysis. Medicine (Baltimore). 2024;103(43):e40152. https://doi.org/10.1097/MD.0000000000040152. PMID: 39470519; PMCID: PMC11521057.
5. Nicholls B, Conn D, Roberts A. The Abbott pocket guide to practical peripheral nerve blockade. Abott Laboratories Ltd.; 2003.

Supraclavicular Block

49

Anju Gupta and Louise Frost

Level of Difficulty Intermediate

Anatomy & Surface Anatomy

Important Anatomical Structures
The brachial plexus trunks descend and move laterally down the neck between the anterior and middle scalene muscles. They are contained in a sheath which posteriorly extends from the posterior tubercles and covers the anterior of the middle scalene muscle. The anterior section of the sheath originates from the anterior tubercle and covers the posterior of the anterior scalene muscle. The plexus descends and moves laterally within this sheath and crosses the base of the posterior triangle of the neck, passing over the first rib and beneath the clavicle. At the level of the clavicle, the three trunks are divided into anterior and posterior divisions.

Surface Landmarks
Interscalene groove, lateral border of sternocleidomastoid, supraclavicular fossa, subclavian artery.

A. Gupta
Anesthesiology Pain and Critical Care, All India Institute of Medical Sciences, New Delhi, India

L. Frost (✉)
Department of Anaesthesia, Waikato Hospital, Hamilton, New Zealand
e-mail: louise.frost@doctors.net.uk

Indications
Anaesthesia & analgesia for elbow, hand and forearm surgery.

If the suprascapular nerve (C5) is still contained in the sheath at this level, the block is suitable for shoulder surgery.

Contraindications

Absolute.
Patient refusal
Contralateral phrenic nerve palsy
Contralateral recurrent laryngeal nerve palsy
Relative.
Severe respiratory disease (phrenic nerve palsy may worsen respiratory function)

Advantages Over Other Techniques

Faster onset of block than infraclavicular or axillary approaches to the brachial plexus. Supraclavicular blocks do not necessitate arm abduction, so it is a valuable option where this is not possible. It gives reliable coverage of the radial nerve, which can be the most difficult to visualise when performing an axillary brachial plexus block.

Nerves Blocked
Brachial plexus at the level of trunks/divisions.

Technique

Ultrasound Techniques

Structures to Identify
Subclavian Artery
Subclavian vein
Brachial plexus
First rib
Pleura

Scanning Protocol

Place the probe transversely in the supraclavicular fossa at the midpoint of the clavicle. Identify the subclavian artery at the supraclavicular fossa. The trunks and divisions of the brachial plexus can typically be found posteriorly and extending superiorly over the artery (a bunch of grapes appearance). The most visible superficial and lateral branches originate from the superior roots (C5-C7), whilst the deeper and more medial ones come from the inferior plexus roots (C8-T1). The probe should be moved medially, laterally, and rotated in a coronal oblique position to obtain a clear picture of the artery and plexus. Tilting the probe caudally may improve the view of the first rib and pleura. An optimal image should include as much of the first rib as possible to protect against pneumothorax. The suprascapular nerve (C5) arises from the superior trunk and leaves the plexus around this level. It may be visible as a flat, oval structure passing laterally and inferiorly to the brachial plexus beneath the omohyoid muscle. Colour doppler should be used to identify vessels crossing the plexus, such as the dorsal scapular artery. The transverse cervical and suprascapular arteries may also be visualised at this level (Fig. 49.1).

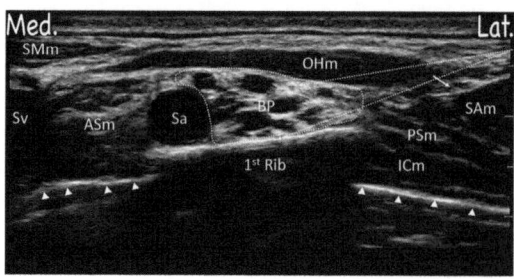

Fig. 49.1 Ultrasound Anatomy for Supraclavicular Brachial Plexus Block. This ultrasound image highlights the anatomy relevant to a supraclavicular brachial plexus block. Key structures include the brachial plexus trunks/divisions (BP), anterior scalene (ASm), Subclavian artery (Sa), Sternocleidomastoid muscle (SMm), Omohyoid muscle (Ohm), Subclavian vein (Sv), Serratus Anterior muscle (SAm), Posterior scalene muscle (PSm), Intercostal muscle (ICm), first rib is an important landmark. Arrow- Supraclavicular nerve branched off from the upper trunk and lies under omohyoid, arrowheads- Pleura

Block Performance

Position/Ergonomics

The patient should be positioned supine or semi-supine with their head turned away from the side of the block (Fig. 49.2). A pillow behind the head and opposite shoulder may optimise conditions. The operator is behind and lateral to the patient, needling in a straight line away from themselves. If using USS, the machine is best placed on the contralateral side for optimal ergonomics.

Probe
Linear transducer 8–14 mHz

Settings
Multibeam resolution

Depth
1–3 cm

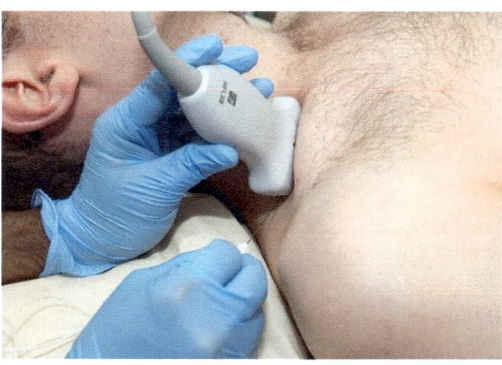

Fig. 49.2 Patient position for Supraclavicular Brachial Plexus Block

Needle Size
22 g short bevel, 50 mm short bevel insulated stimulating needle

Needling Technique

In the plane, needling posterior lateral to anterior medial. Meticulous care must be taken to visualise the needle tip at all times due to the proximity to the pleura and vascular structures at this level.

Optimal Needle Tip Position

Due to the compact nature of the anatomy at this level, once within the sheath (a palpable "pop" may be felt on entering), local ana esthetic spread can be seen throughout the plexus with increasing volume. Septa separate the individual trunks. As described below, multiple injection sites may improve the block's success rate and onset speed, though they may increase the risk of nerve injury. As the divisions move apart with hydro-dissection, the needle can be carefully advanced close to the artery at a 5 o'clock position, also known as the "corner pocket." Generous local anaesthetic volume here (approximately 10–15 ml) may aid adequate coverage of the lower plexus levels, reducing the risk of sparing the ulnar border. Withdrawing the needle almost out of the sheath, then carefully advancing with hydrodissection to inject between the superior and middle trunks at an approximately 1 o'clock position will help

ensure coverage of the plexus's upper divisions. Further infiltration at 3 "may be considered should local anaesthetic spread not be visualised in this area.

Drug Choice

Surgical anaesthesia: 20mls of 1% lignocaine with adrenaline, 0.25–0.5% bupivacaine or 0.375% ropivacaine. Higher volumes, up to 30mls, are described, though this may be associated with an increased rate of phrenic nerve palsy.

Subclavian Perivascular Block (Nerve Stimulator Technique)

The patient is supine or semi-supine, with the head turned to the opposite side, the elbow flexed, and the forearm resting on the lap. They should be encouraged to lower the ipsilateral shoulder.

Palpate the interscalene groove and trace to a point above the clavicle where the skin flattens over the supraclavicular fossa. The subclavian artery is palpable in 50% of patients at this point. The needle is inserted in the posterior part of the groove, posterior to the artery. Directly parallel to the floor (or bed position if semi-supine), caudad. NO MEDIAL ANGULATION due to the risk of pneumothorax.

Alternatively, palpate the lateral insertion of the sternocleidomastoid at the level of the clavicle. Move 2.5 cm laterally along the clavicle to avoid the pleural dome. The needle insertion point is 1.5 cm (approximately one finger breadth) cephalad of this point. Insert the needle through the skin, then advance in a caudal direction, parallel to the midline—NO MEDIAL ANGULATION.

Do not insert more than a 2.5 cm needle if no muscle twitches are noted.

Optimal Current if Nerve Stimulation Is Used
0.9mA or less (injections at higher currents than 0.5mA are only recommended for supraclavicular and lumbar plexus blocks.)

Muscle Responses Acceptable

A motor response to nerve stimulation is unnecessary if a good local anaesthetic spread is visualised on ultrasound in a combined technique.

If using the nerve stimulator only technique:
Wrist extension/flexion
Finger extension/flexion
These imply the needle's proximity to the lower trunks of the plexus, decreasing the likelihood of sparing the ulnar border.

- No twitch- redirect anterior/posteriorly.
- Arterial puncture- redirect posteriorly
- Bone contact (first rib), "walk" needle antero-posteriorly along the rib.

Testing Block Success

Inability to flex the elbow (musculocutaneous)
Failure to extend the elbow and wrist (radial)
Inability to flex wrist and fingers (median)
Failure to oppose the thumb and little finger (ulnar)

Side Effects

The following are possible if there is sufficient cephalad spread of the local anaesthetic within the sheath:

- Horner's Syndrome (ipsilateral ptosis, miosis, and enopthalmia)
- Phrenic nerve blockade
- Recurrent laryngeal nerve blockade

Complications Specific to the Block

Subclavian arterial puncture
Pneumothorax

Continuous Regional Anaesthesia Techniques

Typically, needling in-plane lateral to medial with a similar technique to a single-shot injection. The needle tip is aimed to enter the posterior surface of the sheath, followed by catheter placement.

Indication

Analgesia post elbow, forearm, or hand surgery.

Catheter

Multi-orifice catheter

Regime

5–8 mls/h 0.125% bupivacaine
+/− bolus's of 3–5 mls, reduce continuous infusion to 5 ml/hour for a PCRA regimen

Questions

1. What components of the brachial plexus lie in the supraclavicular area?
2. What is the incidence of pneumothorax with supraclavicular brachial plexus block?
3. What precautions should be undertaken to minimise complications with a supraclavicular block?
4. What is the advantage of a supraclavicular block over an interscalene block for upper limb surgeries?
5. Which trunk is most frequently spared with this approach?
6. What is the selective truncal approach?

Suggested Reading

1. Ellis L. Anatomy for anaesthetists. 9th ed. Wiley Blackwell publishing; 2014.
2. Hazdic A. Hazdic's textbook of regional anaesthesia and pain management. 2nd ed. McGraw-Hill Education; 2017.
3. Bao X, Huang J, Wang X, et al. Effect of local anesthetic volume (20 mL vs 30 mL ropivacaine) on electromyography of the diaphragm and pulmonary function after ultrasound-guided supraclavicular brachial plexus block: a randomized controlled trial. Reg Anesth Pain Med. 2019;44(1)
4. Nicholls B, Conn D, Roberts A. The Abbott pocket guide to practical peripheral nerve blockade. Abott Laboratories Ltd.; 2003.

Lumbar Plexus Block

50

Arunangshu Chakraborty and Amit Dixit

Lumbar plexus block is a proximal approach for providing unilateral anaesthesia or analgesia for hip, thigh, knee, and foot surgeries. It can also be used to manage pain associated with conditions such as chronic pelvic pain, postoperative pain, and chronic regional pain syndrome.

Level of difficulty Advanced

Anatomy

The lumbar plexus is formed by the ventral rami of L1–L4 spinal nerves, along with a contribution from the ventral ramus of the T12 spinal nerve. It is located within the psoas major muscle. The psoas major muscle comprises two portions: an anterior portion that arises from the anterolateral surface of the intervertebral discs and vertebral bodies and a posterior portion that originates from the anterior aspect of the transverse processes. These two portions of the psoas are separated by a fascia, creating, in effect, a "compartment" between them. The lumbar plexus lies in this compartment alongside the lumbar ascending vein and branches of the lum-

bar artery. This plane communicates medially to the lumbar paravertebral space. The component ventral rami of the lumbar plexus exit the neural canal through their respective intervertebral foramen, turn in a steep caudal direction across the lumbar paravertebral space, and enter the psoas muscle one vertebral level below. After forming within the psoas muscle, the branches of the lumbar plexus diverge in separate courses and exit the body of the psoas muscle independently of each other (Fig. 50.1).

The branches of the lumbar plexus include:

1. The **femoral nerve**, the largest terminal branch of the lumbar plexus, emerges from the lower part of the psoas major and iliacus muscles. It then runs deep to the iliacus fascia and provides motor supply to the quadriceps muscle and sensory supply to the anterior thigh and medial lower leg. The nerve first innervates the pectineus muscle before passing under the inguinal ligament and lying lateral to the femoral artery to enter the thigh.

2. The **obturator nerve** descends medially through the psoas major muscle and enters the thigh through the obturator foramen. It divides into anterior and posterior branches and provides motor supply to the obturator externus and adductor muscles, with variable sensory innervation to the hip and knee joints. Adductor muscle weakness is the most reliable sign of obturator nerve block. An acces-

A. Chakraborty (✉)
Sultan Qaboos Comprehensive Cancer Care and
Research Centre, Muscat, Oman

A. Dixit
Department of Anaesthesia, Ruby Hall Hospital,
Pune, India

Fig. 50.1 Lumbar plexus

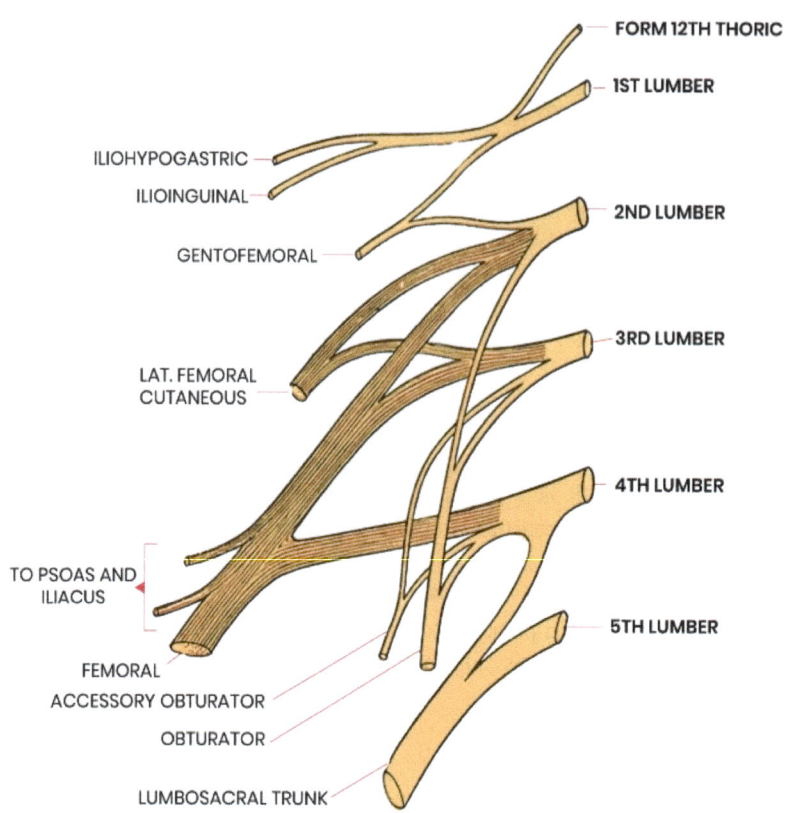

ILIOHYPOGASTRIC

ILIOINGUINAL

GENTOFEMORAL

LAT. FEMORAL
CUTANEOUS

TO PSOAS AND
ILIACUS

FEMORAL

ACCESSORY OBTURATOR

OBTURATOR

LUMBOSACRAL TRUNK

FORM 12TH THORIC

1ST LUMBER

2ND LUMBER

3RD LUMBER

4TH LUMBER

5TH LUMBER

sory obturator nerve is present in about 20–30% of individuals.

3. The **lateral cutaneous nerve of the thigh** arises from the lateral part of the psoas muscle and supplies sensory innervation to the anterior and lateral aspects of the thigh. It passes under the inguinal ligament medial to the anterior superior iliac spines.

4. The **iliohypogastric nerve** divides into anterior and lateral cutaneous branches above the iliac crest. The anterior cutaneous branch provides sensory innervation to the skin over the anterior aspect of the abdomen above the pubis, while the lateral branch supplies the skin over the posterolateral aspect of the gluteal region.

5. The **ilioinguinal nerve** emerges at the lateral border of the psoas muscle and provides sensory innervation to the superomedial thigh and genital region.

6. The **genitofemoral nerve** divides into genital and femoral branches. The genital branch supplies the skin of the scrotum in men and the skin of the mons pubis and labium majus in women, while the femoral branch supplies sensory innervation to the skin over the upper part of the femoral triangle.

Surface Anatomy

L2–L4 Spinous processes, intercristal line, posterior superior iliac spine

Indications

1. Surgical anaesthesia of the lower limb, when performed in combination with a sciatic block, is used in high-risk patients who may not tolerate hemodynamic changes experienced with the central neuraxial blockade.

2. Analgesia following injuries or surgeries of the hip or thigh

3. Chronic pain conditions like Herpes zoster and complex regional pain syndrome.

Contraindications

- Patient refusal
- Allergy to local anaesthetics
- Infection at the site of injection
- As this is a deep block, nearby Systemic anti-coagulation (INR >1.5 or inadequate time since cessation of anticoagulant)

Relative contraindications or where one might consider an alternative technique:

- Presence of intrathecal pump or spinal cord stimulator
- Major lumbar spine deformity
- Prior major spine surgery, implanted hardware, fusion, Pre-existing neurologic deficit

Nerves blocked

Genitofemoral nerve, lateral femoral cutaneous nerve, femoral nerve, obturator nerve, accessory obturator nerve.

Positioning for Block performance

Patients are positioned in lateral decubitus with the side to be blocked facing upward and the ipsilateral knee flexed and hip flexed at 90° and 30°, respectively.

Block Performance

Landmark—Peripheral Nerve Stimulation Technique

Winnie's approach

Using surface landmarks, two lines are drawn on the skin perpendicular to each other—a transverse line at L4/L5 and a vertical line parallel to the spine through the Posterior Superior Iliac Spine (PSIS). The needle is inserted at the intersection of these lines with a slight medial inclination. The needle should be between the transverse processes of L4 and L5. The needle can be redirected caudally if the transverse process of L5 is encountered. Winnie used paresthesia as his end point, but today, the accepted endpoint for the lumbar plexus is stimulation of the femoral nerve

component, observed by contraction of the quadriceps muscle.

Chayen approach

The L4 spinous process is identified (from the intercristal line). Needle insertion is 3 cm caudad and 5 cm lateral. This should elicit contact with the L5 Transverse process; the needle is then re-angled slightly cranially to pass between the L4 and L5 Transverse Processes, advancing 1–2 cm beyond the transverse process. The endpoint is twitching/contraction of the ipsilateral quadriceps.

Dekrey's approach

This more proximal technique described an approach from the L3 vertebrae. The puncture site is 3–4 cm lateral to the spinous process of L3, with the needle directed slightly cephalad to contact the transverse process of L3. The needle is then redirected caudally and advanced approximately 1.5 cm further until the lumbar plexus is reached, seeking quadriceps contraction.

Capdevila's approach

The spinous process of L4 is identified, and a line is drawn horizontally through the centre of the L4 spinous process to intersect with a vertical line that passes through the posterior superior iliac spine parallel to the vertebral column on the side to be blocked. The puncture point is at the junction of the lateral one-third and medial two-thirds of the line joining L4 to the line passing through the PSIS. The needle is advanced at right angles to the skin until the transverse process of L4 is encountered. The needle is then directed caudally for about 2 cm.

Ultrasound-Guided Approaches to Lumbar Plexus Block

Paramedian sagittal approach

The patient is positioned in the same way as described for the landmark technique. The ultrasound probe is placed in a paramedian sagittal plane at the level of L3 and L4 on the side to be blocked. The optimal ultrasound image shows

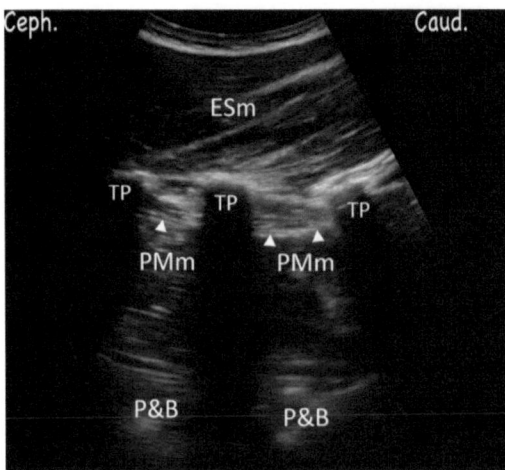

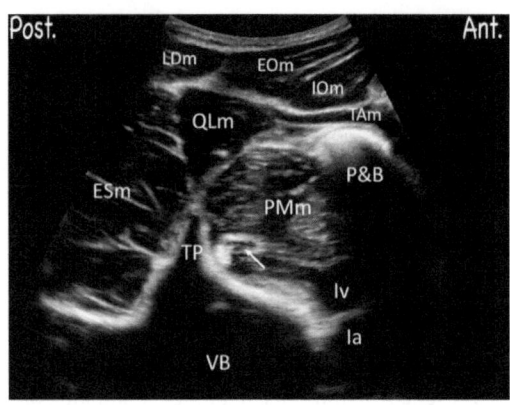

Fig. 50.2 Ultrasound anatomy for lumbar plexus block: trident sign. This ultrasound image demonstrates the "trident sign," a key landmark for performing a lumbar plexus block. The transverse processes (TP) and psoas major muscles (PMm) are visualized, resembling the three-pronged trident configuration, with adjacent posterior structures such as the paravertebral space (P&B) and erector spinae muscle (ESm)

Fig. 50.3 Ultrasound anatomy of the lumbar plexus (Shamrock sign). This ultrasound image depicts the "shamrock sign," a key landmark for identifying the lumbar plexus. Key structures include the quadratus lumborum (QLm), psoas major (PMm), transverse process (TP), and surrounding muscles and fascial planes used in regional anesthesia

the lumbar "trident" sign formed by the transverse processes of the lumbar vertebrae (Fig. 50.2). The aim is to guide the needle (inserted from the caudal end of the transducer) into the posterior aspect of the psoas muscle while monitoring for quadriceps twitch, like the landmark technique. After negative aspiration, the spread of local anaesthetic can be visualized in real-time. During and after injection, the plexus may itself become more prominent.

Shamrock approach (Fig. 50.3)
The patients are positioned in lateral decubitus with the side to be anaesthetised facing upwards. The ultrasound probe is placed on the patient's flank in the transverse plane just above the iliac crest. The "Shamrock sign" is identified by first identifying the transverse process and vertebral body of L4. The psoas muscle appears anterior to the transverse process, the erector spinae muscle posterior to the transverse process, and the quadratus lumborum muscle attached to the apex of the transverse process, an easily recognisable pattern of a shamrock with three leaves. The

plexus will be visualised within the psoas muscle, typically 2 cm anterior to the transverse process. The transducer is then slid slightly caudal until the transverse process of L4 disappears from the ultrasound image. The needle insertion point is 4 cm lateral to the midline in a line representing the intersection of the ultrasound beam with the skin. The needle will be advanced in the plane in the anterior direction. The needle tip must be positioned lateral to the L3 spinal nerve; a dual guidance technique with peripheral nerve stimulation should be used where an electrical nerve stimulation (0.1 ms impulse duration, 2 Hz) would confirm the identification of the plexus and reduce the risk of intraneural needle tip positioning. A threshold below 0.2 mA indicates an intraneural needle position and would require repositioning of the needle tip.

Structures to identify
Transverse process and vertebral body of L4 vertebra, quadratus lumborum muscle, psoas major muscle, erector spinae muscle.

Ergonomics
The operator stands behind the patient with the USG in front of the patient.

Probe

A low-frequency (5–10 Hz) curved array transducer.

Settings

Preset: MSK, with general or penetration mode, Compound imaging/Multibeam.

Depth: Around 6–9 cm, depending on the body habitus.

Needle size: 50–80 mm short bevel nerve block needle.

Drug choice

Surgical anesthesia: stock solution of 0.75% ropivacaine +2% lignocaine with adrenaline, total of 15–20 ml

Analgesia: 0.2% ropivacaine 15–20 ml

Muscle response acceptable Quadriceps twitch

Testing block success

A successful block can be defined as a loss of sensation to touch, temperature, and pinprick in the thigh's anterior, medial, and lateral aspects. Motor blockade success can be described as a reduced muscle power of the hip and knee flexors and the adductors of the hip.

Clinical Pearls

- Dual guidance is advocated for the lumbar plexus block, as it can improve block performance accuracy and detect intraneural needle tip placement (Table 50.1).

Side effects Lower limb weakness.

Complications

1. Direct trauma to nerves.
2. Intra-neural injection
3. Damage to abdominal viscera.
4. Retro-peritoneal haematomas
5. Psoas hematoma
6. Psoas abscess
7. Epidural spread
8. Spinal, or sub-arachnoid, injection
9. Intravascular injection and LA toxicity

Table 50.1 Response to nerve stimulation during lumbar plexus block

Response obtained	Interpretation	Action
Stimulation of the femoral nerve does not occur within 2 cm of the transverse process	The needle is too far away from the plexus	Fan the needle cephalad and caudad from the transverse process Angle the needle slightly more medially Switch to a loss-of-resistance technique
Hamstring or gastrocnemius contraction	The needle is angled too medially. Stimulation of the L4 or L5 component of the sacral trunk at the level of the nerve root	Withdraw the needle from the skin and redirect it laterally
Scrotum or labia electrical paraesthesia	Stimulation of the genitofemoral nerve, which lies anteromedial in the psoas compartment	Redirect the needle more laterally and not as deep
Abdominal wall contraction	Stimulation of the iliohypogastric nerve	Redirect the needle more medially
Contraction of the paraspinal muscle	The needle is too shallow	Advance the needle
Flexion of the hip	Direct stimulation of the psoas muscle	Reduce current flow or pulse width. Try again
Twitching of the opposite limb	Stimulation of nerves to the contralateral leg- needle is likely intrathecal	Withdraw the needle and reinsert/redirect more laterally
After injection of local anaesthetic, the patient notes numbness or weakness in both limbs	Intrathecal or epidural injection	Stop any further injections. Prepare to resuscitate as total spinal may ensue.

Continuous Catheter Technique

Indication: Extended analgesia for unilateral lower limb surgery.

Position: as above for single-shot technique.

Kit: 18G/16G Tuohy echogenic needle is inserted. The final positioning of the catheter should be at a depth of the skin of 4–5 cm more than the depth of the needle at its final positioning. The catheter can be secured with clear, transparent dressings. Despite proper needle placement, there is a small risk of catheter misplacement -intravascular or neuraxial. Therefore, catheters should constantly be tested for negative aspiration for blood or CSF, and local anaesthetic injection should be fractionated and slow. A continuous infusion of 8–10 ml/h of ropivacaine 0.2% has been suggested for analgesia.

The development of foot drop is not a sign of excessive block and should not be mistaken as being due to the block. It is likely a surgical complication (e.g., hematoma, bone fragment, dislocation) causing sciatic compression and should be addressed urgently.

Suggested Reading

1. Karmakar MK. Atlas of sonoanatomy for regional anaesthesia and pain medicine. McGraw-Hill; 2018.
2. Polania Gutierrez JJ, Ben-David B. Lumbar plexus block. In: StatPearls [Internet]. Treasure Island: StatPearls Publishing; 2022.
3. Akkaya T, Comert A, Kendir S, Acar HI, Gumus H, Elhan A. Detailed accessory obturator nerve blockade anatomy. Minerva Anesthesiol. 2008;74(4):119–22.
4. Axel S, et al. The Shamrock lumbar plexus block: a dose-finding study. Eur J Anaesthesiol. 2015;32:764–70.
5. Chakraborty A. Blockmate: a practical guide for ultrasound guided regional anaesthesia. Springer; 2021.

iPACK Block

Namita Sharma, Chetan Mehra, and Kausik Dasgupta

Level of difficulty Intermediate

The iPACK block of precise ultrasound-guided local anaesthetic infiltration targets the space between the popliteal artery and the posterior capsule of the knee (iPACK).

Anatomy & Surface Anatomy

The iPACK block targets a fine meshwork of nerves called the popliteal nerve plexus, which supplies the posterior capsule of the knee joint.

This includes:

- The superomedial and lateral genicular nerves,
- The articular branches of the tibial nerve (major contribution) and common peroneal nerve,
- The articular branches of the obturator nerve in the popliteal region.

The innervation to the anteromedial capsule of the knee joint is by the saphenous nerve, nerve to vastus medialis, obturator nerve, and two nerves

arising from the deep nerve plexus, i.e., the medial and anterior genicular nerves.

Therefore, the anterior capsule, periosteum, and prepatellar fat pads are stripped off during surgery and are not the primary pain generators after TKR.

The posterior capsule of the knee joint is innervated primarily by the articular branches of the tibial nerve. These include the superior and inferior branches of the tibial nerve and the posterior branch of the common fibular nerve. Apart from these, the posterior capsule is also supplied by the genicular branch of the posterior division of the obturator nerve.

The anatomical location of the inferior branch of the tibial nerve and the genicular branch of the posterior division of the obturator nerve is usually consistent, whereas the presence of the superior branch of the tibial nerve and the posterior branch of the common fibular nerve is found to be variable (Fig. 51.1).

Indications

The iPACK block is used in combination with a saphenous nerve block (Adductor canal block/Femoral nerve block) to provide analgesia for the posterior compartment of the knee in case of:

- Total knee arthroplasty
- Arthroscopic anterior cruciate ligament repair

Posterior compartment pain after TKR can be treated with distal adductor canal block, selective tibial nerve block, genicular nerve block,

N. Sharma (✉)
Ashford and St Peter's Hospital, Chertsey, UK

C. Mehra
Department of Anaesthesia, Indraprastha Apollo Hospital, New Delhi, Delhi, India

K. Dasgupta
NHS, Leicester, UK

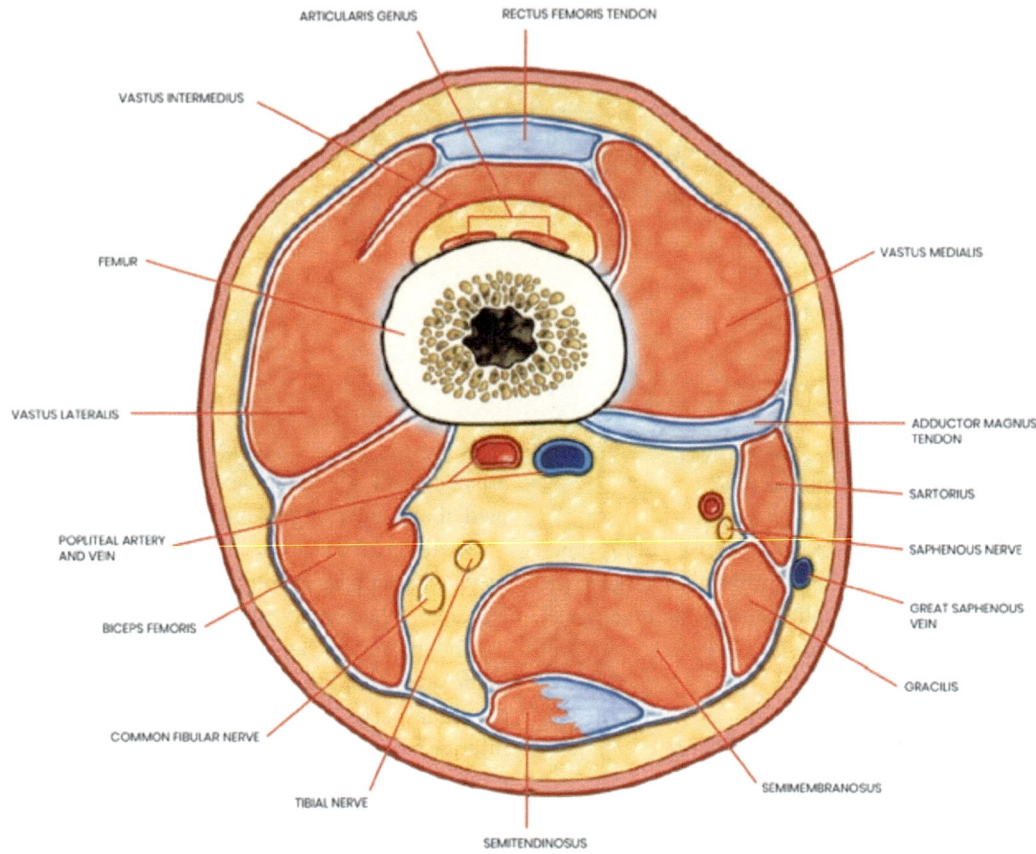

Fig. 51.1 Cross-sectional anatomy

surgical LIA, and iPACK. Due to the least level of complexity and consistent outcome, iPACK is the most commonly performed block for posterior compartment analgesia.

Contraindications

- **Absolute**
  - Patient refusal
  - Infection at the site of injection
  - Allergy to local anaesthetics
- **Relative**
  - Prior knee surgery or trauma leading to distortion of anatomy
  - Deranged coagulation profile
  - Sepsis

Advantages of sciatic nerve block approaches
It provides analgesia for the posterior compartment of the knee without affecting the motor nerves. Hence, it prevents distal muscle weak-

ness and post-block foot drop caused by sciatic nerve block at the popliteal level.

Aim
The iPACK block aims to deposit local anaesthetic drugs in the fatty space just posterior to the femur, which envelops the knee joint capsule.

Ultrasound Technique

Scanning protocol
iPACK block is performed by scanning the popliteal fossa (iPACK space) by placing an ultrasound transducer either

- *Posterior:* over the popliteal crease
- *Anterior:* over the medial thigh, roughly one finger-breadth above the patella, to obtain a posteromedial acoustic window

Posterior probe: the popliteal fossa is scanned to identify the popliteal vessels and the femur shaft. The femoral condyles can be identified as two discrete humps on either side of the popliteal vessels. Sliding the probe cephalad until the condylar humps disappear *to* bring the flat femoral shaft (metaphysis) in view.

Anterior probe: identify femur shaft and popliteal artery. In this view, the femur shaft appears as a diagonal-sloping hyperechoic line when placed over the medial thigh.

Colour flow Doppler can locate the popliteal artery *in both probe positions*.

Relevant Sonoanatomy

Structures to identify
- Bone: Femoral condyles and shaft
- Vessels: Popliteal artery and vein
- Nerves: Sciatic nerve with its tibial and common peroneal (*common fibular is the new terminology*) branches within their circum-neural sheath, located superficial to popliteal vessels
- Muscles: Sartorius, Vastus medialis, Semitendinosus, Semimembranosus, Biceps femoris (Fig. 51.2)

Block Performance

Position/Ergonomics
Supine anterior probe: The patient is placed in a supine position with the knee flexed at 45° or in a frog leg position (leg supported with external rotation and flexion).

Lateral posterior probe: The patient can also be placed in a lateral decubitus position, with the operative side being non-dependent, which improves ergonomics.

Supine posterior probe: The straight leg is elevated, and the ankle is supported on an elevated stand.

Probe selection
A low-frequency curvilinear ultrasound transducer (2–5 MHz) is preferred because it allows visualization of all the structures of the knee and the needle in a single window by sliding the probe.

A linear transducer can also be used in a slim-built patient, although one must slide it on either side to identify the anatomical structures.

Settings
Multibeam resolution

Fig. 51.2 USG image demonstrating iPACK (infiltration between popliteal artery and capsule of the knee) block. The popliteal artery (PA) and popliteal vein (PV) are visualised posterior to the femur with the injection target area between the femur and these vessels; the tibial nerve (TN) and common peroneal nerve (CPN) lie more posteriorly and are to be avoided

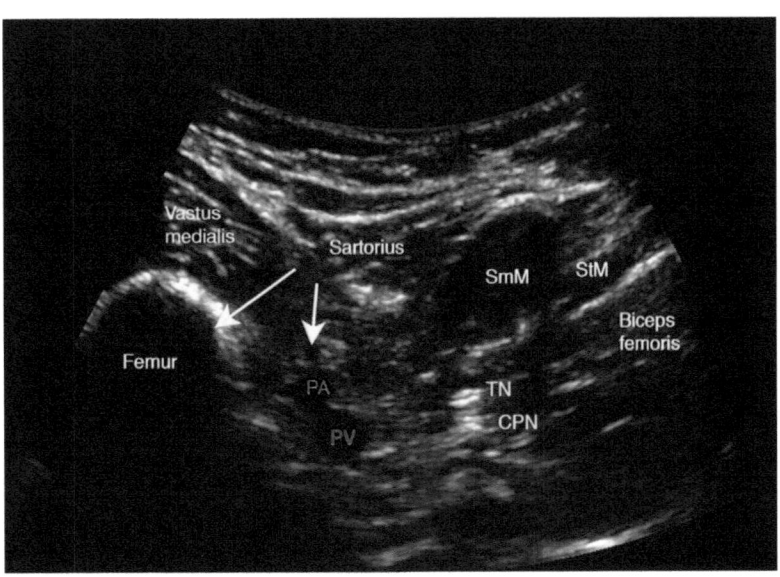

Depth

In supine anterior probe placement: Approximately 3.5–4.5 cm from skin to femoral shaft (metaphysis).

In supine posterior and lateral decubitus posterior probe placement, the depth of the popliteal artery from the skin surface is noted, and the needle is inserted at the same distance from the edge of the transducer.

Needle size

22G short bevel, 100 mm insulated stimulating needle.

Needling technique

Anterior probe: The needle is inserted in a plane from the medial aspect of the knee between the popliteal artery and the femur (iPACK space). The needle is advanced from the anteromedial to the posterolateral direction.

Posterior probe: The needle is advanced parallel to the femoral metaphysis in the fat-filled space between the popliteal artery and shaft. Needle entry points can be medial or lateral.

Posterior probe: Medial to lateral needle insertion: *Caution: saphenous vein puncture causing haematoma.*

Posterior probe: Lateral to medial needle insertion· *Caution: iPACK done at the condylar level risks blocking the common fibular nerve.*

The lateral-to-medial approach is commonly preferred in the posterior probe position.

Saline hydrodissection can help negotiate the needle through the iPACK space. However, contact with popliteal vessels or the femur should be avoided.

Optimal needle tip position

Anterior probe: The tip of the needle is placed 1–2 cm beyond the lateral edge of the popliteal artery.

Posterior probe: The tip of the needle and the shaft are placed in the fatty tissue between the popliteal artery and the femoral shaft, with three zonal injections at the lateral, middle, and medial areas while the needles are withdrawn.

Drug dosing

After confirmation of negative blood aspiration, 20 ml of 0.2% ropivacaine is injected incrementally as the needle is withdrawn to fill the iPACK space.

Proximal iPACK versus Distal iPACK block

Block can be performed at two potential sites:

- Proximal iPACK:
  - It is performed above the level of the patella (i.e., at the level of the femoral shaft).
  - The common peroneal nerve (CPN) is not entirely separated from the sciatic nerve's main trunk at this level.
  - CPN becomes more vulnerable to being blocked by local anaesthetic deposited at this level. This may cause foot drop and hinder mobilisation in the post-operative period.
  - The medial and lateral genicular nerves are possibly targeted at this level rather than the popliteal plexus.
  - The needle manoeuvrability is found to *be* easy with this approach.
- Distal iPACK block:
  - It is performed at the distal portion of the popliteal fossa at the femoral condyle level (intercondylar area), the popliteal plexus site.
  - CPN runs superficially and away from the posterior capsule at this level. This allows it to be spared by the local anaesthetic deposited in this area.

iPACK versus LIA

The LIA technique delivers the local anaesthetic around the knee, covering pericapsular and periosteal tissues, ligaments, and subcutaneous tissues. Posterior capsular infiltration is limited to a certain extent because of the fear of accidental neurovascular injury.

A high volume of LA (100–150 mL of 0.2% Ropi) with variable adjuncts has been used, viz. adrenaline, NSAIDS, opioids, steroids, and liposomal bupivacaine.

iPACK block involves ultrasound-guided drug delivery near the posterior capsule of the knee to target the popliteal plexus and nerve while preventing an unintentional needle tip injury to the popliteal vessels and sciatic nerve. The volume used is around 15–20 mL, 0.2% ropivacaine LA, and fewer adjuncts, *viz. adrenaline.*

Present Evidence for the Use of iPACK Block
Along with adductor canal block (single shot or continuous) with or without LIA (local infiltration analgesia), iPACK block may provide superior analgesia and improve functional outcomes. Compared with tibial nerve block, it reduces the occurrence of foot drop.

Adding the iPACK block does not provide superior analgesia to the LIA technique for posterior knee pain following total knee arthroplasty. A medial spread of local anaesthetic to the medial and lateral genicular nerves may account for an additional effect on other parts of the knee that are not covered by LIA or adductor canal block.

Complications
Generic: for all nerve blocks: failure, nerve damage, infection, bleeding, LAST
Specific:
- **Popliteal vessel puncture/ hematoma**
- Sciatic nerve (tibial/ common peroneal) blockade, causing foot drop/ motor weakness of foot muscles
- *Saphenous vein puncture*

Clinical Pearls
- *In posterior probe position*: The distance from the transducer to the iPACK space gives a rough estimation of the needle insertion distance from the edge of the transducer. This avoids repeated adjustments of needle direction to stay within the iPACK space and also helps prevent unintentional sciatic nerve contact or vascular puncture.
- Higher volumes of local anaesthetic drugs can track superficially to block sciatic nerve branches (tibial and common peroneal), which is undesirable for early mobilisation.
- While injecting near the lateral femoral condyle, one should make sure that the drug is spreading laterally rather than superficially to avoid an unintentional peroneal nerve blockade. For the same reason, the needle tip should

not venture more than 1.5 cm beyond the lateral margin of the popliteal artery.
- To ensure a uniform deposition of local anaesthetic, the total drug volume can be divided into three equal parts, and each part sequentially deposited over the lateral, middle (intercondylar groove), and medial aspects of the posterior surface of the femoral shaft.
- Proximal versus distal iPACK block: according to a Systematic Review of Randomized Controlled Trials, an anteromedial dye spread (involving superior medial genicular nerve) was seen in cadavers where proximal iPACK block was performed, whereas an anterolateral dye spread was seen with distal iPACK block (involving superior lateral genicular nerve and anterior branch of common fibular nerve). A better motor-sparing effect was observed with the distal approach. Pain scores were slightly worse with the proximal approach.

Questions
- What will be your anaesthesia protocol to provide post-operative analgesia after Total Knee Arthroplasty while incorporating iPACK as a component of multi-modal analgesia?
- How can one prolong the duration of analgesia provided by iPACK block?
- Which superficial vein puncture can lead to a hematoma while inserting a needle from the medial side of the femur?
- How can one assess the effectiveness of the iPACK block?
- How is the iPACK block different from the LIA (local infiltration analgesia) technique?
- What are the issues with using the larger volume of LA for the iPACK block?
- What are the possible advantages and disadvantages of performing iPACK block proximally at the level of a femoral shaft or distally at the femoral condyles?

Suggested Reading

1. Burckett-St Laurant D, Peng P, Girón Arango L, et al. The nerves of the adductor canal and the innervation of the knee: an anatomic study. Reg Anesth Pain Med. 2016;41:321–7.

2. Tran J, Giron Arango L, Peng P, et al. Evaluation of the iPACK block injectate spread: a cadaveric study. Reg Anesth Pain Med. 2019;44:689–94.

3. Chan E, Howle R, Onwochei D, et al. Infiltration between the popliteal artery and the capsule of the knee (IPACK) block in knee surgery: a narrative review. Reg Anesth Pain Med. 2021;46:784–805.

4. Vichainarong C, Kampitak W, Tanavalee A, et al. Analgesic efficacy of infiltration between the popliteal artery and capsule of the knee (iPACK) block added to local infiltration analgesia and continuous adductor canal block after total knee arthroplasty: a randomised clinical trial. Reg Anesth Pain Med. 2020;45:872–9.

5. Et T, Korkusuz M, Basaran B, Yarımoğlu R, Toprak H, Bilge A, Kumru N, Dedeli İ. Comparison of iPACK and periarticular block with adductor block alone after total knee arthroplasty: a randomised clinical trial. J Anesth. 2022;36(2):276–86.

6. Kampitak W, Tanavalee A, Ngarmukos S, Tantavisut S. Motor-sparing effect of iPACK (interspace between the popliteal artery and capsule of the posterior knee) block versus tibial nerve block after total knee arthroplasty: a randomised controlled trial. Reg Anesth Pain Med. 2020;45(4):267–76.

7. Wang F, Ma W, Huang Z. Analgesia effects of IPACK block added to multimodal analgesia regiments after total knee replacement: a systematic review of the literature and meta-analysis of 5 randomised controlled trials. Medicine (Baltimore). 2021;100(22):e25884.

8. D'Souza RS, Langford BJ, Olsen DA, Johnson RL. Ultrasound-guided local anesthetic infiltration between the popliteal artery and the capsule of the posterior knee (IPACK) block for primary total knee arthroplasty: a systematic review of randomized controlled trials. Local Reg Anesth. 2021;14:85–98.

Ankle Block

Namita Sharma and Chetan Mehra

Level of difficulty Basic

Anatomy

The ankle block involves five basic level blocks targeting the nerves around the ankle joint. Four of the target nerves (the superficial and deep peroneal, tibial, and sural nerves) are branches of the sciatic. The saphenous nerve is the terminal extension of the femoral nerve (Fig. 52.1).

The superficial peroneal, saphenous, and sural nerves have a superficial orientation relative to the 'deep' nerves: the tibial and deep peroneal.

The tibial nerve (posterior tibial nerve, TN)
A terminal branch of the sciatic nerve, the tibial nerve, courses behind the gastrocnemius in the lower leg before entering the foot. In the ankle, the posterior tibial nerve travels behind the medial malleolus between the posterior tibial vessels anteriorly and the flexor hallucis longus muscle and tendon posterolaterally.

The nerve finally divides to form the medial and lateral plantar nerves, supplying the plantar aspect of the foot.

N. Sharma (✉)
Ashford and St Peter's Hospital, Chertsey, UK

C. Mehra
Department of Anaesthesia, Indraprastha Apollo Hospital, New Delhi, Delhi, India

The deep peroneal nerve (DPN)
The DPN is a deep branch of the common peroneal nerve (CPN) lying deep to the extensor hallucis longus tendon and extensor digitorum longus tendon in the distal leg. The nerve is anterior to the tibia and interosseous membrane and typically situated lateral to the anterior tibial artery just above the ankle joint.

The nerve finally divides in the dorsum of the foot, with its medial branch supplying cutaneous innervation to the web space between the first and second toes and a lateral branch providing motor innervation to the middle toes.

The superficial peroneal nerve (SPN)
The SPN is a second branch of the CPN. The SPN travels deep to the peroneal muscles of the lateral leg, which become superficial at the leg's midpoint. The nerve sends cutaneous branches anteriorly to the foot's dorsum at the ankle's level.

The sural nerve
The sural nerve typically forms around the middle leg from cutaneous branches of the tibial and common peroneal nerve. The nerve travels in deep fascia in the lower lateral leg before becoming superficial and coursing around the posterior portion of the lateral malleolus.

The sural nerve provides cutaneous innervation to a portion of the lateral foot and ankle.

S. Phillips et al. (eds.), *Regional Anaesthesia*, https://doi.org/10.1007/978-3-032-05165-3_52

Fig. 52.1 US/S showing tibial nerve. FDL flexor digitorum longus, FHL flexor hallucis longus, TP tibialis posterior, PT posterior tibial, a artery, v vein, nerve

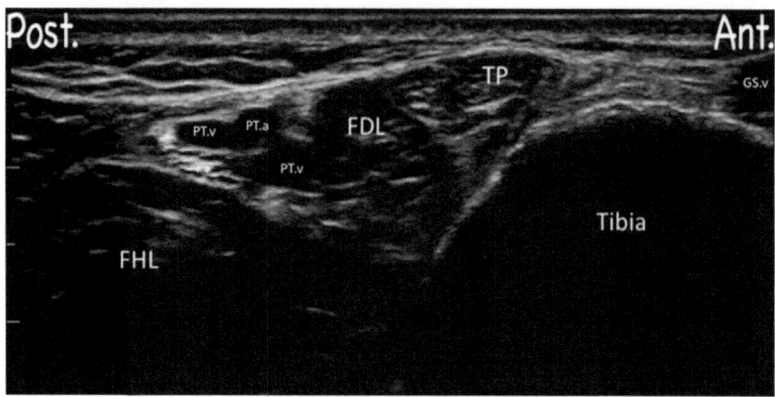

The saphenous nerve

The saphenous nerve and its cutaneous branches are the terminal extensions of the femoral nerve. The nerve provides sensory innervation to the medial ankle and foot in the distal leg.

Surface Landmarks

Dorsalis pedis artery, posterior tibial artery, medial malleolus, lateral malleolus, calcaneum, sustentaculum tali.

Indications

Perimalleolar: Foot and ankle surgery

Mid-tarsal block: Forefoot surgery

Combined tibial, superficial peroneal, deep peroneal, sural, and saphenous nerve blocks provide complete foot anesthesia.

Contraindications

Absolute

- Patient refusal
- Infection at the site of needle insertion
- Allergy to local anesthetics

Advantages over other techniques

- Ankle block causes minimal motor blocks compared with other lower limb blocks.

Landmark Techniques (Ankle and Midtarsal)

Tibial Nerve

- **Position:** The patient is supine, lower extremity to be blocked to be elevated on a blanket with external rotation at the hip to maximize exposure to the medial aspect of the foot
- **Depth:** 10–25 mm
- **Needle size**: 22–25G hypodermic needle
- **Needling technique**:

  Peri malleolar approach: Draw a line joining the medial malleolus to the posterior inferior border of the calcaneum. If the posterior tibial pulse cannot be felt, inject at a point halfway along this line. If the pulse can be felt, insert the needle at 45° towards the tibia to contact the posterior tibial pulse. Withdraw the needle a few millimeters, and after negative aspiration, inject the local anesthetic.

  Mid-tarsal approach: Identify the tibial artery distal to the medial malleolus on the calcaneus or the sustentaculum tali (ST, the prominence directly inferior to the medial malleolus). Insert the needle towards the calcaneus under the ST or on either side of the artery, contact the bone, then withdraw the needle 2 mm and inject.

- **Drug choice**: 0.25–0.5% Levobupivacaine

- **Drug volume**: 3–5 ml
- **Stimulation:** Plantar-flexion of the toes, paraesthesia to the sole/toes

Deep Peroneal Nerve
- **Position:** The patient is supine, lower extremities to be blocked and elevated on a blanket
- **Depth:** 10–25 mm
- **Needle size:** 22–25G hypodermic needle
- **Needling technique:**

  Peri-malleolar approach: The patient is asked to extend their great toe to tense and identify the extensor hallucis longus tendon at the level of the intermalleolar line. The needle is inserted lateral to the tendon, perpendicular to the tendon, and advanced until the bone is contacted. The needle is withdrawn 2 mm, and after negative aspiration, LA is injected.

  Mid-tarsal approach: The extensor hallucis tendon and pulse of the dorsalis pedis artery are identified more distally on top of the foot. The needle is inserted lateral to the tendon and medial to the artery, and after negative aspiration, the LA is injected.
- **Drug choice:** 0.25–0.5% Levobupivacaine
- **Drug volume:** 3–5 ml

Superficial Peroneal Nerve
- **Position:** supine, lower extremity to be blocked and elevated on a blanket
- **Depth:** 10–25 mm
- **Needle size:** 22–25G hypodermic needle
- **Needling technique:**

  Peri-malleolar approach: Infiltrate subcutaneously medially and laterally from the insertion point described for the DPN peri-malleolar block (above). **Mid tarsal approach:** infiltrate subcutaneously laterally and medially across the dorsum of the foot to the dorsum/plantar junction block from the insertion point described for the DPN mid tarsal block (above).
- **Drug choice:** 0.25–0.5% Levobupivacaine
- **Drug volume:** 3–5 ml

Sural
- **Position:** supine, lower extremity to be blocked elevated on a blanket
- **Depth:** 10–25 mm

- **Needle size:** 22–25G hypodermic needle
- **Needling technique:** Infiltrate subcutaneously from the lateral malleolus to the lateral border of the Achilles tendon.
- **Drug choice:** 0.25–0.5% Levobupivacaine
- **Drug volume:** 3–5 ml

Saphenous
- **Position:** supine, lower extremity to be blocked to be elevated on a blanket with external rotation at the hip to maximize exposure to the medial aspect of the foot
- **Depth:** 10–25 mm
- **Needle size:** 22–25G hypodermic needle
- **Needling technique:** Infiltrate LA subcutaneously and posteriorly to the level of the medial malleolus.
- **Drug choice:** 0.25–0.5% Levobupivacaine
- **Drug volume:** 3–5 ml

Ultrasound-Guided Block Technique

Tibial Nerve

Ultrasound anatomy
Scanning protocol: Place the transducer transversely 2–3 cm above the medial malleolus. Scan from the tibia to the Achilles tendon. Identify all the structures mentioned below by scanning up and down the leg. Approach the nerve from posterior to anterior (to avoid tibialis posterior and flexor digitorum longus tendons and vascularity) at a level where the nerve is most visible, which may be 10 cm proximal to the ankle.

Structures to identify: medial malleolus; tibialis posterior; flexor digitorum longus; posterior tibial artery and two veins (typically); tibial nerve; soleus; Achilles tendon; flexor hallucis longus (FHL) lying deep to these structures (Fig. 52.1).

Block performance
- **Position:** patient supine with leg externally rotated and knee slightly flexed to allow access to the medial malleolus
- **Probe:** High frequency linear (8–12 MHz) or 25 mm hockey stick probe

- **Settings:** Nerve setting, MB resolution, low depth
- **Depth:** 10–25 mm
- **Needle size:** 50 mm, 22G echogenic block needle
- **Needling technique:** In-plane (anterior or posterior) or out-of-plane
- **Needle endpoint:** Aim to deposit LA at a 6 o'clock position, then a 12 o'clock position to get a circumferential spread of LA
- **Drug choice:** 0.25–0.5% Levobupivacaine
- **Drug volume:** 2–5 ml

Deep Peroneal Nerve
- **Structures to identify:** tibia, anterior tibial vein, anterior tibial artery, extensor digitorum longus (EDL), extensor hallucis longus (EHL), and deep peroneal nerve
- **Scanning protocol:** Place the transducer in the transverse axis over the ankle joint. Identify the pulsatile anterior tibial artery. Be aware not to put too much pressure on the probe so as not to compress the artery. Two veins, one on either side, usually accompany the artery. Scanning up and down the leg, the DPN is seen as a small hypoechoic structure rolling over the top of the vessels from medial to lateral (Fig. 52.2).

Block performance
- **Position:** Patient supine
- **Probe:** High frequency linear (8–12 MHz) or 25 mm hockey stock probe

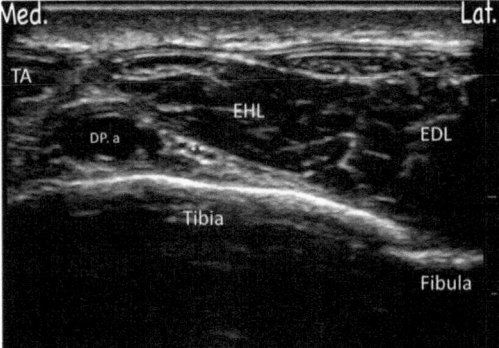

Fig. 52.2 Deep peroneal nerve on USG scanning. EDL extensor digitorum longus, EHL extensor hallucis longus, DP.a deep peroneal artery

- **Settings:** Nerve setting, MB resolution, low depth
- **Depth:** 10–25 mm
- **Needle size:** 50 mm, 22G echogenic block needle
- **Needling technique:** In-plane. Insert the needle from either medial or lateral, depending on the position of the nerve, and try to avoid tendons and periosteum. If you cannot see the nerve, carefully inject LA on either side of the anterior tibial artery.
- **Needle endpoint:** Above the DPN
- **Drug choice:** 0.25–0.5% Levobupivacaine
- **Drug volume:** 1–2 ml

Superficial Peroneal Nerve
- **Structures to identify:** Extensor digitorum longus (EDL), peroneus brevis (PB), peroneus longus tendon (PLT), fibula, superficial peroneal nerve (SPN) (Fig. 52.3).
- **Scanning protocol:** Place the transducer on the anterolateral aspect of the distal third of the leg in the transverse axis and scan proximally from the lateral malleolus. The fibula moves deeper as the probe moves proximally up the leg, and two muscle groups can be seen. The anterior muscle is EDL, and the posterior is PB. The PLT appears hyperechoic and often lies superficial to PB. The SPN (hyperechoic) lies in the groove between EDL and PB.

Block performance
- **Position:** Patient supine with leg internally rotated
- **Probe:** High frequency linear (8–12 MHz) or a 25 mm hockey stick probe
- **Settings:** Nerve setting, MB resolution, low depth
- **Depth:** 5–25 mm
- **Needle size:** 50 mm, 22G echogenic block needle
- **Needling technique:** In-plane, it is usually easier to needle from medial to lateral
- **Needle endpoint:** above the SPN and deep to the fascia of the lower leg
- **Drug choice:** 0.25–0.5% Levobupivacaine
- **Drug volume:** 1–2 ml

Fig. 52.3 USG scan showing superficial peroneal nerve. PL peroneus longus, PB peroneus brevis, EDL extensor digitorum longus, TA tibial artery

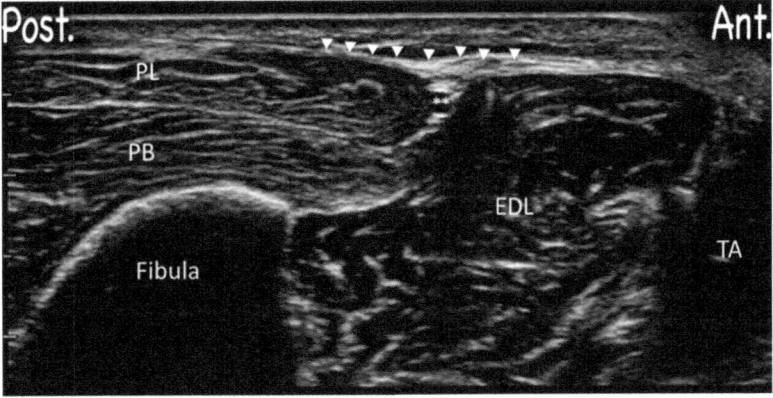

Fig. 52.4 USG scan showing sural nerve. AT Achilles tendon, PL peroneus longus, PB peroneus brevis, SS.v saphenous vein

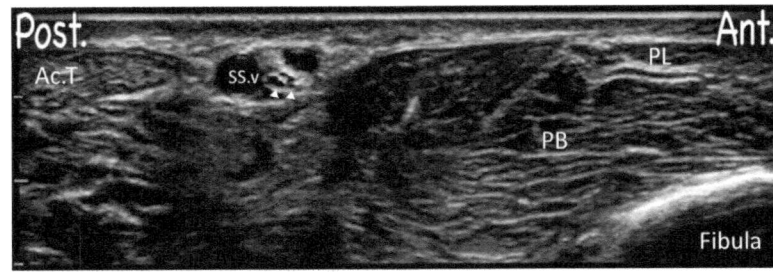

Sural

- Structures to identify: Achilles tendon (AT), lateral malleolus, peroneus brevis, peroneus longus tendon (PLT), short saphenous vein (SSV), sural nerve
- Scanning protocol: Place the transducer just proximal to the lateral malleolus of the ankle. Scan up and down and from anterior to posterior. Identify the AT posteriorly with the peroneus brevis muscle anterior to this. Both the AT and PB are posterior to the fibula. The short saphenous vein runs between the AT and PB, and the sural nerve can be identified as a round or triangular hyperechoic structure that is either anterior or posterior to the SSV (Fig. 52.4).

Block performance

- **Position:** supine with the leg internally rotated or in the lateral decubitus position
- **Probe:** High frequency linear (8–12 MHz) or 25 mm hockey stock probe

- **Settings:** Nerve setting, MB resolution, low depth
- **Depth**: 5–25 mm
- **Needle size:** 50 mm, 22G echogenic block needle
- **Needling technique:** In-plane. The needle can be brought in from the anterior or posterior. Avoid the AT using the posterior approach and PLT using an anterior approach.
- **Needle endpoint:** Above the sural nerve
- **Drug choice:** 0.25–0.5% Levobupivacaine
- **Drug volume:** 1–2 ml

Saphenous

- **Structures to identify:** Tibia, great saphenous vein (GSV), and saphenous nerve
- **Scanning protocol:** Place the transducer on the anteromedial aspect of the ankle in the transverse axis without compressing the GSV. Scan up and down the ankle, looking for the nerve near the vein. The nerve can be small

Fig. 52.5 USG scan showing saphenous nerve. FDL flexor digitorum longus, FHL flexor hallucis longus, TP tibialis posterior, PT posterior tibial, a artery, v vein, n nerve, GS.v great saphenous vein

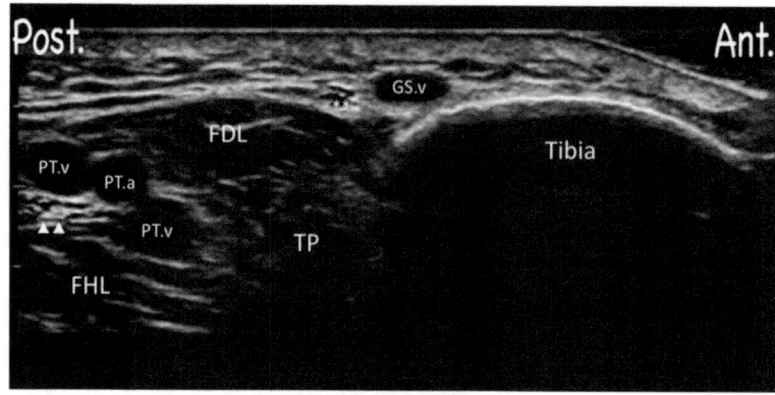

and best visualized 10–15 cm proximal to the medial malleolus. A proximal calf tourniquet can assist in increasing the size of the GSV as a landmark (Fig. 52.5).

Block performance
- **Position:** Patient supine with leg externally rotated
- **Probe:** High frequency linear (8–12 MHz) or a 25 mm hockey stick probe
- **Settings:** Nerve setting, MB resolution, low depth
- **Depth:** 5–25 mm
- **Needle size:** 50 mm, 22G echogenic block needle
- **Needling technique:** Depending on the position of the nerve about the GSV, the method can be in-plane, anterior, or posterior.
- **Needle endpoint:** above the saphenous nerve
- **Drug choice:** 0.25–0.5% Levobupivacaine
- **Drug volume:** 1–2 ml

Ankle Block
Complications: falls risk following block placement until resolution; vessel disruption/hematoma; nerve damage.

Clinical Pearls
- Ankle block is well suited for ambulatory foot surgery; success rates are higher with midtarsal blocks owing to the superficial nature of

TN and DPN, so it is the preferred approach for forefoot surgery.
- A saphenous nerve block can be omitted in 97% of patients undergoing forefoot or toe surgery, as innervation does not extend beyond the midfoot in these patients.
- Redirection of the needle to achieve a circumferential spread of LA around the nerve is unnecessary in such small nerves, and the LA diffuses quickly through the neural tissue.
- When using veins as landmarks, as little pressure as possible on the transducer allows the veins to fill. A proximal calf tourniquet can also assist in identifying veins used as landmarks to fill.

Questions
1. Commencing at a level proximal to the medial malleolus and moving posteriorly toward the Achilles tendon?
2. What is the correct order of structures?

Suggested Reading

1. Sort R, Brorson S, Gögenur I, Hald LL, Nielsen JK, Salling N, Hougaard S, Foss NB, Tengberg PT, Klausen TW, Møller AM. Peripheral nerve block anaesthesia and postoperative pain in acute ankle fracture surgery: the AnAnkle randomised trial. Br J Anaesth. 2021;126(4):881–8. https://doi.org/10.1016/j.bja.2020.12.037. Epub 2021 Feb 2. PMID: 33546844.

2. Gianakos AL, Romanelli F, Rao N, Badri M, Lubberts B, Guss D, DiGiovanni CW. Combination lower extremity nerve blocks and their effect on postoperative pain and opioid consumption: a systematic review. J Foot Ankle Surg. 2021;60(1):121–31. https://doi.org/10.1053/j.jfas.2020.08.026. Epub 2020 Sep 3. PMID: 33168443.

3. Lee M, Lee C, Lim J, Kim H, Choi YS, Kang H. Comparison of a peripheral nerve block versus spinal anesthesia in foot or ankle surgery: a systematic review and meta-analysis with a trial sequential analysis. J Pers Med. 2023;13(7):1096. https://doi.org/10.3390/jpm13071096. PMID: 37511709; PMCID: PMC10381348.

53

Namita Sharma and Chetan Mehra

Sciatic Nerve

Anatomy

The sciatic nerve, the largest peripheral nerve in the human body, is formed by the ventral roots of the lumbosacral plexus (L4–S3).

The sciatic nerve leaves the pelvis by coursing distally through the greater sciatic foramen, under the piriformis muscle. It passes midway between the ischial tuberosity (IT) and greater trochanter (GT) of the femur before entering the posterior thigh between the gluteus maximus muscle (posterior) and the quadratus femoris muscle (anterior).

At this point, the sciatic nerve provides some motor innervation to the posterior hip capsule's external rotators and articular branches.

In the proximal thigh, the nerve remains between the adductor muscles of the hip (anterior) and the gluteus maximus muscle (posterior) before coursing behind the long head of the biceps femoris muscle. The nerve continues deep to the hamstring muscles as it travels through the thigh, providing motor innervation to the adductor magnus and hamstring muscles.

Proximal Sciatic Blocks

Indications (in combination with femoral nerve block)

- Operations on the knee, lower leg, and foot (e.g., Knee replacement, tibial head osteotomy, arthrodesis)
- Fixation of fractures of the lower leg and foot
- Amputations of the thigh, lower leg, and foot
- Regional sympathetic block

Contraindications
Absolute
- Patient refusal
- Infection at the site of needle insertion
- Allergy to local anaesthetics

Relative
- Ipsilateral neuromuscular disease
- Contralateral neuromuscular disease
- Anticoagulation or bleeding disorder

Complications
- Motor blockade of the foot and ankle for the duration of the local anaesthetic effect
- The patient is at risk for the duration of the local anaesthetic effect
- Intravascular injection
- Perforation of pelvic viscera
- Urinary retention (parasacral approaches, rare)

N. Sharma (✉)
Ashford and St Peter's Hospital, Chertsey, UK

C. Mehra
Department of Anaesthesia, Indraprastha Apollo Hospital, New Delhi, Delhi, India

Clinical Pearls
- When first learning these ultrasound-guided approaches, use a nerve stimulator to confirm the nerve's position.
- The skin of the posterior thigh is innervated by the posterior femoral cutaneous nerve (S1–S3). To block this nerve requires large volumes of LA placed around the proximal sciatic nerve (infra gluteal). Sparing of this nerve and thus the skin of the posterior thigh can occur when the subgluteal or anterior block approaches are undertaken.

Landmark techniques
Parasacral Block (Mansour)
- **Surface landmarks**: posterior superior iliac spine, ischial tuberosity
- **Position:** patient lies in the lateral position with the side to be blocked uppermost and hip flexed. The leg underneath can be extended
- **Depth:** 40–100 mm (depending on the body habitus)
- **Needle size:** 80–100 mm, 22G echogenic block needle (150 mm may be needed in obese patients)
- **Needling technique:** Draw a line between the PSIS and IT. Six centimetres caudal to the PSIS is the puncture site—advance needle perpendicular to the skin to elicit a motor response at a minimal current of 0.3 mA. If contact with bone (likely sacral ala or ileum), redirect the needle caudally, advancing no more than 2 cm.
- **Drug choice:** 0.25% Levobupivicaine
- **Drug volume:** 20–40 ml
- **Stimulation:** Plantar flexion of the foot/toes (tibial nerve), can accept dorsiflexion of the foot (common peroneal nerve)
- **Catheter technique:** Using the puncture site of the Mansour technique and redirecting the needle towards the middle third of the line connecting the GT and IT. The catheter is advanced 4–5 cm caudally past the needle.

Landmark techniques
Dorsal Sciatic Nerve Block (Raj)
- **Surface landmarks:** greater trochanter and ischial tuberosity
- **Position:** patient lies supine with the hip and knee flexed to 90°.

- **Depth:** 40–100 mm (depending on the body habitus)
- **Needle size:** 80–100 mm, 22G echogenic block needle (150 mm may be needed in obese patients)
- **Needling technique:** Draw a line connecting the GT and IT. Halfway across this line should correspond to the groove between the hamstring and adductor muscles. Insert the needle perpendicular to the skin with slight medial intent to elicit correct stimulation.
- **Drug choice:** 0.25% Levobupivicaine
- **Drug volume:** 20–40 ml
- **Stimulation:** Plantar flexion of the foot/toes (tibial nerve), can accept dorsiflexion of the foot (common peroneal nerve)
- **Catheter technique:** The catheter is advanced 4–5 cm beyond the needle tip following the injection.
- **Advantages over other techniques**: the patient can lie supine

Landmark techniques
Anterior Proximal Sciatic Nerve Block (Beck)
- **Surface landmarks:** greater trochanter, anterior superior iliac spine, pubic tubercle
- **Position:** patient lies supine with the leg to be anaesthetised extended
- **Depth:** 80–100 mm (depending on the body habitus)
- **Needle size:** 100–150 mm, 22G echogenic block needle
- **Needling technique:** draw a line joining the ASIS to the pubic tubercle (inguinal ligament) (line A) and another line parallel to this through the greater trochanter (line B). A perpendicular line is drawn from line A's middle/medial third down to Line B. The intersection of this vertical line marks on line B larks the puncture site. Insert a needle at the puncture site with lateral intent towards the medial side of the femur. Once the bone is in contact, note the needle's depth, withdraw the needle, and direct the needle vertically past the femur by 50 mm.
- **Drug choice:** 0.25% Levobupivicaine
- **Drug volume:** 20–40 ml
- **Stimulation:** Plantar flexion of the foot/toes (tibial nerve), can accept dorsiflexion of the foot (common peroneal nerve)

- **Advantages over other techniques:** minimal patient movement is required as the block is supine.

Landmark techniques
Lateral Approach Proximal Sciatic Block
- **Surface landmarks:** greater trochanter, ischial tuberosity
- **Position:** patient lies supine with the leg to be anaesthetised extended
- **Depth:** 40–100 mm (depending on the body habitus)
- **Needle size:** 80–100 mm, 22G echogenic block needle (150 mm may be needed in obese patients)
- **Needling technique:** draw a line parallel to the femur distally from the posterior border of the greater trochanter. Insert the needle 3–5 cm distal to the GT along this line. Direct the needle dorsally (15–30°) and cranially. Muscular contractions at the back of the thigh are frequent. Redirect the needle anteriorly if no response is elicited. The common peroneal nerve (CPN) is often stimulated first, initially causing dorsiflexion of the foot.
- **Drug choice:** 0.25% Levobupivicaine
- **Drug volume:** 20–40 ml
- **Stimulation:** Plantar flexion of the foot/toes (tibial nerve), can accept dorsiflexion of the foot (common peroneal nerve)

Landmark techniques
Posterior/Trans Gluteal Proximal Sciatic Nerve Block (Labat)
- **Surface landmarks:** posterior superior iliac spine, greater trochanter, ischial tuberosity, and sacral hiatus
- **Position:** the patient lies laterally with the side to be blocked uppermost. The leg underneath can be extended. The leg to be blocked is flexed at the hip at 30–40° and the knee flexed at 70°
- **Depth:** 50–100 mm (depending on the body habitus)
- **Needle size:** 80–100 mm, 22G echogenic block needle (150 mm may be needed in obese patients)
- **Needling technique:** draw a line connecting the PSIS to the GT (line A) and another con-

necting the GT to the sacral hiatus (line B). Drop a perpendicular line down from the midpoint of line A. Where this line intersects line B is the needle puncture site. The needle is directed perpendicular to the skin, and the direction of the needle can be corrected in a fan pattern along the line A until a motor response is elicited.
- **Drug choice:** 0.25% Levobupivicaine
- **Drug volume:** 20–40 ml
- **Stimulation:** Plantar flexion of the foot/toes (tibial nerve), can accept dorsiflexion of the foot (common peroneal nerve)
- **Advantages over other techniques:** It can be combined well with a psoas compartment block, as the patient's position does not have to be changed further.

Ultrasound-guided block technique
Parasacral Block

Level of difficulty
Difficult

Ultrasound anatomy (Fig. 53.1)
Scanning protocol: Place the transducer between the posterior iliac spine (PSIS) and the midpoint of the line connecting the PSIS and the greater trochanter. The image identifies the iliac bone line, gluteus maximus, and medius.

Moving the transducer infero-medially (parasacral parallel shift) from the above line identifies a discontinuity in the iliac bone line signifying the greater sciatic notch. This is where the sacral plexus exits the pelvis. Tilting the transducer caudad at this point can help visualise the hyperechoic sacral plexus between the ischial and sacral bones and beneath the piriformis muscle.

A secondary technique relies upon identifying the posterior border of the ilium (PBI). A transducer is placed in the axial plane 8 cm lateral to the natal cleft to locate the PBI.

When the probe is slid cranially, the continuous hyperechoic area of the ilium can be seen. When slid caudally, a gap in the bony structure (the greater sciatic foramen) appears. With the probe tilted caudally at this point, the hyperechoic sciatic nerve can be seen (Fig. 53.2).

Fig. 53.1 (a–d) Figure showing sonoanatomy of the location of the sacral plexus

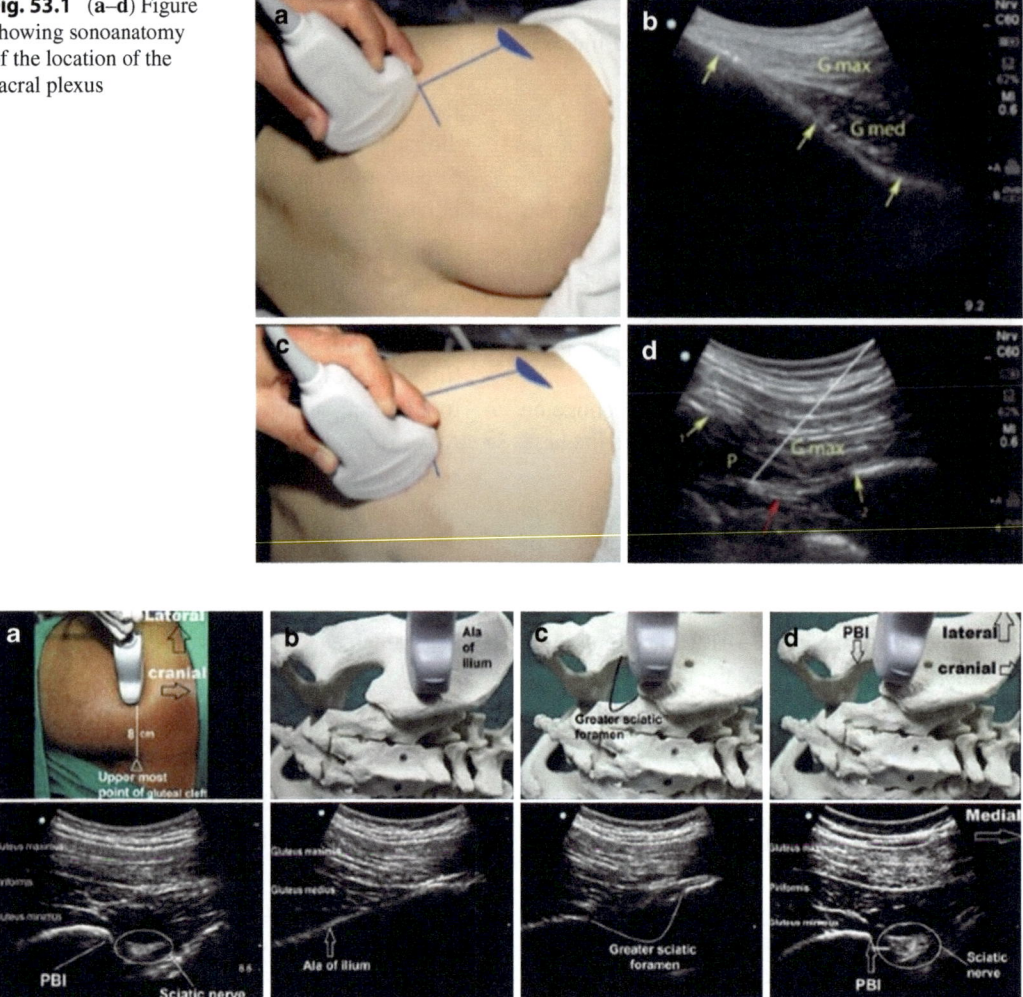

Fig. 53.2 (a–d) Ultrasound-guided anatomical approach for sciatic nerve localization in the gluteal region

Structures to identify: Iliac bone line; gluteus maximus, gluteus medius, piriformis muscle; sacral plexus; greater sciatic foramen

Posterior border of ilium (Taha approach)

Landmarks to palpate Posterior superior iliac spine; greater trochanter of the femur

- **Position:** Lateral position with the side to be blocked uppermost. Flex the hip and knee of the side to be blocked.
- **Ergonomics:** Place the ultrasound machine at the head of the bed with the operator standing on the side of the patient's back (patient facing away from them)
- **Probe:** Linear or curved (2–5 Hz) array depending on body habitus
- **Settings:** Nerve setting, high depth
- **Depth:** 40–100 mm (depending on the body habitus)
- **Needle size:** 80–100 mm, 22G echogenic block needle (150 mm may be needed in obese patients)
- **Needling technique:** In-plane, needling lateral to medial. Out of plane is also possible, but it relies on seeing only the needle tip at more considerable depths.

- **Needle endpoint:** Deposit LA perineurally around sacral plexus incrementally, only repositioning the needle under ultrasonographic guidance.
- **Drug choice**: 0.25% Levobupivicaine
- **Drug volume**: 20–40 ml
- **Catheter technique:** After injection of half the volume of LA, thread the chosen catheter through or over the needle into the hypoechoic area created by LA injection. Aim to leave 5 cm of catheter adjacent to the nerve. Inject the remaining LA and secure the catheter in place.

Transgluteal Approach

Level of difficulty
Difficult

Ultrasound anatomy (Fig. 53.3)
Scanning protocol: Place the transducer at the midpoint between an imaginary line between the greater trochanter and ischial tuberosity, perpendicular to the expected course of the sciatic nerve.

The gluteus maximus muscle is striped in appearance. The fascial planes are hyperechoic and extend from GT to IT. The sciatic nerve is within this fascial plane, midway between the GT and IT, appearing as an oval hyperechoic structure.

Structures to identify: Greater trochanter; quadratus femoris muscle, the fascia separating the muscle bellies of the gluteus maximus muscle and the ischial tuberosity, sciatic nerve.

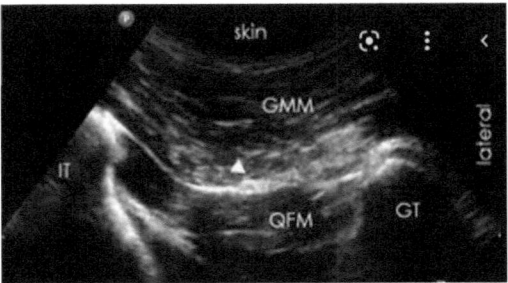

Fig. 53.3 Ultrasound image of greater trochanter (GT) and ischial tuberosity (IT) with fascia separating and position of probe

Block performance
- **Position:** Lateral position with side to be blocked facing up. Flex the hip and knee of the side to be blocked.
- **Ergonomics:** Place the ultrasound machine at the head of the bed with the operator standing on the side of the patient's back (patient facing away from them)
- **Probe:** Linear or curved (2–5 Hz) array depending on body habitus
- **Settings:** Nerve setting, high depth
- **Depth:** 40–50 mm
- **Needle size:** 80–100 mm, 22G echogenic block needle (150 mm may be needed in obese patients)
- **Needling technique:** In-plane, needling lateral to medial. Out-of-plane is also possible, but relies on seeing only the tip of the needle at more considerable depths.
- **Needle endpoint:** Pierce through the surrounding fascia, and as LA is incrementally injected, the nerve will hydrodissect away from the muscle
- **Drug choice:** 0.25% Levobupivicaine
- **Drug volume:** 10–20 ml (depending on the size of the patient)
- **Catheter technique:** After injection of half the volume of LA, thread the chosen catheter through or over the needle into the hypoechoic area created by LA injection. Aim to leave 5 cm of catheter adjacent to the nerve. Inject the remaining LA and secure the catheter in place.

Subgluteal Approach

Level of difficulty
Difficult

Ultrasound anatomy (Fig. 53.4)
Scanning protocol: Place the transducer transversely on the posterior thigh just caudal to the gluteus maximus muscle (buttock crease). Identify two muscle planes. Biceps femoris (laterally) and semitendinosus (medially) should be identified. Deep to these muscles lies the adductor magnus muscle. The sciatic nerve can be found running between these two muscle groups.

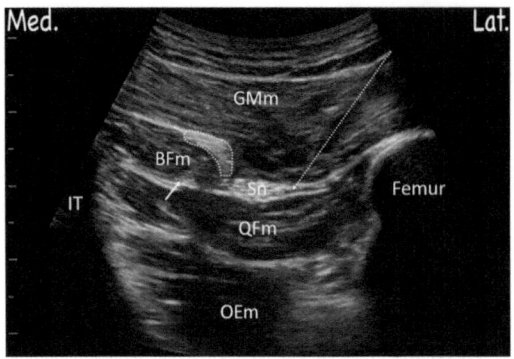

Fig. 53.4 Ultrasound image of sciatic nerve via the subgluteal approach

Structures to identify: semitendinosus, biceps femoris, adductor magnus muscles, and sciatic nerve.

Block performance
- **Position:** Lateral position with side to be blocked facing up. Flex the hip at 30–40° and the knee at 30–40° of the side to be blocked.
- **Ergonomics:** Place the ultrasound machine at the head of the bed with the operator standing on the side of the patient's back (patient facing away from them)
- **Probe:** Linear or curved (2–5 Hz) array depending on body habitus
- **Settings:** Nerve setting, high depth
- **Depth:** 40–80 mm
- **Needle size:** 80–100 mm, 22G echogenic block needle (150 mm may be needed in obese patients)
- **Needling technique:** In-plane, needling lateral to medial. Out-of-plane is also possible, but relies on seeing only the needle tip at more considerable depths.
- **Needle endpoint:** Pierce through the surrounding fascia and position the needle tip at either 3 or 9 o'clock to the nerve, and as LA is incrementally injected, the nerve will hydrodissect away from the muscle
- **Drug choice:** 0.25% Levobupivicaine
- **Drug volume:** 10–20 ml (depending on the size of the patient)
- **Catheter technique:** After injection of half the volume of LA, thread the chosen catheter through or over the needle into the hypoechoic

area created by LA injection. Aim to leave 5 cm of catheter adjacent to the nerve. Inject the remaining LA and secure the catheter in place.

Anterior Proximal Sciatic Approach

Level of difficulty
Advanced

Ultrasound Anatomy (Fig. 53.5)
Scanning protocol: Place the transducer transversely approximately 4–8 cm below the inguinal crease. Move the probe medially, laterally, superiorly, and inferiorly to identify the lesser trochanter of the femur. The edge of the hyperechoic lesser trochanter appears medially; externally rotating the lower limb can aid its identification. The flattened hyperechoic sciatic nerve can lie adjacent to or below the lesser trochanter in a fascia layer separating the gluteus maximus muscle and adductor muscles. The femoral artery and vein may be noted above the femur.

Structures to identify: Lesser trochanter of the femur, fascia separating gluteus muscle from adductor muscle, adductor magnus muscle, gluteus maximus muscle, and possibly femoral vessels.

Block performance
- **Position:** Supine
- **Ergonomics:** Place the ultrasound machine at the foot of the bed, with the operator facing the machine

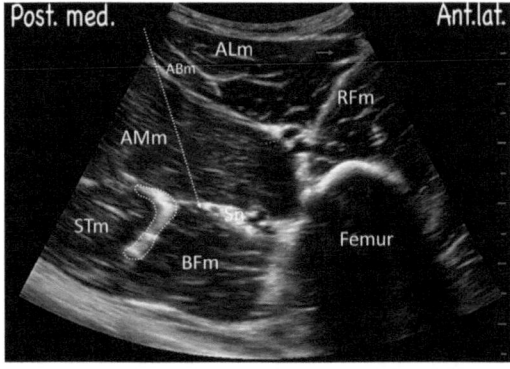

Fig. 53.5 Ultrasound image of sciatic nerve via the anterior approach

- **Probe:** Curved (2–5 Hz) array
- **Settings:** Nerve setting, high depth
- **Depth:** 60–100 mm
- **Needle size**: 80–100 mm, 22G echogenic block needle (150 mm may be needed in obese patients)
- **Needling technique**: The in-plane lateral to medial technique may require needling with the right or left hand, depending on the laterality of the block. Out-of-plane using hydro dissection can be a more practical way to accomplish this block compared to in-plane.
- **Needle endpoint:** Pierce through the surrounding fascia, and as LA is incrementally injected, the nerve will hydrodissect away from the muscle
- **Drug choice**: 0.25% Levobupivicaine
- **Drug volume**: 220–40 ml (depending on the size of the patient)
- **Catheter technique:** After injection of half the volume of LA, thread the chosen catheter through or over the needle into the hypoechoic area created by LA injection. Aim to leave 5 cm of catheter adjacent to the nerve. Inject the remaining LA and secure the catheter in place.

Thoracic Paravertebral Block

54

Arunangshu Chakraborty and Amit Dixit

First described by Sellheim in 1905. Thoracic paravertebral block (TPVB) is the technique by which local anaesthetic is injected in a wedge-shaped paravertebral space alongside the vertebral body called the thoracic paravertebral space (TPVS). This provides unilateral somatic and sympathetic blockade at selective thoracic segmental regions.

Level of difficulty Advanced

Anatomy

The TPVS is a wedge-shaped space bordering the vertebral bodies extending from T1 to T12 on either side of the vertebral column (Fig. 54.1).

The parietal pleura forms the anterolateral boundary. The base is formed by the vertebral body, intervertebral disc, intervertebral foramen, and its contents. The transverse process and the superior costotransverse ligament form the posterior boundary. Lying in between the parietal pleura anteriorly and the superior costotransverse ligament posteriorly is the endothoracic fascia, the thorax's deep fascia.

The endothoracic fascia is attached to the periosteum of the vertebral body. A layer of loose areolar connective tissue, the subserous fascia, lies between the parietal pleura and the endothoracic fascia (Fig. 54.2). Therefore, there are two potential fascial compartments in the TPVS: the anterior extra pleural paravertebral compartment and the posterior sub-endothoracic paravertebral compartment.

The TPVS contains adipose tissue within which lie the intercostal (spinal) nerve, the dorsal ramus, intercostal vessels, rami communicantes, and anteriorly, the sympathetic chain.

The spinal nerves are segmented into small bundles and lie freely in the TPVS's adipose tissue, which makes them accessible to local anaesthetic solutions injected into the TPVS. The TPVS communicates medially with the epidural space and intercostal space laterally.

Surface anatomy

C7 spinous process, Tips of thoracic spinous processes, the spine of the scapula, and the inferior angle of the scapula.

Indications
- Mastectomy
- Thoracotomy, Video-assisted thoracoscopic surgery & other chest wall surgery
- Analgesia for rib fractures
- Unilateral upper abdominal surgery- nephrectomy, cholecystectomy, hepatectomy, hernia repair, minimally invasive cardiac surgery
- Chronic chest wall neuropathic pain- post-thoracotomy, herpes & cancer pain, CRPS.

A. Chakraborty (✉)
Sultan Qaboos Comprehensive Cancer Care and
Research Centre, Muscat, Oman

A. Dixit
Department of Anaesthesia, Ruby Hall Hospital,
Pune, India

Fig. 54.1 Anatomy of thoracic paravertebral space: SCTL superior costotransverse ligament

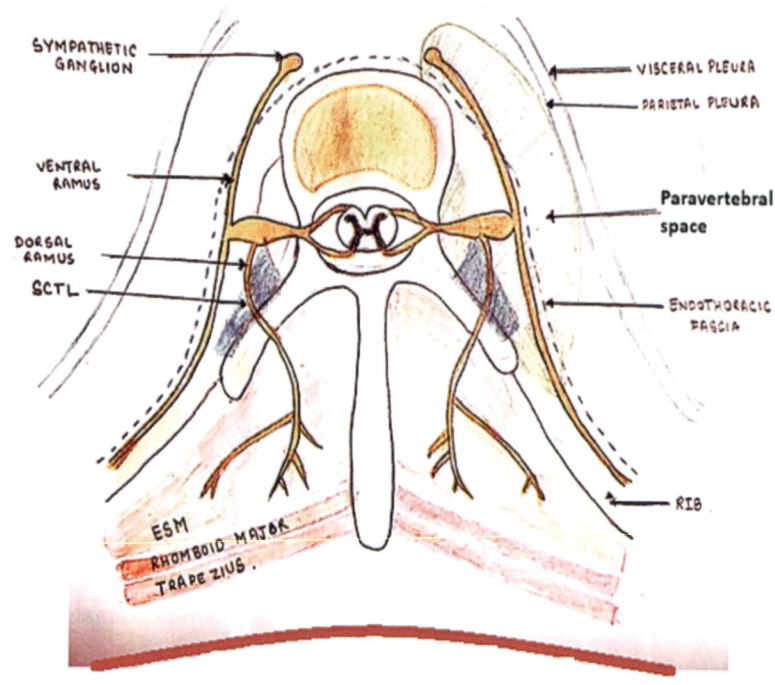

Fig. 54.2 Sagittal section through the paravertebral space

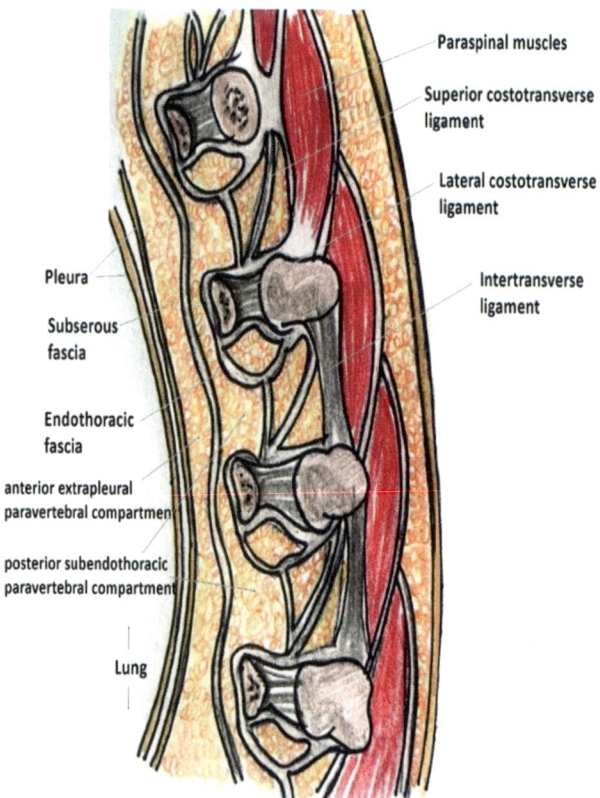

Nerves blocked

Thoracic sympathetic ganglia, multi-level thoracic spinal nerves.

Positioning

Patient sitting, lateral decubitus (sedated or under general anaesthesia), or prone (chronic pain procedures).

Structures to identify

Spinous process, transverse process, superior costo-transverse ligament, inner intercostal membrane, paravertebral space, ribs, pleura, paraspinal muscles.

Methods to perform a TPVB

There are three approaches to perform a TPVB

1. Landmark Based Technique: At the appropriate level, either a 20G/22G Tuohy or B bevel block needle can be used for single-shot injection. An 18G/16G Tuohy needle is used for catheter insertion. The needle is introduced 2.5 cm lateral to the highest spine level and perpendicularly to hit the transverse process. Then, the needle is removed and introduced again in the cephalad direction until loss of air resistance is elicited as soon as the needle traverses the superior costotransverse ligament. The depth of the space is 1–2 cm from the transverse process.

2. Ultrasound Assisted Technique: This is similar to the landmark technique, but a pre-procedure scan is done to assess the distance of the transverse process and TPVS from the skin. The ultrasound screening can be performed with either the transverse or parasagittal scans. In most patients, a high-frequency linear probe (6–13 MHz) may be sufficient; in obese patients, low-frequency USG with 2–5 MHz and lower depth settings may have to be used.

3. Ultrasound Guided Technique.

Scanning technique

1. PARASAGITTAL SCANNING: With the patient in sitting, lateral decubitus, or prone position, the probe is placed in the parasagittal plane 5–6 cm away from the midline. The hyperechoic curved shadow of the ribs with the bony drop-out shadow and the sharp hyperechoic pleura sliding beneath in the intercostal space are observed. The probe is then moved medially to observe the ribs diving more profoundly. At a transition point, 2–3 cm away from the midline, the deeper hyperechoic curved shadow of the ribs is replaced by the square top (square pattern) shaped transverse process shadow. Angling the foot end of the probe slightly obliquely and tilting the beam laterally in the window between the transverse processes shows, from below upwards, pleura, the triangular paravertebral space, the superior costotransverse ligament, the external intercostal muscles, and the paraspinal muscles (Fig. 54.3).

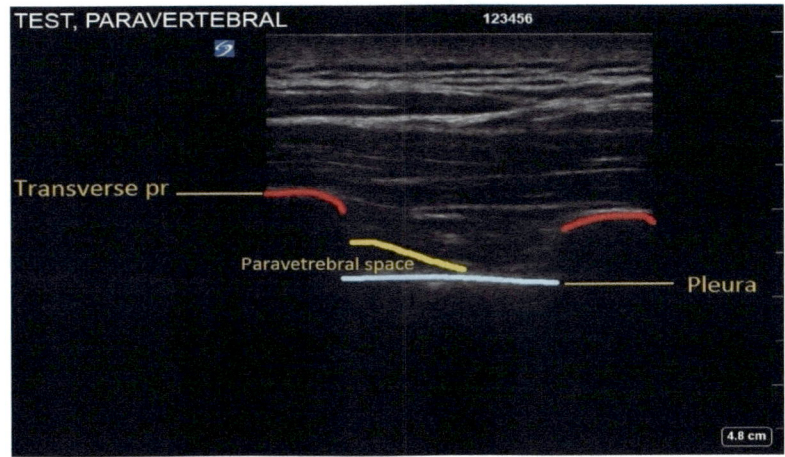

Fig. 54.3 Sonographic appearance of the parasagittal approach to the paravertebral space

Needling:

Parasagittal approach:

An in-plane (Fig. 54.4a) or out-of-plane (Fig. 54.4b) approach can be used for needle insertion. For the in-plane technique, keeping the lower transverse process at the edge of the screen where the needle is inserted allows for a steep insertion angle. Needle visualisation may be difficult because of the oblique position of the probe. If this approach is used, the needle should be contacted with the transverse process, and then it should be withdrawn and readvanced under the transverse process. If there is any doubt in finding the tip of the needle, hydrodissection should be done with 2–3 mL of saline. Once the superior costotransverse ligament is penetrated and local anaesthetic is injected, the pleura depresses, and the real-time spread of local anaesthetic can be seen. Extension of local anaesthetic can also be seen in other paravertebral spaces better with this view (Fig. 54.4a, b).

2. TRANSVERSE SCANNING

As the USG probe is placed transversely on the spinous process in the midline, the spinous process is visualized as a bright hyperechogenic dot with acoustic shadow anteriorly (Fig. 54.5). In the thoracic region, the spinous process is more angulated caudally than in the lumbar area. Hence, the lamina and transverse process lie above the spinous process. As the probe is placed laterally on the transverse process hyperechogenic lamina, the transverse process and the rib

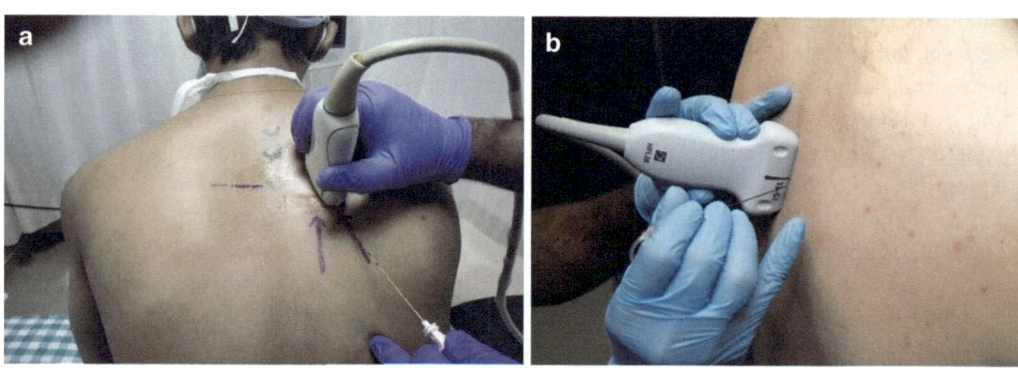

Fig. 54.4 (**a**) Parasagittal in plane TPVB. (**b**) Parasagittal out of plane TPVB

Fig. 54.5 Transverse midline scanning-spinous process view

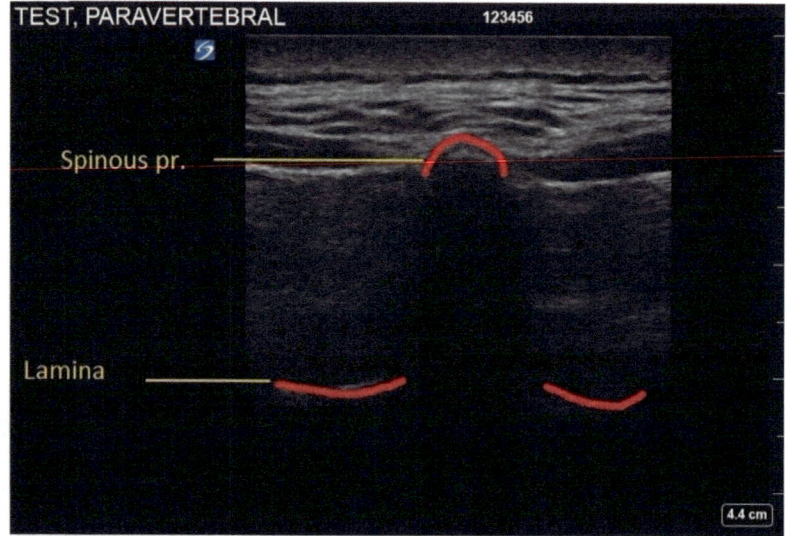

are identified (Fig. 54.6). After sliding it more caudally, only the hyperechogenic outline of the lamina and transverse process with their acoustic shadow are seen (Fig. 54.7). Lateral to transverse process anteriorly, hyperechogenic pleura and lung are visualized. Posteriorly lies the superior costotransverse ligament. A hypoechogenic paravertebral space is visualized between the two. Now, sliding the probe slightly caudally, the hyperechogenic articular process is seen medially with its acoustic shadow, and the superior costotransverse ligament, parietal pleura, lung, and apical part of paravertebral space are clearly defined. This view is between the transverse processes.

Needling:

The needle is inserted either in-plane (Fig. 54.8a–c) or out-of-plane (Fig. 54.8b) approach, either in the sitting position (Fig. 54.8a, b) or lateral decubitus position (Fig. 54.8c). Once the transverse process is contacted, the needle is withdrawn slightly and directed under the transverse process. After confirming negative aspiration for blood and CSF, local anaesthetic is injected. The pleura is depressed, and a rim of hypoechogenic fluid surrounds it.

Block performance

- Position/Ergonomics:
  - Patient sitting, the operator behind the patient, US machine in front of the patient & operator
  - Patient lateral decubitus, operator in front or behind the patient, machine facing operator
  - Patient prone, operator by the side to be blocked, machine in front of operator
- Probe: High-frequency   linear   probe (15–6 MHz, 25–38 mm) or Curvilinear C35 or C60 (2–5 MHz) probe

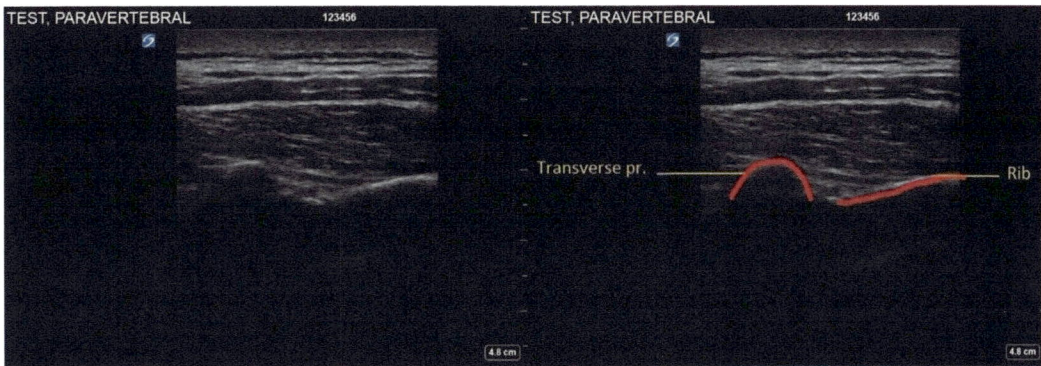

Fig. 54.6 Transverse scanning- transverse process and rib shadows

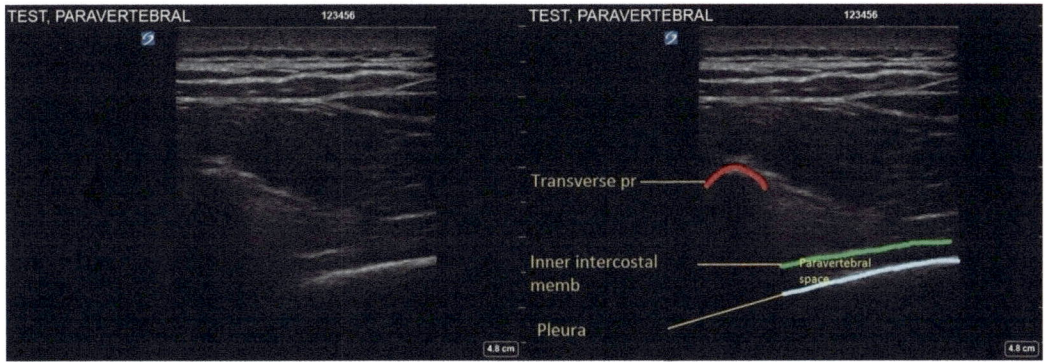

Fig. 54.7 Transverse scanning of TPVS

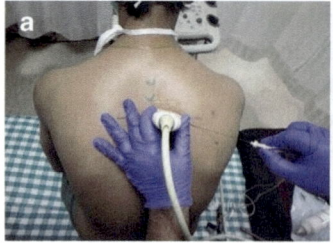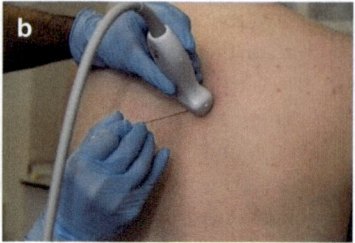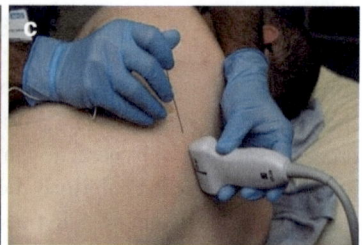

Fig. 54.8 Needling approaches (**a**) Sitting position, transverse in-plane technique, (**b**) Sitting position, transverse, out-of-plane technique, (**c**) Lateral position, transverse, in-plane technique

- Settings: Nerve/MSK, General/penetration, Compound imaging/Multibeam
- Depth: 3–8 cm
- Needle size: 50–80 mm short-bevel nerve block stimulating needle or 50–100 mm echogenic Tuohy needle
- Needling technique: As above
- Optimal needle tip position:
  - Parasagittal approach: Needle penetrates superior costotransverse ligament and enters paravertebral space; injection of LA produces depression of pleura
  - Transverse approach: Needle penetrates internal intercostal membrane and enters paravertebral space; injection of LA produces depression of pleura

Drug choice

1. Surgical Anaesthesia: 0.375–0.5% Ropivacaine or Levobupivacaine in the dose of 3–5 mL at each level. Multilevel injections with or without a catheter are preferred methods.
2. Post-operative analgesia: 0.3 mL/kg or 15–20 mL of 0.2% ropivacaine or 0.125–0.25% levobupivacaine
   - Volume: single level injection of 10 mL produces 3–4 dermatome spread, 20 mL produces 4–6 dermatome spread, 2 level injection of 10 mL each produces between 4 and 8 dermatome cover.
   - Optimal current if NS used: <0.5 mA at 2 Hz
   - Muscle responses acceptable: contraction of corresponding intercostal muscles

Clinical Pearls
- In the parasagittal approach, at the level of the transverse process, the pleura curves around the vertebral bodies to enter the mediastinum; hence, the visibility of the pleura is poor as the ultrasound beam is scattered and not reflected by the angulating probe laterally, the ultrasound beam is more perpendicular to the pleura and hence visibility improves.
- During needling in the parasagittal approach, keeping the inferior transverse process towards the edge of the screen allows a steeper insertion angle.
- Using echogenic needles allows for steep insertion angles and better needle visibility.
- Pleural drop may not always be seen in patients having a pre-existing pneumothorax.
- Although TPVB can provide excellent analgesia for thoracic surgeries, the manipulation of chest wall muscles such as pectoralis major, minor, serratus anterior and latissimus dorsi evoke pain as these muscles are innervated by branches of brachial plexus, which have a much higher (C5–T1) origin compared to the level of the paravertebral block (T3–T6).
- A higher volume of LA injected in TPVB on one side can theoretically block the other as the prevertebral space connects the two spaces.
- The sympathetic chain is also blocked as a part of TPVB, which is responsible for the superior quality of visceral analgesia.
- Interfascial plane blocks like erector spinae plane block, serratus anterior plane block, retrolaminar block, MTP (midpoint transverse

process to pleura), etc., are some of the newly emerging safer alternatives to paravertebral block.

- These blocks are easy to perform and have less chance of hematoma formation, hemodynamic fluctuations, and pneumothorax than TPVB.
- Prospect guidelines recommend TPVB as the first choice for postoperative analgesia in VATS and open thoracotomies as complications are less with TPVB when compared with thoracic epidural.

Side effects
- Epidural spread & hypotension
- Horner's syndrome

Complications
- Pneumothorax
- Inadvertent vascular injection
- LA toxicity
- Intercostal nerve injury
- Haemothorax
- High epidural/Total spinal

Contraindications
Absolute:
- Local infection
- Allergy to local anaesthetics
- Empyema
- Neoplasms in paravertebral space
- Coagulopathy

Relative:

- Severe kyphoscoliosis/chest wall deformity
- Previous chest wall surgery

Continuous techniques
- Indication:
  - Mastectomy
  - Rib fractures
  - Nephrectomy, Cholecystectomy, Liver surgery
- Kit: 16–18G Tuohy 50–100 mm, Echogenic needle with 17/19G multi orifice catheter

- Catheter: After the needle enters the paravertebral space, a catheter is inserted for 3–5 cm, surgical glue is applied to the puncture site, and the catheter is secured with a clip device and semi-permeable dressings.
- Pearls: Use of self-retaining catheters prevents intrapleural or accidental epidural migration after threading a catheter
- Regime:
  - Boluses 20 mL of 0.25% Bupivacaine eighth hourly
  - Infusion of 0.125% Bupivacaine at a rate of 8–12 mL/h
  - PCRA- 4 mL/h infusion, 20–30 mL 0.125% Bupivacaine bolus with 4 h lockout

Questions
1. What level of paravertebral block would you perform for a mastectomy, nephrectomy, or thoracotomy?
2. How many dermatomes will be reliably covered with a single-shot paravertebral block, and when would you consider a two-level paravertebral block?
3. What are the risks and benefits of a multilevel paravertebral block?
4. In addition to a TPVB, what other nerves need to be blocked for complete surgical anaesthesia for a mastectomy?
5. How could negative or positive pressure ventilation affect the spread of local anaesthetic in the paravertebral space?
6. What are the complications of TPVB?
7. What are newer approaches to block described?

Suggested Reading

1. Chakraborty A. Blockmate: a practical guide for ultrasound guided regional anaesthesia. Springer Nature; 2020.
2. Karmakar MK, et al. Atlas of sonoanatomy for regional anaesthesia and pain medicine. McGraw Hill Professional; 2017.
3. Hadzic A. Hadzic's peripheral nerve blocks and anatomy for ultrasound guided regional anaesthesia. 3rd ed. McGraw-Hill; 2021.

Serratus Plane Block

55

Arunangshu Chakraborty and Amit Dixit

The serratus plane block provides a multilevel dermatomal block from T2 to T9, involving the lateral divisions of the intercostal nerves.

Level of difficulty Basic

Anatomy

The spinal nerves exit the vertebral foramen; the ventral ramus becomes an intercostal nerve passing between the innermost and internal intercostal muscle. At the midaxillary line, the lateral cutaneous branch of each intercostal nerve pierces the intercostal and serratus anterior muscles. It divides into anterior and posterior branches to supply the anterolateral aspect of the chest wall.

The lateral cutaneous branch of the intercostal nerves travels in the fascial plane between the serratus anterior and latissimus dorsi. The thoracodorsal artery (branch of a subscapular artery) delineates the plane between the muscles. The nerve to the serratus anterior (the long thoracic) and the nerve to latissimus dorsi (thoracodorsal nerve) also travel in this plane.

Serratus Anterior Muscle (Fig. 55.1)

Origin: First eight ribs.

Insertion: Superior angle of the scapula (first slip), medial border of the scapula (next 3), inferior angle of the scapula (last 4).

Nerve: The long thoracic nerve is a branch of the upper trunk of the brachial plexus, which passes under the clavicle and over the first and second rib.

Action: Lateral rotation of the scapula.

Indications

- Mastectomy with or without reconstruction/subpectoral implant insertion
- Wide local excision of the breast.
- Sentinel node biopsy.
- Axillary clearance.
- Rib fractures are mainly anterolateral.
- Thoracotomy and VATS
- Unilateral subcostal incisions: Nephrectomy/Cholecystectomy

Nerves blocked [3]

1. Lateral branches of intercostal nerves T3–T9
2. Intercostobrachial nerve
3. Long thoracic nerve
4. Thoracodorsal nerve

Positioning

Patient supine, arm abducted, or patient in the lateral position.

A. Chakraborty (✉)
Sultan Qaboos Comprehensive Cancer Care and Research Centre, Muscat, Oman

A. Dixit
Department of Anaesthesia, Ruby Hall Hospital, Pune, India

Fig. 55.1 Anatomy of
serratus anterior block

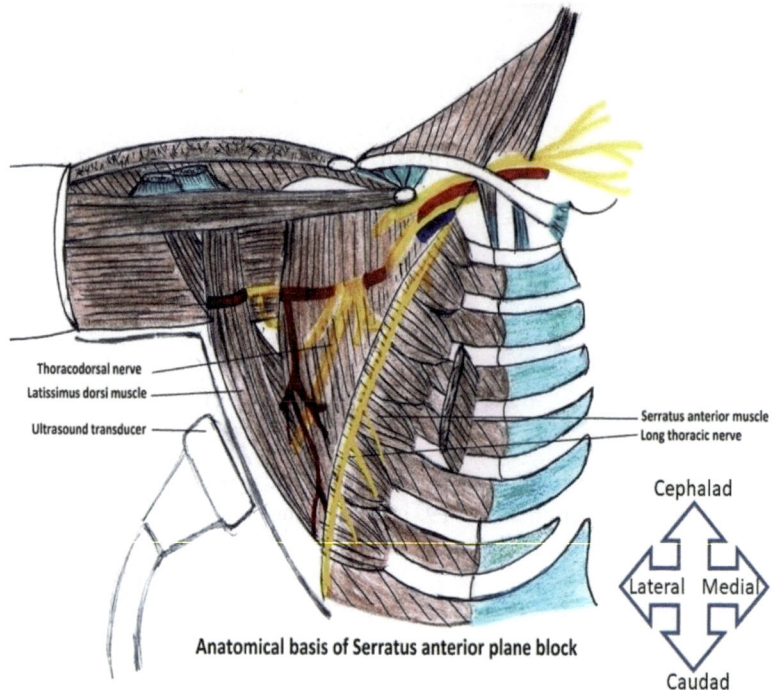

Thoracodorsal nerve
Latissimus dorsi muscle
Ultrasound transducer

Serratus anterior muscle
Long thoracic nerve

Cephalad

Lateral Medial

Caudad

Anatomical basis of Serratus anterior plane block

Scanning technique

Method 1: Patient supine, scanning as for Pec's 1
& 2 blocks with the probe continued in an inferolateral direction to identify the latissimus dorsi
and serratus anterior in the mid-axillary line at
the level of the fifth rib.

Method 2: Patient in the lateral position, probe
placed in the coronal plane in the posterior axillary line at the level of the fifth rib to identify the
latissimus dorsi and serratus muscle (Figs. 55.2,
55.3, and 55.4).

Structures to identify (Fig. 55.5)

Latissimus dorsi, serratus anterior, teres major,
thoraco-dorsal vessels, fourth or fifth rib, pleura.

Block performance

- Position/Ergonomics: Patient supine and arm
  abducted, operator coming from the patient's
  side (ipsilateral or contralateral), machine in
  front of operator. The patient is lateral and the
  probe is laced in the transverse or coronal
  plane.
- Probe: High-frequency linear probe
  (15–6 MHz, 25–38 mm)

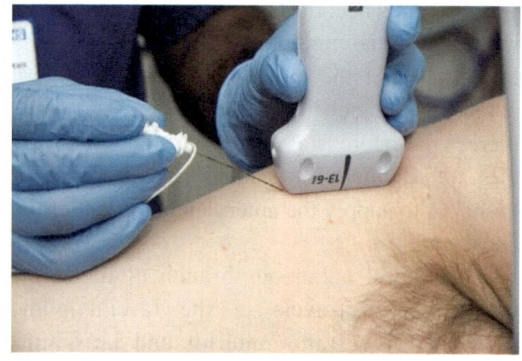

Fig. 55.2 Scanning and needling technique in coronal
plane

- Settings: Nerve/MSK, Resolution, Compound
  imaging/Multibeam
- Depth: 1–4 cm
- Needle size: 50–100 mm B-bevel nerve block
  needle
- Needling technique:
  - In plane anterior to posterior if the patient
    is in the supine position.
  - In plane caudad to cephalad in a coronal
    plane or in plane anteroposterior or pos-
    teroanterior with probe positioned trans-

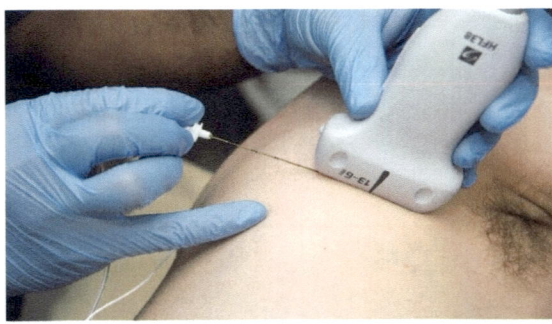
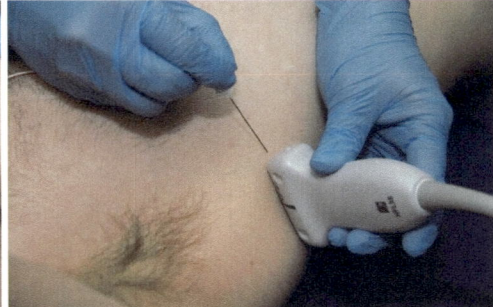

Fig. 55.3 and 55.4 Probe positioning and needling technique in lateral position with the probe placed transversely

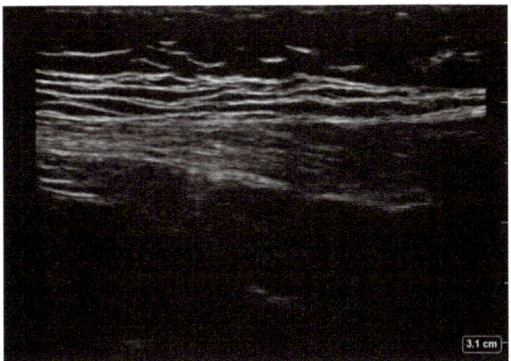

Fig. 55.5 Sonoanatomy of SAP block showing thoracodorsal artery as landmark between serratus anterior and latissimus dorsi

versely if the patient is in a lateral position.

- Optimal needle tip position: In the fascial plane between latissimus dorsi and serratus anterior, the thoracodorsal vessels serve as a landmark to delineate the paircraft Fig. 55.5 Injection above the serratus (superficial SAP block) or below the serratus, making contact with the rib (deep SAP block) produces a similar spread pattern and sensory analgesia. Two-level injections above (superficial) or below (deep) the serratus anterior muscle produce a spread from T2 to T9 (Fig. 55.6)
- Drug choice: 0.25% levobupivacaine or 0.2% ropivacaine.
- Volume: 20 ml injected at two levels, either above or below the serratus; total volume 40 ml.

Clinical Pearls

- The needle endpoint between serratus and latissimus dorsi reduces the likelihood of loss of the needle tip and the occurrence of pneumothorax.
- Injection into the plane above the serratus has a higher likelihood of intramuscular injection than injection between the serratus anterior and rib.
- Lifting off the serratus anterior muscle from the rib may be more painful in the awake patient.
- A deep serratus anterior plane block can be effectively administered to scarred or cicatrised chest walls e.g., thoracotomy pain syndrome, post-chemo and radiotherapy, when superficial serratus anterior plane block is not possible.
- The lateral cutaneous branch of the intercostal nerve will pierce the serratus anterior muscle at the midaxillary line. The opening of the serratus anterior plane should happen at the mid or posterior axillary line. A block performed anterior to the midaxillary line may produce inadequate analgesia.
- Deep serratus anterior plane block can be effectively administered using 2a 2G hypodermic needle over the fifth rib in the midaxillary line using the landmark method [5]. This technique is beneficial in resource-poor areas. Landmark-guided serratus anterior plane block can rescue breakthrough pain in wards after thoracic surgery e.g., accidental dis-

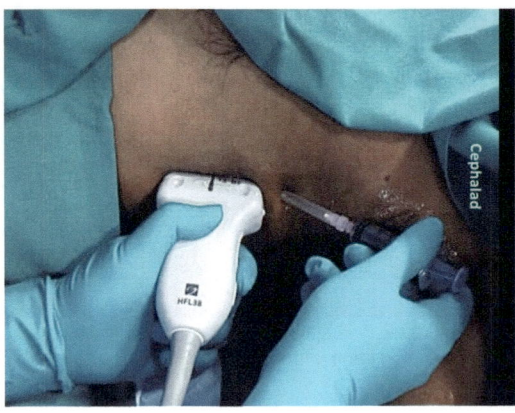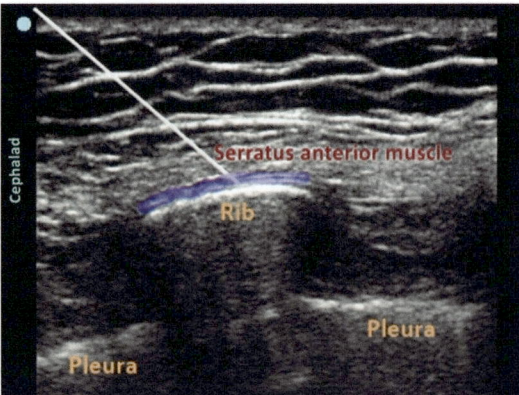

Fig. 55.6 Deep serratus anterior block

lodgement of epidural or paravertebral catheter post-surgery.

- Intensive care, emergency medicine, and surgery residents can be trained to perform serratus anterior plane blocks.
- Serratus anterior plane block with catheter insertion can aid weaning from ventilation in patients who have chest trauma and pain.
- This block can be utilised to alleviate pain due to intercostal drain (ICD)

Side effects

- Block of the long thoracic nerve and nerve to the serratus anterior can cause motor weakness
- DA dragging sensation or heaviness is noted on the anterolateral aspect of the chest wall.

Complications

- Pneumothorax
- Intramuscular injection
- LAST
- Infection
- Vascular injury
- Nerve injury (Thoracodorsal and long thoracic nerves)

Continuous techniques

The catheter can be inserted in the serratus plane for the management of pain following mastectomy & rib fractures.

The 18G Tuohy needle is inserted into the serratus plane in either the anteroposterior or caudo-cephalad direction. Hydrodissection should be done to create the fascial plane between latissimus dorsi and serratus, and the catheter should be inserted 3–5 cm beyond the needle tip. The catheter was secured with surgical glue and semipermeable dressings. A multi-orifice catheter is preferred as it's a fascial plane block.

Regime

- 20–30 ml 0.25% levobupivacaine or 0.375% ropivacaine eighth hourly
- Infusion of 0.125% levobupivacaine or 0.2% ropivacaine at a rate on 5–12 ml/h
- Patient controlled regional anaesthesia, PCRA- 4 ml/h infusion, 20–30 ml 0.125% levobupivacaine or 0.2% ropivacaine bolus with 4 h lock out
- A bolus regime would be preferred as this is a fascial plane block, and local anesthetic spread will be superior to a low volume hourly infusion.

Contraindications

1. Patient refusal
2. Patient on anticoagulants, low platelets, etc.
3. Local site infection
4. Drug allergy

Questions

1. If you are asked to perform an SAP block and insert a catheter for a patient with a rib fracture, what further information would you want to know before performing the block?

2. What vessels can be seen running between the latissimus dorsi and serratus anterior muscle?

3. A patient has lateral rib fractures in ribs 3–10; how can you manage this with a SAP block/catheter?

4. What is the difference between the pectoserratus and the serratus anterior plane block

5. What additional blocks would need to be performed for a mastectomy if a serratus anterior plane block is to provide complete analgesia

6. What are the advantages and disadvantages of a serratus anterior plane block over an erector spinae block for rib fractures

7. What are the advantages and disadvantages of a serratus anterior plane block over a paravertebral block for rib fractures

8. What would happen if a serratus anterior plane block is performed above the anterior axillary line?

Suggested Reading

1. Karmakar MK. Atlas of sonoanatomy for regional anesthesia and pain medicine. McGraw-Hill; 2018.

2. Hadzic A. Hadzic's peripheral nerve blocks and anatomy for ultrasound guided regional anesthesia. 3rd ed. McGraw-Hill; 2021.

3. Datu MD, et al. Serratus anterior plane block in modified radical mastectomy surgery; a case series. JA Clin Rep. 2020;6:82.

4. de Oliveira Camacho FC, et al. Continuous serratus anterior plane block provides analgesia in multiple rib fractures; a case report. Rev Bras Anesthsiol. 2019;69(1):87–90.

5. Vadera HK, et al. Serratus anterior plane block: anatomical landmark-guided technique. Saudi J Anaesth. 2020;14(1):134–5.

Interpectoral and Pecto-Serratus Block (PECs1 and PECs 2)

56

Arunangshu Chakraborty and Amit Dixit

Level of difficulty Basic

Anatomy

The muscles involved in the pectoral region are pectoralis Major, pectoralis Minor, serratus anterior, and latissimus Dorsi.

Pectoralis Major (Fig. 56.1)

Origin: Medial half of clavicle, anterior surface of sternum, first six costal cartilages.

Insertion: External oblique muscle, the lip of the bicipital groove of the humerus.

Nerve: Medial and lateral pectoral nerves. The lateral pectoral nerve is seen near the pectoral branch of the thoracoacromial artery, between the pectoralis major and pectoralis minor at the midclavicular line.

Action: Adduction of the extended limb, medial rotation of the arm, flexion of the upper limb, depression of the arm and shoulder, elevation of the rib.

Pectoralis Minor

Origin: Third–fifth ribs, fascia covering intercostal muscles.

Insertion: Coracoid process of the scapula

Nerve: Medial pectoral nerve

Action: Shoulder depression draws the scapula forward along with the serratus anterior.

Nerves

- Brachial plexus: Lateral and medial pectoral nerves arise from the brachial plexus's lateral and medial cords, respectively. The lateral Pectoral nerve (C5–C7) runs between the major and minor to supply the pectoralis major. The medial pectoral nerve (C8–T1) runs deep to the pectoralis minor to supply the pectoralis major and minor.
- Thoracic intercostal nerves arise from the anterior rami of the spinal nerves T1–T11. After emerging from the intervertebral foramen, the nerves travel in the paravertebral space between the parietal pleura and posterior intercostal membrane. The nerves then enter the intercostal space between the innermost and internal intercostal muscles and the intercostal vessels in the subcostal groove.
- The intercostal nerves at the midaxillary line give a lateral branch which pierces the external intercostal and serratus anterior muscles and then divides into the anterior and posterior divisions. The lateral branch of the second intercostal, the intercostobrachial nerve, innervates the skin and subcutaneous tissue of the axilla and proximal medial side of the arm.
- Near the sternum, the intercostal nerves pierce the pectoralis major muscle and emerge as the anterior cutaneous branches of the thorax.

A. Chakraborty (✉)
Sultan Qaboos Comprehensive Cancer Care and
Research Centre, Muscat, Oman

A. Dixit
Department of Anaesthesia, Ruby Hall Hospital,
Pune, India

S. Phillips et al. (eds.), *Regional Anaesthesia*, https://doi.org/10.1007/978-3-032-05165-3_56

Surface anatomy

The transducer is placed in sagittal orientation near the midclavicular line just below the clavicle.

Indications

1. Breast surgeries
2. Subpectoral prosthesis/breast expanders/ implant insertion
3. In addition to the paravertebral block following mastectomy or for awake breast surgeries to improve the functional movement of the arm and reduce opioid consumption
4. Thoracotomies
5. Analgesia for device insertions like subpectoral pacemaker or ICD (implantable cardioverter defibrillator) and subpectoral chemoport insertion.
6. Ribs and clavicle fractures
7. Axillary lymphadenopathy, sentinel node biopsy, shoulder surgery involving the armpit, high AV fistula near axilla .
8. Herpes Zoster infection, involving anterior dermatomes of the chest wall.

Nerves blocked

1. Medial and lateral pectoral nerves
2. Lateral cutaneous branches of intercostal nerves
3. Intercostobrachial nerve
4. Long thoracic nerve

Positioning This block is performed in the supine position with the arm abducted at 90 degrees and the elbow flexed.

Scanning technique

The probe is initially placed along the midclavicular line with parasagittal orientation just below the clavicle to identify the pectoral major and minor muscles. Later, the probe is moved caudally and laterally to determine the lateral border of pectoralis minor and to identify the serratus anterior just over the third and fourth rib.

Structures to identify

Pectoralis major, pectoralis minor and its lateral border, a pectoral branch of the thoracoacromial

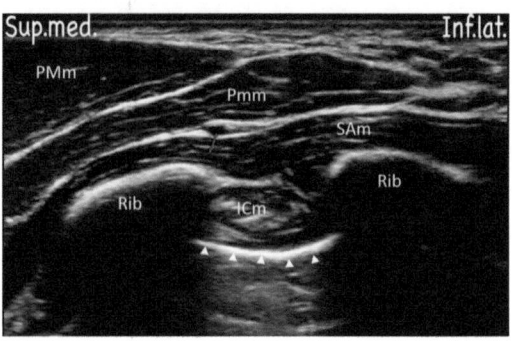

Fig. 56.1 PEC block

artery between two pectoral muscles, serratus anterior, ribs (third, fourth), pleural sliding, Gerdy's ligament (Fig. 56.1).

Block performance

- Position/Ergonomics: patient supine, operator standing by the head end, machine in front of patient & operator
- Probe: High-frequency linear probe (15–6 MHz, 25–38 mm)
- Settings: nerve, resolution, compound imaging/multibeam
- Depth: 1–4 cm
- Needle size: 50–100 mm B bevel nerve block stimulating needle
- Needling technique: In-plane, cephalad to caudad
- Optimal needle tip position:
- The needle is advanced medial to lateral.
  1. Interpectoral block (PECs 1 and the first injection of PECs 2): The local anaesthetic is injected between the major and minor pectoralis muscles. Separation of the fascial layer between the pectoralis major and minor is noted.
  2. Pecto-serratus block (second injection of PECs 2): The LA is injected between the pectoralis minor and serratus anterior.
- Surrogate structures: The pectoral branch of thoracoacromial vessels helps in delineating the plane between the two muscles for PECs 1 (interpectoral block)
- Drug choice & volume: 0.125%–0.25% Levobupivacaine or 0.2%–0.375% Ropivacaine with or without 4 mg dexametha-

sone. Usually 10 in interpectoral and around 15–20 ml in pecto-serratus plane block

Clinical Pearls

- Intramuscular injection is seen as a localised globular spread, and interfascial spread is seen as the local anaesthetic splitting the layers and spreading beyond the needle tip.
- Interfascial spread is seen as the local anaesthetic splitting the layers and spreading beyond the needle tip.
- It is always desirable to perform this block preoperatively, as postoperative air pockets will make sonoanatomy challenging.
- This block causes paralysis of pectoral nerves and is, therefore, better than LIA for surgeries involving stretching of pectoral muscles. e.g. subpectoral breast implant
- Multilevel TPVB with interpectrol blocks. It can be utilised for awake breast surgery. The intercostobrachial nerve (T2) blockade may be inconsistent in some patients and require additional infiltration by the surgeon.
- Reassurance and pre-procedural sedation with midazolam and fentanyl is desirable to allay anxiety if block is performed in awake patients. Deeply situated Pecto-serratus block injection is performed first, followed by superficial interpectoral Block while withdrawing the needle.
- Checking the block action with hot or cold saline for cutaneous mapping after block performance is essential.
- Using a colour Doppler to identify vessels before the block starts is essential.
- To avoid inadvertent pneumothorax, the needle tip must be visualised during slow and gradual needle advancement.
- These are interfascial plane blocks, so they are helpful for postoperative analgesia. However, unlike epidural or TPVB, they cannot provide predictable dermatomal coverage, so they cannot be utilised as the sole technique for surgical anaesthesia.
- Blockade of the lateral cutaneous branch of intercostal nerves via pesto block is inconsis-

tent, and it will not cover the whole hemithorax, making this block a poor choice for rib fractures.

Side effects

1. Pre-operative block sometimes distorts anatomical structures in the axillary area and can increase challenges in the surgical field.
2. Pectoral muscle paralysis causes a heaviness and dragging sensation over the anterior chest, which can be annoying to some patients.

Complications

1. Pneumothorax
2. Hematoma formation due to bleeding from the thoracoacromial vessels
3. Infections
4. LAST

Continuous techniques

- Indication: Analgesia following mastectomy
- Kit: 18G Tuohy echogenic needle
- Approach: similar to single shot technique, in-plane, cephalad to caudad
- Catheter: inserted 3–5 cm in the plane between pectoralis minor and serratus anterior.
- Regime:
  - 20–30 ml 0.25% levobupivacaine or 0.2% Ropivacaine eighth hourly
  - Infusion of 0.125% levobupivacaine or 0.2% Ropivacaine at the rate of 5–12 ml/h via balloon elastomeric pump [5]
  - e.g.
    PCRA (patient-controlled regional anaesthesia) with PIB (programmed intermittent bolus)
    20–30 ml 0.125% levobupivacaine bolus with 4 h lockout and 8–10 ml programmed intermittent bolus every hour with no background infusion.

Contraindications

1. Patient refusal
2. Patient on anticoagulants, low platelets, etc.
3. Local site infection
4. Drug allergy

Questions

1. Compare and contrast PECs 1, PECs 2, SAP, and ESP
2. Role of these blocks in patients with LD flap
3. Prevention and management of pneumothorax.
4. Can these blocks be used as a sole technique for surgical anaesthesia in procedures like subpectoral placement of pacemakers, chemoport, etc?

Suggested Reading

1. Karmakar MK. Atlas of sonoanatomy for regional anaesthesia and pain medicine. McGraw-Hill; 2018.
2. Zhang N, Wang T, Wei P, Zhou J, Li J. Ultrasound-guided regional anesthesia under sedation for radical mastectomy in an SAS patient: a case report. Front Oncol. 2021;11:631003.
3. Luo G, Zhu J, Ni H, et al. pretreatment with pectoral nerve block II is effective for reducing pain in patients undergoing thoracoscopic lobectomy: a randomised, double-blind, placebo-controlled trial. Biomed Res Int. 2021;2021:8. Article ID 6693221.
4. Hadzic A. Hadzic's peripheral nerve blocks and anatomy for ultrasound guided regional anesthesia. 3rd ed. McGraw Hill; 2021.
5. Shakuo T, et al. Continuous Pecs II block for postoperative analgesia in patients undergoing transapical transcatheter aortic valve implantation. JA Clin Rep. 2017;3:65.

Arunangshu Chakraborty and Amit Dixit

Quadratus Lumborum Block (QLB) is an emerging proximal interfascial plane block in the posterior abdominal wall postulated to provide somatic and visceral analgesia for abdominal surgery. It originated as a variation of the posterior TAP block; thereafter, various technique modifications have been described.

Level of difficulty Advanced

Anatomy

The quadratus lumborum (QL) muscle originates from the iliac crest and attaches to the inferior border of the 12th rib and the transverse process of L1–L4 vertebrae. The QL muscle is enclosed by the thoracolumbar fascia (TLF), which is the key structure determining the spread of injected LA. The TLF is a cylindrical fibrous connective tissue layer enclosing the paraspinal muscles; it has three layers: the anterior, middle, and posterior. The psoas major (PM) lies anterior to the anterior layer of TLF; the anterior and middle layers enclose the QL, and the erector spinae is enclosed between the middle and posterior layers of the TLF. The TLF medially is attached to the thoracic and lumbar vertebrae, continues cranially with the endothoracic fascia, and caudally with the fascia iliaca. The anterior layer blends medially with the fascia covering the psoas and laterally with the transversalis fascia. The middle layer of the TLF joins the deep lamina of the posterior layer at the lateral border of the erector spinae to form the fascial structure called the lumbar interfascial triangle (LIFT).

The fascial plane between the QL and PM is thought to be continuous with the paravertebral plane, which is why a QL block, unlike any other muscle plane block of the abdominal wall, is considered to produce autonomic blockade and resultant visceral analgesia.

Indications

- Procedures requiring bilateral blocks:
  - Lower abdominal surgery: Caesarean section, gynaecologic laparoscopic surgery
  - Midline/upper abdominal surgery: bowel resection (small/extensive), gastrectomy
- Procedures requiring unilateral blocks
  - Colostomy, appendicectomy, inguinal hernia repair, nephrectomy (laparoscopic or open)

Nerves blocked: T6–L1 spinal nerves (possibly higher if paravertebral spread), sympathetic trunk.

Positioning

- Lateral decubitus (for all approaches to QLB)
- Supine with a wedge under the hip (only lateral QLB)
- Supine position for the anterior approach of the QLB

A. Chakraborty (✉)
Sultan Qaboos Comprehensive Cancer Care and Research Centre, Muscat, Oman

A. Dixit
Department of Anaesthesia, Ruby Hall Hospital, Pune, India

Scanning technique

With the patient in a lateral position (anterior or transmuscular) (Fig. 57.3b) or supine position (lateral or posterior), linear/curvilinear ultrasound transducer (UST) placed in the transverse plane above the iliac crest, the three layers of the abdominal wall, external oblique (EOM), internal oblique (IOM), transversus abdominis (TAM) are identified and traced backwards until TAM can be seen tapering into an aponeurosis. The QL is a boat-shaped muscle generally seen attached to the transverse process of the lumbar vertebra (L1). The psoas major (PM) muscle is anterior to the QL, and posterior to the erector spinae (ES). The retroperitoneal fat, the kidney, and the layers of the TLF can be identified anterior to QL and PM.

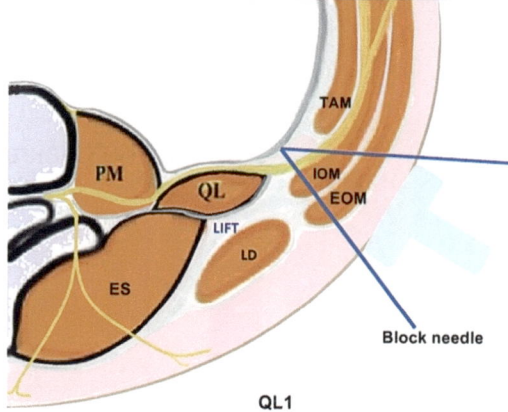

Fig. 57.1 QL1 Block: Note the linear UST, needle approach in plane and injection endpoints. PM Psoas major, QL QL, IOM Internal oblique muscle, EOM External oblique muscle, LD Latissimus dorsi muscle

Structures to identify

Muscles: External oblique, internal oblique, transversus abdominis, QL, PM, latissimus dorsi

Fasciae: thoracolumbar fascia

Bony surface: transverse process (of L1), body of lumbar vertebra (L1)

Others: retroperitoneum with kidney, intrabdominal contents (bowel loops)

Types of QLB (Figs. 57.1, 57.2, and 57.3)

1. Lateral QLB (QLB 1)

For the type 1 QL (QL1) block, a linear transducer is placed in the axial plane in the midaxillary line and moved posteriorly until the posterior aponeurosis of the TAM becomes visible as a strong specular reflector. The injection endpoint is deep to the aponeurosis but superficial to the TF at the lateral margin of the QL muscle. This is just lateral to the pararenal fat compartment. The needle is inserted from either the anterior or the posterior end of the transducer and advanced until the needle tip penetrates the posterior aponeurosis of the TAM. Local anaesthetic (LA) is injected between the aponeurosis and the TF at the lateral margin of the QL muscle. The main effect is the anaesthesia of the lateral cutaneous branches of the iliohypogastric, ilioinguinal, and subcostal nerves (T12–L1).

A catheter can be inserted in the QL1 technique for continuous analgesia.

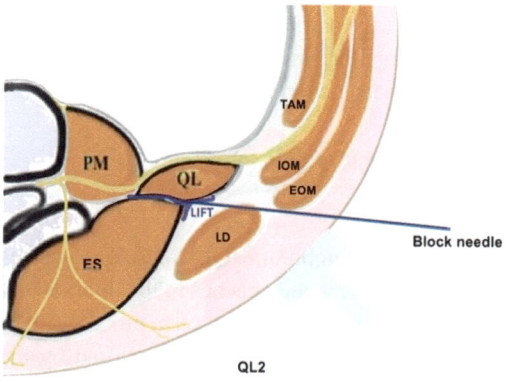

Fig. 57.2 QL2 Block: Note the linear UST, needle approach in plane and injection endpoints. PM Psoas major, LIFT Lumbar interfascial triangle

QL1 block is identical to the fascia transversal plane block.

2. Posterior QLB (QLB 2)

In the type2 of QL (QL2) block, a linear/curvilinear transducer is placed transversely in the mid-axillary line and moved posteriorly as in the QL1 nerve block, until the lumbar interfascial triangle (LIFT), bound posteriorly by latissimus dorsi (LD), medially by erector spinae and anteriorly by QL can be imaged. The needle is inserted from the lateral end of the transducer. The needle tip is advanced until it is

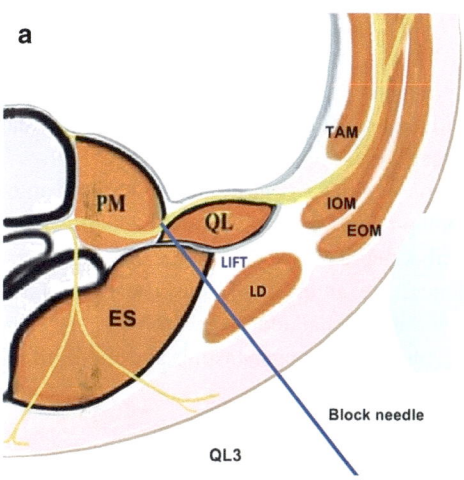
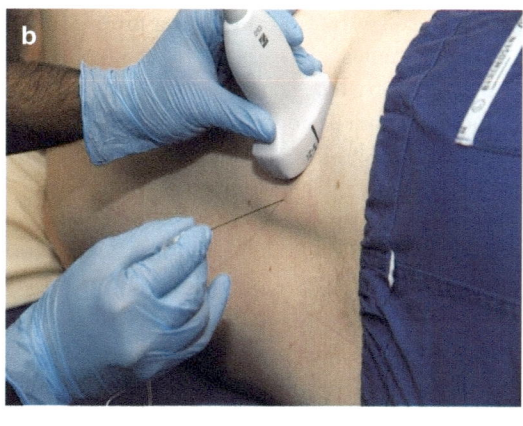

Fig. 57.3 (**a**) QL3 Block: Note the curvilinear UST, needle approach in plane and injection endpoint between the QL and the PM. LIFT Lumbar interfascial triangle. (**b**) Position for QL3

inside the middle layer of the TLF close to the LIFT. The local anesthetic is injected intrafascially. QL2 has been reported to provide analgesia equivalent to TQL nerve block but with a faster onset.

As a variation of the technique, the LIFT can be injected and expanded with LA at first, following which the needle can be directed medially to enter the middle layer of the TLF between QL and ES.

3. Anterior QLB/Transmuscular QLB/QLB 3

The transmuscular QL block, known as TQL, anterior QL, and QL3, employs a curved array transducer. UST is placed in the axial plane on the patient's flank, just cranial to the iliac crest. The "shamrock sign" is visualised: The transverse process of vertebra L4 is the stem, whereas the erector spinae posteriorly, QL laterally, and psoas major anteriorly represent the three leaves of the trefoil. The target for injection is the fascial plane between the QL and psoas major muscles. The needle is inserted using an in-plane technique from the posterior end of the transducer through the QL muscle (Fig. 57.3b). The injectate should ideally spread from the injection site inside the fascial plane between the QL and psoas major muscles to the thoracic paravertebral space to

accomplish segmental somatic and visceral analgesia from T4 to L1.

4. Intramuscular QLB (QLB 4)

For the Intramuscular QLB, the patient should be placed supine or lateral decubitus. Following identification of QL, the practitioner inserts the needle in an in-plane approach and an anterolateral to posteromedial direction with an injection of LA directly into the muscle.

Block performance
- Position/Ergonomics: For lateral and posterior QLB, the patient is supine with a wedge under the hip, with the operator on the same side of the patient and the machine in front of the operator. Depending on operator dexterity, the setup can be moved around or done from the same side for bilateral blocks. Anterior and intramuscular QLB is performed with the patient placed in the lateral position with the side to be blocked uppermost, the operator facing the patient's back, and the US machine in front of the patient and operator. The patient position and set-up can be changed for bilateral blocks, or the block could be done from the same position as the operator, only turning the patient to the respective sides.

- Probe: 2–5 MHz C60 curvilinear probe (anterior, intramuscular), high-frequency linear probe (15–6 MHz, 38 mm) in thin patients and for lateral and posterior QLB)
- Settings: MSK, General/Resolution, Compound imaging/Multibeam
- Depth: 5–8 cm in general, 3–5 cm in thin patients
- Needle size: 50–80 mm short bevel nerve block needle
- Needling technique:
  - Lateral QLB: Transverse, in-plane, lateral to medial approach
  - Posterior QLB: Transverse, in-plane, lateral to medial approach
  - Anterior & Transmuscular QLB: Transverse, in plane, posteromedial to anterolateral
- Optimal needle tip position
  - Lateral QLB: In this block, the injection is done laterally to the QL at contact with the transversal fascia, where the TAM tapers off as aponeurosis.
  - Posterior QLB: the injection is done posteriorly, between the QL and the middle layer of the TLF, i.e., between QL and erector spinae muscle
  - Anterior QLB: The injection is done between the QL and the psoas major.
  - Intramuscular QLB: injection done into the body of the QL muscle.
- Drug choice: 0.25% Bupivacaine or 0.375% Ropivacaine
- Volume: 20 ml per side blocked has been commonly used in all trials. The optimal volume and concentration of LA are yet to be determined.
- Testing block success: loss of sensation to touch, temperature, and pinprick in the T7–L1 dermatomal distribution.

Clinical Pearls

- Angulating the probe caudally improves the visibility of the QL muscle
- The anterior QL is the most technically challenging approach; the other approaches are still intermediate-level blocks.
- The spread patterns for the different approaches vary posterior (T7–L1), lateral

(T7–L1), intramuscular (T7–T12), anterior T10–L4
- Lateral and posterior QL have the current best evidence to be recommended for abdominal surgery.
- Motor weakness is more likely with the anterior approach due to the involvement of the lumbar nerve roots between the QL and psoas. Hence, the anterior QL may be helpful for lower abdominal and lower limb surgery.
- QL blocks are longer-lasting and more effective than TAP blocks.

Side effects

- Lower limb weakness & mechanical falls

Complications

- Visceral injury (bowel, kidney)
- LAST
- Bleeding/hematoma

Continuous techniques

- Indication: Extended abdominal surgery analgesia, predominantly somatic and visceral analgesia. This is also indicated in situations where, in addition to midline incision, the presence of stomas and drains complicates pain management. Bilateral blocks are needed for midline incisions.
- Position: as above for single-shot technique
- Kit: 18G/16G Tuohy echogenic needle is inserted into the QL plane either in the posteroanterior (Anterior or Transmuscular QL) or anteroposterior direction (lateral or posterior QL). Hydrodissection should be done to create the fascial plane depending on the type of QLB, and a 17/19G catheter should be inserted for 3–5 cm. The catheter was secured with surgical glue and semi-permeable dressings. A splitter device can attach both catheters to a single pump.
- Regime
  - If inserted bilaterally, 20 ml 0.25% Bupivacaine or 0.375% Ropivacaine eighth hourly **via each catheter**.
  - Infusion of 0.125% Bupivacaine or 0.2% Ropivacaine at a rate of 10–14 ml/h via splitter device

– PCRA-4 ml/h infusion, 20–30 ml 0.125% Bupivacaine or 0.2% Ropivacaine bolus via splitter device with 4 h lockout

Contraindications

- Local inflammation/infection/skin disease
- Known allergy to LA
- As transmuscular QL is a deep block, it is advisable to use caution in coagulopathic patients. Though thrombocytopenia or coagulopathy are not absolute contraindications, caution must be applied.

Suggested Reading

1. Blanco R. TAP block under ultrasound guidance: the description of a 'non pops technique. Reg Anesth Pain Med. 2007;32(1):130.
2. Kadam VR. Ultrasound-guided quadratus lumborum block as a postoperative analgesic technique for laparotomy. J Anaesthesiol Clin Pharmacol. 2013;29:550–2.
3. Blanco R, Ansari T, Girgis E. Quadratus lumborum block for postoperative pain after caesarean section: a randomised controlled trial. Eur J Anaesthesiol. 2015;32:812–8.
4. Hebbard PD. Transversalis fascia plane block, a novel ultrasound-guided abdominal wall nerve block. Can J Anesth. 2009;56:618–20.
5. Abrahams M, Derby R, Horn J-L. Update on ultrasound for truncal blocks: a review of the evidence. Reg Anesth Pain Med. 2016;41:275–88.
6. Blanco R, McDonnell JG. Optimal point of injection: the quadratus lumborum type I and II blocks. 2013. http://www.respond2articles.com/ANA/forums/post/1550.aspx.
7. Murouchi T, Iwasaki S, Yamakage M. Quadratus lumborum block: analgesic effects and chronological ropivacaine concentrations after laparoscopic surgery. Reg Anesth Pain Med. 2016;2016(41):146–50.
8. Willard FH, Vleeming A, Schuenke MD, Danneels L, Schleip R. The thoracolumbar fascia: anatomy, function and clinical considerations. J Anat. 2012;221:507–36.
9. El-Boghdadly K, Elsharkawy H, Short A, Chin KJ. Quadratus lumborum block nomenclature and anatomical considerations. Reg Anesth Pain Med. 2016;41(4):548–9.
10. Elsharkawy H. Quadratus lumborum block with paramedian sagittal oblique (subcostal) approach. Anaesthesia. 2016;71:241–2.
11. Blanco R, Ansari T, Riad W, Shetty N. Quadratus lumborum block versus transversus abdominis plane block for postoperative pain after cesarean delivery. Reg Anesth Pain Med. 2016;41:757–62.
12. Lin J-A, Chuang T-Y, Yao H-Y, Yang S-F, Tai Y-T. Ultrasound standard of peripheral nerve block for shoulder arthroscopy: a single-penetration double-injection approach targeting the superior trunk and supraclavicular nerve in the lateral decubitus position. Br J Anaesth. 2015;115:932–4.
13. Carline L, McLeod GA, Lamb C, Colvin L. A cadaver study comparing the spread of dye and nerve involvement after three different quadratus lumborum blocks. Br J Anaesth. 2016;117:387–94.
14. Baidya DK, Maitra S, Arora MK, Agarwal A. Quadratus lumborum block: an effective method of perioperative analgesia in children undergoing pyeloplasty. J Clin Anesth. 2015;27:694–6.
15. Spence NZ, Olszynski P, Lehan A, Horn J-L, Webb CAJ. Quadratus lumborum catheters for breast reconstruction requiring transverse rectus abdominis myocutaneous flaps. J Anesth. 2016;30:506–9.
16. Ueshima H, Yoshiyama S, Otake H. The ultrasound-guided continuous transmuscular quadratus lumborum block is an effective analgesia for total hip arthroplasty. J Clin Anesth. 2016;31:35.

Transversus Abdominis Plane Block

58

Arunangshu Chakraborty

A. Chakraborty (✉)
Sultan Qaboos Comprehensive Cancer Care and
Research Centre, Muscat, Oman

Level of difficulty Basic

Anatomy

Transversus abdominis plane (TAP) block is a fascial plane block described first by Rafi as an anatomical landmark-guided abdominal field block with the potential to provide somatic post-operative analgesia from dermatomes T7-L1.

Innervation
The somatic innervation of the anterior abdominal wall is from thoracoabdominal nerves (T7-L1). The anterior rami of the lower thoracic nerves (T7–11), which are a continuation of intercostal nerves and run in between the transversus abdominis (TAM) and internal oblique (IOM) muscles- the "TAP" plane (Fig. 58.1). Each thoraco-abdominal nerve gives off branches as posterior, lateral, and anterior cutaneous branches to supply the skin of the abdomen and back. The Lateral cutaneous nerves supply the lateral abdominal wall after passing through the TAP plane, and terminal branches pierce the rectus sheath and rectus muscle to continue as anterior cutaneous nerves. Aberrant nerves may arise from the lateral aspect of the linea semilunaris and may cause block sparing.

The Ilioinguinal (IL) & Iliohypogastric (IH) nerves arise from the anterior primary rami of L1 originating in the lumbar plexus. Both these nerves emerge from the lateral border of the psoas and travel over the quadratus lumborum and iliacus. The IL nerve penetrates TAM near the anterior part of the iliac crest and travels in the TAP plane. This nerve then penetrates the internal oblique, enters the inguinal canal, travels along with the spermatic cord in males (round ligament in females), and emerges through the superficial inguinal ring to supply the upper and medial thigh skin.

Nerves blocked
T 7- T12 lateral & anterior divisions of spinal nerves, Ilioinguinal & Iliohypogastric nerves.

Indications
- Lower abdominal incisions (midline, Pfannenstiel)- require bilateral block
  Gynaecologic surgery- hysterectomy, caesarean section.
  Urologic surgery- prostatectomy.
  General surgery-large bowel resection, laparoscopic cholecystectomy
- Unilateral abdominal surgery
  Inguinal hernia repair, appendicectomy.
  Nephrectomy.

Types of TAP block
- **Landmark-based TAP block**
- **Ultrasound-guided - Lateral, posterior, and anterior approaches**

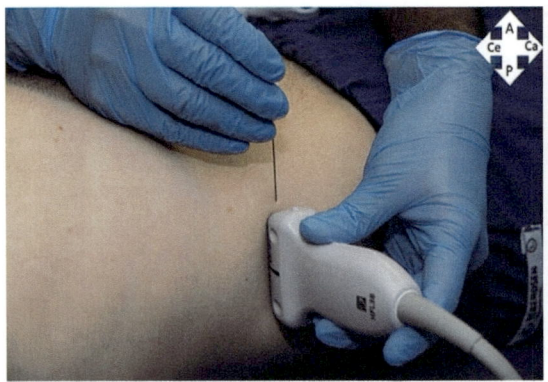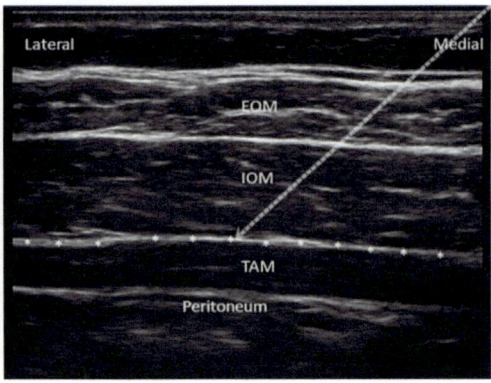

Fig. 58.1 Lateral TAP: Note that the needle (dotted line) enters from a medial to lateral direction, LA deposited in the plane between IOM and TAM. Asterisks denote the TAP plane. EOM = External oblique muscle, IOM = Internal oblique muscle, TAM = Transversus abdominis muscle

Surface anatomy

Iliac crest, a triangle of petit, latissimus dorsi (LD), inferior costal margin, lateral border of rectus abdominis, mid-clavicular, mid-axillary, and posterior axillary lines.

Landmark Technique

In this technique, the landmark is the lumbar triangle of Petit (LTP), a triangular space bound anteriorly by the lateral/ posterior border of the EOM, posteriorly by the anterior border of LD, and caudally by the iliac crest. The advantage of this area is that there is only one muscle above the TA plane here, i.e., the IOM.

Position and ergonomics The patient is positioned laterally, with the side to be blocked uppermost. The operator stands behind the patient. The supine position may be more straightforward for bilateral blocks, with the operator on the ipsilateral side of the block.

Technique LTP is identified by palpating the iliac crest posterior to the mid-axillary line and then palpating the anterior border of LD. A short bevel or blunt-tipped 22 G needle is entered perpendicularly through the skin and gradually introduced deeper. Two distinct "pops" (loss of resistance) will be appreciated when the needle tip traverses the anterior and posterior epimysium

of IOM. After the second "pop," the needle tip should lie in the TAP plane. Upon negative aspiration for blood, LA solution is slowly injected. The injection pressure typically should be less than 10 psi.

Ultrasound technique

The TAP block is one of the most versatile fascial plane blocks. As the effect of any fascial plane block depends on the nerves affected by the local anaesthetic (LA) solution, the clinical impact depends on the choice of the LA, volume injected, and the injection site. Presumably, a site of interfascial injection closer to the surgical incision provides more potent analgesia compared with a site further away. Based on this hypothesis, various modifications of the TAP block have been described, each employing a different injection site, but ultimately targeting the same interfascial plane, i.e., the "TAP" plane. Four approaches were described for ultrasound-guided TAP block: lateral, posterior, anterior, and oblique subcostal.

Scanning technique

Lateral TAP block: A high-frequency linear probe is placed in the transverse plane in the lateral abdominal wall between the costal margin and the iliac crest in the mid-axillary line (lateral approach). The three muscular layers of the abdominal wall, namely EOM, IOM, and TAM, are identified. Deeper to the TAM, the transversalis fascia (TF), peritoneum, and bowel contents can be seen. Further posterior movement of the probe, the TA tapers, becomes an aponeurosis, and merges with the thoracolumbar fascia covering the quadratus lumborum (QL) (posterior approach).

Subcostal TAP block A high-frequency linear probe is placed in the transverse oblique subcostal plane and moved inferolaterally. At the level of the xiphoid, the rectus muscle and linea alba can be seen, as the probe is moved laterally, the first muscle to be seen under the rectus abdominis (RAM) is the TAM, further laterally, the division of the IO to form the two layers of the rectus sheath and the EO aponeurosis are visualised. Further inferolateral movement demonstrates the same three layers of abdominal muscles in the subcostal region. Needle entry is usually from a medial to lateral direction, and LA is injected at the plane between the RAM and the TAM.

Structures to identify
EOM, IOM, TAM, RAM, Linea semilunaris (LS) TF, QL, peritoneum, intraabdominal contents.
1. **Lateral TAP:** It is also known as the classical TAP block. LA is injected in the "TAP" plane with the ultrasound transducer (UST) placed transversely in the mid-axillary line, between the iliac crest and the costal margin (Fig. 58.1). The block needle enters a plane from the anterior axillary line aimed inferolaterally. This is the most used variant of the TAP block and one of the easiest to master. The needle should enter the skin a few centimetres away from the near end of the UST footprint, making the angle less acute and thus the needle easily observable with ultrasound. This technique is also one of the safest, as the needle tip has a minimal chance of entering the abdomen (Fig. 58.1).
2. **Posterior TAP:** Injection in the lumbar triangle of Petit. Usually employed in the landmark-based technique. The drug is injected between the TAM aponeurosis/fascia transversalis and the internal oblique muscle. This technique is considered the precursor of the quadratus lumborum block. The UST is held transversely in the posterior axillary line (Fig. 58.2). Compared with the other varia-

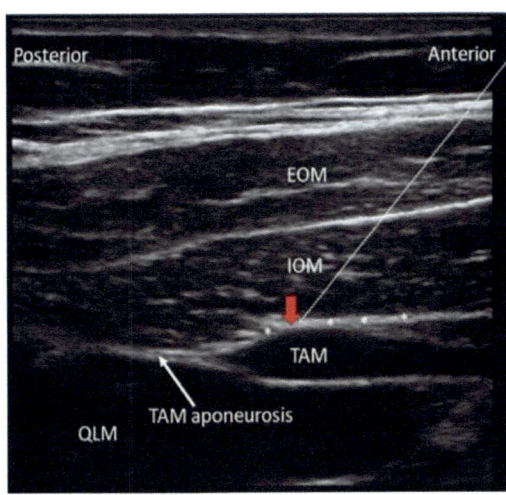

Fig. 58.2 Posterior TAP: asterisks denote the TAP plane; the red arrow indicates the ideal injection point and the dotted line represents the block needle

tions, the posterior TAP block is challenging technically. The patient position and technical details are described below.
3. **Anterior TAP:** The ultrasound transducer is held transversely in the mid-clavicular line and scanned laterally until the three abdominal muscles are seen. The needle is inserted from medial to lateral, and LA is deposited in the TAP plane.
4. **Oblique subcostal TAP:** Injection in the subcostal area, LA is injected between the posterior rectus sheath and TAM (Fig. 58.3).

Patient positioning Supine, hip & knee extended, arms by the side or on the chest.

Block performance
- Position/Ergonomics: operator on ipsilateral or contralateral side, machine facing operator.
- Probe: High-frequency linear probe (15–6 MHz, 25–38 mm)
- Settings: Nerve/MSK, Resolution, Compound imaging/ Multibeam
- Depth: 3–5 cms
- Needle size: 50–80 mm B-bevel nerve block needle
- Needling technique:
  - Transverse in plane- anterior to posterior

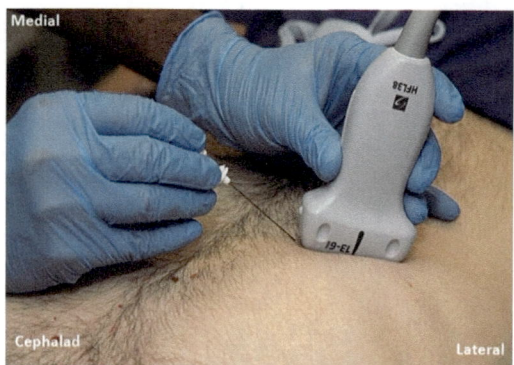 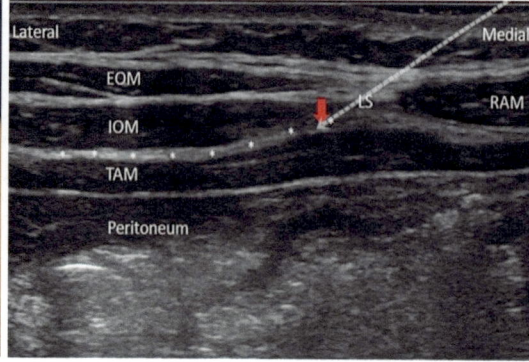

Fig. 58.3 Oblique subcostal TAP: asterisks define the subcostal TAP plane, the red arrow denotes the ideal injection point, and the dotted line is the block needle.

(EOM = External oblique muscle, IOM = Internal oblique muscle, TAM: Transversus abdominis muscle, RAM: Rectus abdominis muscle, LS: Linea semilunaris)

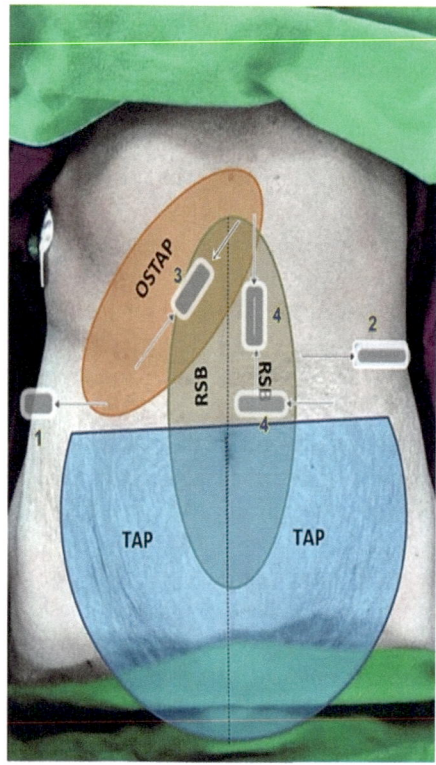

Fig. 58.4 Probe position, needle trajectory, and sensory distribution of anterior abdominal wall blocks: the grey box represents the probe position and the arrow the block needle. 1: lateral TAP, 2: anterior TAP, 3: OSTAP and 4: RSB. The shaded areas represent the extent of the sensory effect of the blocks as mentioned

- Optimal needle tip position (Fig. 58.4):
  - Anterior TAP block: Needle tip in the plane between IOM and TAM at the midaxillary line
  - Posterior TAP block: Needle tip in the plane between IOM & TAM aponeurosis
  - Subcostal TAP block: Needle tip in the plane between RAM & TAM in the mid-clavicular line
- Drug choice: 0.25% Bupivacaine or 0.375% Ropivacaine
- Volume: 20 ml per side
- Testing block success: sensory anaesthesia to touch, pin prick, and thermal testing in the T7-L1 dermatomes
- Pearls:
  - The block can be very superficial in the paediatric population and thin patients.
  - The spread of the block is more extensive and provides better dermatomal coverage with a greater volume and a more posterior deposition of the drug (close to the quadratus lumborum).
  - The classical anterior TAP block rarely provides spread above the T10 dermatome as opposed to the initial reports; greater spread can be achieved by placing the needle tip as posterior as possible (posterior TAP).
  - The IO is thicker closer to the iliac crest, and the TA is closer to the subcostal margin. As the direction of fibres of the EO & IO are in opposite directions, rapidly moving the probe cephalo-caudad shows the muscle fibres moving in opposite directions (Highway sign)

- For upper abdominal surgery, subcostal TAP achieves better coverage, especially for unilateral surgery.
- TAP blocks are somatic blocks and opioid sparing, and do not cover deep visceral pain.
- **Complications**
  - Vascular injection/LAST
  - Hematoma
  - Bowel injury
- **Contraindications**
  - Local infection,
  - Allergy to LA
  - Patient refusal
  - Anatomically difficult conditions such as scarring of the abdomen from previous surgery/ burn, incisional hernia, etc.

Continuous techniques
- Indication: for abdominal surgery (as above) for extended analgesia
- Kit: 18G Tuohy echogenic needle, 17G catheter
- Catheter: Needle-inserted anteroposterior, in-plane into the TAP plane, and space created by hydrodissection with saline: The catheter is threaded into the plane posteriorly for 3–5 cm. The catheter should be secured with surgical glue and semi-permeable dressings.
- Single catheter for unilateral surgery (nephrectomy, cholecystectomy) and bilateral catheters for midline or Pfannenstiel incisions.
- Regime:
  - 20 mls 0.25% Bupivacaine via each TAP catheter eighth hourly
  - Infusion of 0.125% Bupivacaine or 0.2% Ropivacaine 5–10 ml/hr. for unilateral catheters or 10–14 ml/hr. for bilateral catheters (via single pump & splitter device)
  - PCRA- 4mls/hour infusion, 20-30mls 0.125% Bupivacaine or 0.2% Ropivacaine bolus with 4 hr. lockout
  - Programmed intermittent bolus (PIB) with baseline infusion regimen: In this regimen, 1–2 ml/hr. infusion is administered along with 4–6 hourly boluses of 15–20 ml LA on each site. This regimen is

based on the hypothesis that continuous injection of a small volume of 4–5 ml/hr in the fascial plane may not spread as intended and may get absorbed by the local blood vessels and tissue. The baseline infusion in this regimen is designed to keep the catheters patent. In contrast, the larger volume of the intermittent bolus is expected to spread farther and reach more dermatomes for a widespread analgesic effect.

Clinical Use

The spread of the injectate in fascial plane blocks, particularly the deeper ones such as TAP and QLB, has been explored through imaging studies and cadaveric dissections. These studies have revealed that quite a few variables determine the spread of LA, the most notable among them being the injection site, injection volume, and anatomical variations. The larger the volume, the larger the spread is, a good rule for all fascial plane blocks. However, while injecting a large volume in the fascial plane, one must know that the fascial planes are rich in vascularity and there is a potential risk of local anaesthetic systemic toxicity (LAST). So, to reduce the risk of toxicity while maintaining a larger injection volume, the LA solution concentration must be reduced. Various adjuvants have been experimented with to augment the clinical analgesia and extend the duration of a single bolus. The most notable among them is adrenaline, which, when injected in a concentration of 1:100000, can cause local vasoconstriction, slowing down the absorption of the injectate, thereby prolonging the duration of the block and reducing systemic absorption and toxicity. Dexamethasone, opioids, and alpha two agonists have been used to prolong the duration of TAP block, which is reported as 6–24 hrs otherwise. Liposomal bupivacaine holds the promise of extending the duration of a single-shot TAP block to 48–72 hrs. In some systematic reviews, the TAP block is "non-inferior" to thoracic epidural infusion. In abdominal surgeries, on the other hand, one systematic review has found the analgesic effect of TAP block comparable to local wound infiltration for laparoscopic surgeries. The decision to put the block is a clinical judgement of the anaesthesiologist, based on the clinical requirement on a case-by-case basis. TAP block remains one of the most popular truncal blocks practised worldwide.

Questions

1. What are the disadvantages of the TAP block?
2. How would you prolong the duration of action of a single-shot TAP block?
3. What is a 4-quadrant TAP block, and why is it done?
4. How would you be able to identify the layers of the abdominal wall accurately? What is the highway sign?
5. How does a TAP block differ from a Rectus sheath block?
6. How does the TAP block differ from the Quadratus Lumborum block?

Suggested Reading

1. Rozen WM, Tran TM, Ashton MW, Barrington MJ, Ivanusic JJ, Taylor GI. Refining the course of the thoracolumbar nerves: a new understanding of the innervation of the anterior abdominal wall. Clin Anat. 2008;21:325–33.
2. Rafi A. Abdominal field block: a new approach via the lumbar triangle. Anaesthesia. 2001;56:24–6.
3. Hebbard P, Fujiwara Y, Shibata Y, Royse C. Ultrasound-guided TAM plane (TAP) block. Anaesth Intensive Care. 2007;35:616–7.
4. McDonnell JG, O'Donnell B, Curley G, Heffernan A, Power C, Laffey JG. The analgesic efficacy of TAM plane block after abdominal surgery: a prospective randomized controlled trial. Anesth Analg. 2007;104:193–7.
5. Qin C, Liu Y, Xiong J, et al. The analgesic efficacy compared ultrasound-guided continuous transverse abdominis plane block with epidural analgesia following abdominal surgery: a systematic review and meta-analysis of randomized controlled trials. BMC Anesthesiol. 2020;20:52. https://doi.org/10.1186/s12871-020-00969-0.
6. Weihua W, Lishan W, Yan G. A meta-analysis of randomized controlled trials concerning the efficacy of transversus abdominis plane block for pain control after laparoscopic cholecystectomy. Front Surg. 2021;8 https://doi.org/10.3389/fsurg.2021.700318.

Median Nerve Block

59

Louise Frost

Level of difficulty Easy.

Anatomy and Surface Anatomy

The median nerve originates from all brachial plexus roots (C5-T1). The medial and lateral cords of the plexus join in front of the axillary artery to form the median nerve, and stay near the artery as it travels into the antecubital fossa. Initially located superficial and lateral to the artery, the nerve crosses to the medial side at the coracobrachialis insertion level. The nerve crosses the antecubital fossa on the brachialis, then moves deep between the two proximal heads of pronator teres.

The nerve descends in the median plane in the forearm. It passes between the muscle bellies of flexor digitorum superficialis and profundus and through the flexor retinaculum at the wrist.

Supplies
Cutaneous
- The palmar aspect of the thumb, index, middle finger, and medial half of the ring finger, plus the dorsal aspect of the corresponding distal phalanges.

Muscular:
- Pronator teres
- Flexor carpi radialis
- Palmaris longus
- Flexor digitorum superficialis
- 3 muscles of thenar eminence
- Lateral 2 lumbricals
- Anterior intra-osseus branch
  - Flexor pollicis longus
  - Lateral half flexor digitorum profundus
  - Pronator quadratus

Indications
- Anaesthesia for surgery to the forearm and hand, where upper arm tourniquet analgesia is not required and often used in combination with radial/ulnar nerve blocks.
- "Rescue" technique for a failed proximal block
- Could be considered in isolation for minimal surgery to the lateral palm.

Contraindications

Absolute
Patient refusal.

Relative
Coagulopathy.

L. Frost (✉)
Department of Anaesthesia, Waikato Hospital,
Hamilton, New Zealand
e-mail: louise.frost@doctors.net.uk

Advantages over other techniques

Using isolated nerve and forearm blocks enables surgery to the distal forearm and hand whilst allowing the patient to use their upper arm. They are superficial and easily compressed, which makes them lower-risk blocks to perform in patients with impaired coagulation.

Ultrasound-guided block
Surface landmarks:

Medial to the brachial pulsation in the antecubital fossa.

Approximate midline of flexor compartment of mid-forearm.

Techniques

Ultrasound Techniques

Scanning protocol

Place the probe transversely over the pulse of the brachial artery (Fig. 59.1). The median nerve is usually found just medial to the brachial artery and is often oval or tear-shaped at this level. As you scan distally, the nerve moves away from the artery, passing deep through the superficial flexors of the hand and giving off the anterior interosseous nerve. Scanning into the mid-forearm, the nerve runs between the superficial and deep flexors and is often a more triangular or rounded shape.

Structures to identify
Brachial artery.
Pronator teres.

Brachialis muscle.
Medial epicondyle of humerus.
Flexor digitorum superficialis.
Flexor digitorum profundus.

Position/Ergonomics
Patient lying supine, arm abducted and extended, palm upwards.

Probe
Linear transducer 8–14 mHz.

Settings
Multibeam resolution.

Depth
1–2 cm.

Needle size
22 g short bevel, 50 mm insulated stimulating needle.

Needling technique, USS
Can be in plane or out of plane. In plane, the needle passes medial to lateral in the antecubital fossa to avoid the brachial artery. The transverse plane in either direction can be used for the block in the mid-forearm.

Optimal needle tip position
Proximity to the nerve, often at the "tips" of the more oval structures, ensures a visual spread around the nerve as local anaesthetic is deposited.

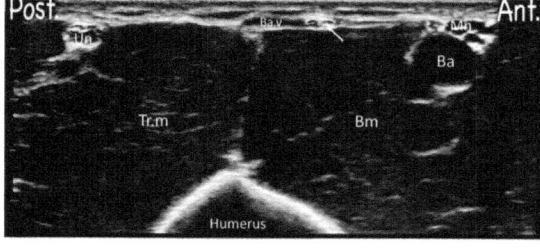
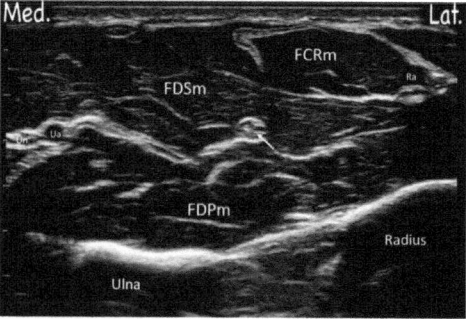

Fig. 59.1 Median nerve block

Needling Technique, Nerve Stimulator

Elbow

Flex the elbow and insert the needle at a medial point to the brachial arterial pulse, aiming 45 degrees proximally—acceptable motor response-finger flexion. Do not accept pronation alone.

Wrist

Identify the flexor carpi radialis and palmaris tendons, which are longer (may be made easier by asking a patient to make a fist). Insert the needle 3–5 cm proximal to the palmar crease between these tendons, 45 degrees to the skin, aiming distally. If no palmaris longus, insert a needle 1 cm medial to FCR.

Accept paraesthesia to the first three digits.

Drug choice

Surgical anaesthesia: 2–5 mls of 0.5% bupivacaine or 0.75% ropivacaine.

Optimal current if nerve stimulation is used

0.2 mA–0.5 mA.

Testing block success

Inability to flex the wrist or the first three digits.

Loss of sensation to the lateral palmar surface and first three digits.

Side effects

Nil specific to block.

Complications specific to the block

Nil specific to block.

Suggested Reading

1. Dufour E, Jaziri S, Novillo MA, Aubert L, Chambon A, Kutz R, Vallée A, Fischler M. A randomized trial to determine the minimum adequate lidocaine volume for median nerve block using hydrodissection. Sci Rep. 2022;12:52.
2. Liu W, Liu J, Tan X, Wang S. Ultrasound-guided lower forearm median nerve block in open surgery for trigger thumb in 1- to 3-year-old children: a randomized trial. Paediatr Anaesth. 2018;28:134–41.
3. Men X, Wang Q, Hu WS, Chai Y, Ni TT, Shou HY, Zhou ZF. Median nerve block increases the success rate of radial artery cannulation in women with gestational hypertension undergoing cesarean section. BMC Anesthesiol. 2022;22(1):248.

Radial Nerve Block

60

Louise Frost

Level of difficulty Easy.

Anatomy and Surface Anatomy

The radial nerve is a continuation of the posterior cord of the brachial plexus, containing fibres from C5-T1. It lies posterior to the artery in the lower third of the axillary artery and descends across the muscle bellies of subscapularis, teres major, and latissimus dorsi. It passes between the triceps' long and medial heads into the arm's posterior compartment, accompanied by the brachii profundus vessels. At the level of the axilla, the radial nerve lies on the conjoined tendon of teres major and latissimus dorsi, situated deep to the axillary artery, and sometimes obscured on ultrasound by its' acoustic shadow.

Moving distally, the radial nerve descends with the profunda brachii artery, giving off motor branches to the triceps' long and lateral heads, and the arm's posterior cutaneous nerve. It lies deep to the long, then lateral head of the triceps, and superficial to its medial head, passing through the triangular interval and into the spiral groove. As it wraps around the humerus, it gives off a motor branch to the lateral head of the triceps and two sensory nerves- the inferior lateral cutaneous nerve of the arm, and the posterior cutaneous nerve of the forearm. In the lower third of the arm, the nerve pierces the intermuscular septum into the anterior compartment, lying between the brachialis and brachioradialis. At the elbow, the nerve moves anteriorly to the lateral epicondyle of the humerus, dividing it into superficial and deep radial nerves.

The superficial radial nerve is purely sensory. It passes with the radial artery and runs deep to the brachioradialis muscle. It then moves dorsally over the anatomical snuff box and divides into medial and lateral branches. The deep branch of the radial nerve is a motor nerve, passing deep to the heads of the supinator to become the posterior interosseus nerve. It supplies all the muscles of the posterior compartment of the forearm.

Supplies
Cutaneous
- Cutaneous strip to the posterior and anterolateral arm, and posterior forearm.
- The superficial radial nerve supplies the dorsal aspect of the lateral hand, including the thumb, index, middle finger, and lateral half of the ring finger, except the areas over the distal phalanges (median nerve).

L. Frost (✉)
Department of Anaesthesia, Waikato Hospital,
Hamilton, New Zealand
e-mail: louise.frost@doctors.net.uk

Muscular:
- Triceps
- Anconeus
- Brachialis (also supplied by musculocutaneous nerve)
- Brachioradialis
- Extensor carpi radialis longus
- All muscles of the extensor compartment of the forearm.

Indications:
- Anaesthesia for surgery to the forearm and hand, where upper arm tourniquet analgesia is not required. Often used in combination with median/ulnar nerve blocks.
- "Rescue" technique for a failed proximal block
- Could be considered in isolation for minimal surgery to the lateral dorsum of the hand.

Contraindications

Absolute
Patient refusal.

Relative
Coagulopathy.

Advantages over other techniques
Using isolated nerve and forearm blocks enables surgery to the distal forearm and hand whilst enabling the patient to use their upper arm. They are superficial and easily compressed, which makes them lower-risk blocks to perform in patients with impaired coagulation.

Ultrasound-guided block
Surface landmarks:
Lateral aspect of the lower third of the arm.
Alternatively, the lateral epicondyle of the humerus is in the antecubital fossa.

Techniques

Ultrasound techniques
Scanning protocol: arm.

Place the probe transversely over the lateral aspect of the lower third of the arm. The radial nerve can be visualised as a triangular or teardrop-shaped structure, which may be seen to give off a small branch (posterior cutaneous nerve of the forearm) at this level. Scanning distally, the radial nerve moves over the humerus, then drops deeper and away from the bone. This point often provides an optimal point for insertion of the block. Alternatively, the nerve can be traced further into the antecubital fossa and blocked at that level, as described below.

In the antecubital fossa, the radial nerve can be found by placing the probe transversely over the lateral epicondyle of the humerus, locating the median nerve next to the brachial artery, and then scanning laterally. As you scan distally, the radial nerve passes from the artery, moving deep to pass under the brachioradialis. You may visualise the separation into superficial and deep branches, which may have already occurred more proximally. Take care to visualise any adjacent blood vessels typically found just deep to the nerve at this level.

Structures to identify:
Brachial artery
Pronator teres
Brachialis muscle
Medial epicondyle of humerus
Flexor digitorum superficialis
Flexor digitorum profundus

Position/Ergonomics
Patient lying supine, arm abducted and extended, pal upwards.

Probe
Linear transducer 8–14 mHz or higher.

Settings
Multibeam resolution.

Depth
1–2 cm.

Needle size
22 g short bevel, 50 mm insulated stimulating needle.

Needling technique, USS
It can be on or off the plane. In-plane, the needle is inserted lateral to medial in the antecubital fossa to avoid the brachial artery. The transverse plane in either direction can be used for the block in the mid-forearm.

Optimal needle tip position
Proximity to the nerve, often at the "tips" of the more oval structures, ensures a visual spread around the nerve as local anaesthetic is deposited. At the level of the distal arm, ideally, a needle is used once the nerve has moved away from the humerus, to avoid damage to the nerve against the bone. (Fig. 60.1).

In the anticubital fossa, identify the brachial artery, noting the position of the median nerve. Slide the probe laterally to determine the radial nerve as it moves anterior to the lateral epicondyle. (Fig. 60.2).

Needling technique, Nerve Stimulator
See "Midhumeral block".

Drug choice
Surgical anaesthesia: 2–5 mls of 0.5% bupivacaine or 0.75% ropivacaine.

Optimal current if nerve stimulation is used
0.2 mA–0.5 mA

Testing block success
Inability to extend the wrist or first three digits.

Loss of sensation to the dorsum of the first three digits.

Side effects
Nil specific to block.

Complications specific to the block
Nil specific to block.

Continuous regional anaesthesia techniques Indication

Catheter
Multi-orifice catheter.

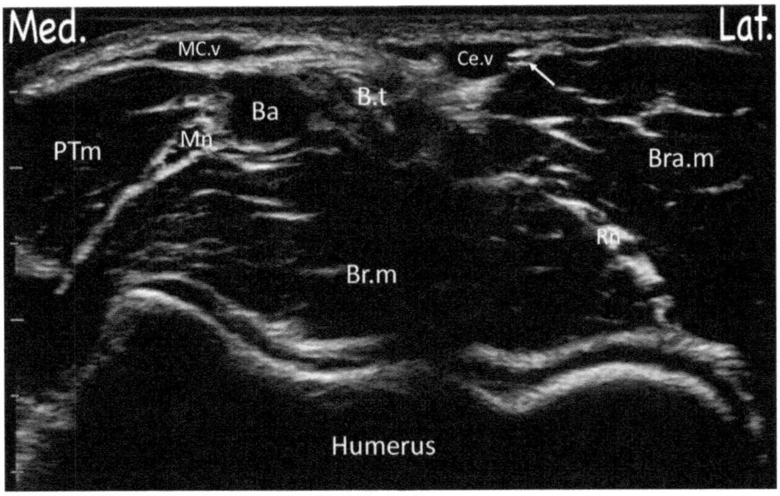

Fig. 60.1 Radial Nerve ACF

Fig. 60.2 Radial nerve

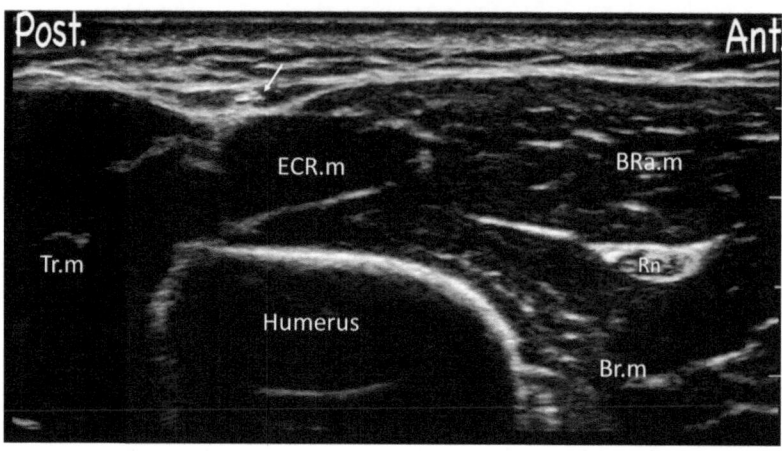

Suggested Reading

1. Glover NM, Murphy PB. Anatomy, shoulder and upper limb, radial nerve. StatPearls 2023;22.

Ulnar Nerve Block

61

Anju Gupta and Louise Frost

Level of Difficulty Easy

Anatomy & Surface Anatomy

The ulnar nerve arises from the medial cord of the brachial plexus (C8-T1). Initially found near the axillary artery, the nerve moves away from the artery and pierces the medial intermuscular septum in the upper arm, where it runs fairly superficially and posteriorly down the arm to enter the cubital tunnel at the posteromedial elbow. It runs between the olecranon process and the medial epicondyle of the humerus, then into the flexor compartment of the forearm between the ulnar and humeral heads of flexor carpi ulnaris. As it travels through the forearm, it is typically found deep to flexor carpi ulnaris, and lateral to flexor digitorum profundus, joining the ulnar artery approximately one-third down the forearm. The ulnar nerve moves with the artery, giving off a superficial palmar cutaneous branch just above the wrist. It passes superficial to the flexor retinaculum at the wrist, entering the palm through Guyon's canal. (Fig. 61.1).

Supplies

Cutaneous
Forearm:

- Palmar and dorsal cutaneous branches provide sensation to the skin of the medial (ulnar) side of the forearm.

Hand:

- Dorsal cutaneous branch: Innervates the dorsum of the hand and the medial side of the dorsum of the ring finger and the little finger.
- Superficial branch: Supplies sensation to the skin of the palm, the little finger, and the medial half of the ring finger.
- Other: The deep branch provides sensation to the hypothenar eminence.

Muscular
Forearm

- Flexor carpi ulnaris
- Flexor digitorum profundus

A. Gupta
Anesthesiology Pain and Critical Care, All India Institute of Medical Sciences, New Delhi, India

L. Frost (✉)
Department of Anaesthesia, Waikato Hospital, Hamilton, New Zealand
e-mail: louise.frost@doctors.net.uk

© The Author(s), under exclusive license to Springer Nature Switzerland AG 2026
S. Phillips et al. (eds.), *Regional Anaesthesia*, https://doi.org/10.1007/978-3-032-05165-3_61

STRUCTURE AT FRONT OF RIGHT WRIST

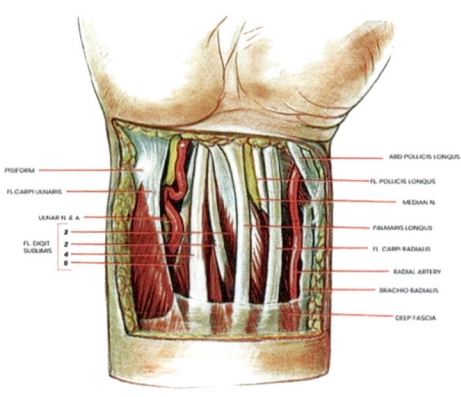

Fig. 61.1 Anatomical relation of the Ulnar nerve

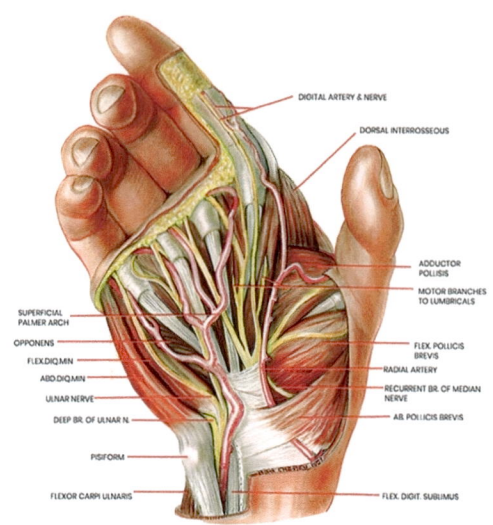

Hand

- Hypothenar muscles: abductor digiti minimi, opponens digiti minimi, and flexor digiti minimi brevis.
- Palmaris brevis
- Interossei muscles: palmar and dorsal.
- Lumbricals 3 and 4
- Adductor pollicis
- Flexor pollicis brevis (deep head)

Indications

- Anaesthesia for surgery to the forearm and hand, where upper arm tourniquet analgesia is not required. Often used in combination with median and radial nerve blocks.
- "Rescue" technique for a failed proximal block

Contraindications

<u>Absolute:</u> Patient refusal.
<u>Relative:</u> Coagulopathy.

Advantages Over Other Techniques

Using isolated nerve and forearm blocks enables surgery to the distal forearm and hand whilst enabling the patient to use their upper arm. They are superficial and easily compressed, which makes them lower-risk blocks to perform in patients with impaired coagulation.

Ultrasound Techniques

Mid-Arm Level

Patient position: Supine, arm abducted and externally rotated, elbow extended or slightly flexed.
Transducer position: Transverse (short-axis) scan on the medial aspect of the mid-arm. (Fig. 61.2).

Landmarks & Anatomy
The ulnar nerve lies in the posterior compartment, near the medial intermuscular septum (MIS). It is positioned posterior to the brachial

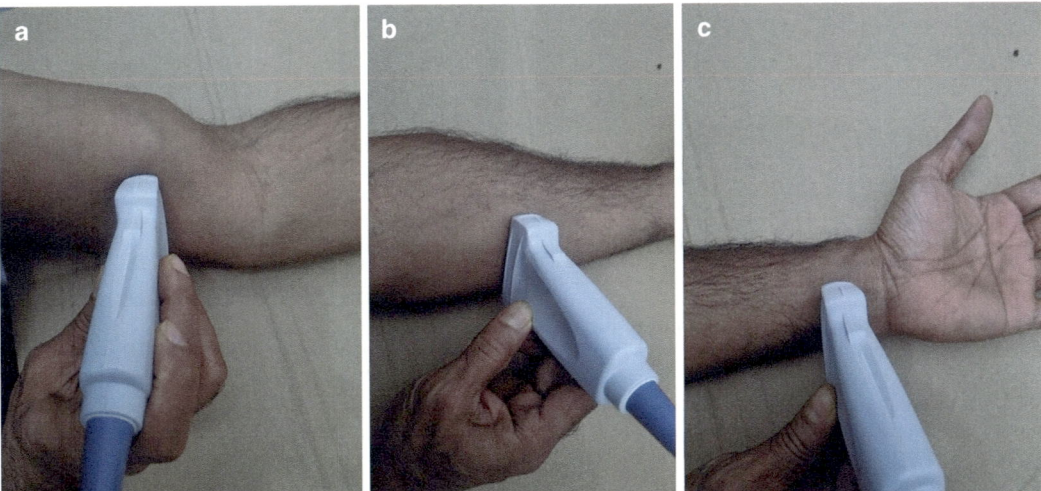

Fig. 61.2 Probe position for scanning ulnar nerve (**a**). Distal arm (**b**). Mid forearm (**c**). Wrist

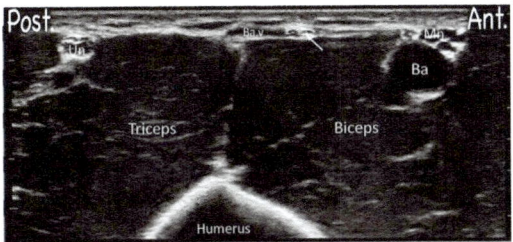

Fig. 61.3 USG image of the ulnar nerve at the mid-arm level. Brachial artery (Ba) along with the median nerve (Mn), Basillic vein (Ba.v), Ulnar nerve (Un) along with the ulnar collateral artery

artery and vein, and anterior to the medial head of triceps. The septo-fascial plane between biceps and triceps helps locate it. In more distal mid-arm, the ulnar nerve moves posteriorly toward the medial epicondyle as it approaches the cubital tunnel.

Ultrasound Appearance
The ulnar nerve appears as a hyperechoic, honeycomb-like oval or round structure (Fig. 61.3). Located adjacent to a bright, linear MIS, separating anterior and posterior compartments. In long-axis view, it appears as a linear fibrillar structure coursing toward the medial epicondyle.

Mid-Forearm Level

Patient position: Forearm supinated and resting on a flat surface.
Transducer position: Transverse over the ulnar aspect of the forearm, midway between elbow and wrist (Fig. 61.2).

Landmarks & Anatomy
The ulnar nerve runs between the flexor carpi ulnaris (FCU) and the flexor digitorum profundus (FDP). It lies deep to the FCU muscle belly. The ulnar artery usually joins the nerve at the proximal third of the forearm, running lateral (radial) to it distally.

Ultrasound Appearance
The ulnar nerve appears as a flattened oval hyperechoic structure between the two muscle bellies (FCU and FDP). The ulnar artery (anechoic circular structure with Doppler flow) is visible just lateral to the nerve in most individuals. When followed distally, the nerve maintains its fascicular pattern and may slightly increase in cross-sectional area (Fig. 61.4).

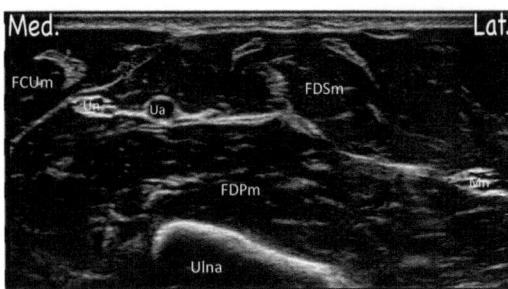

Fig. 61.4 USG image of the ulnar nerve at the mid-forearm level. Ulnar nerve (Un) along with the ulnar artery (Ua) lies under the flexor carpi ulnaris muscle (FCUm). Flexor digitorum superficialis muscle (FDSm), flexor digitorun profundus muscle (FDPm), median nerve (Mn)

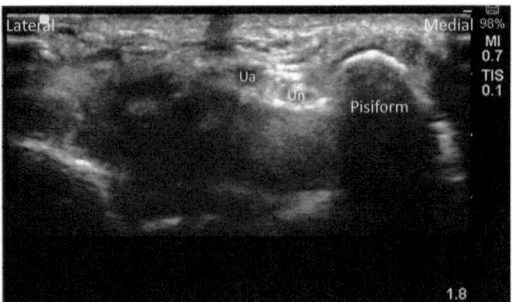

Fig. 61.5 USG image of the ulnar nerve at the wrist level. Ulnar artery (Ua), ulnar nerve (Un)

Wrist Level (Guyon's Canal)

Patient position: Wrist supinated and extended slightly on a support.

Transducer position: Transverse on the ulnar aspect of the volar wrist, just proximal to the pisiform (Fig. 61.2).

Landmarks & Anatomy
The ulnar nerve and artery enter Guyon's canal, located superficial to the flexor retinaculum and between the pisiform and hook of hamate. The canal is roofed by the palmar carpal ligament.

Ultrasound Appearance
The ulnar nerve is seen ulnar (medial) to the ulnar artery, both lying superficial and lateral to the pisiform. Within the canal, the nerve divides into superficial sensory and deep motor branches. The nerve remains hyperechoic with fascicular architecture, smaller than at the forearm. Doppler helps confirm the adjacent ulnar artery (Fig. 61.5).

Position/Ergonomics
Patient lying supine, arm abducted and extended, palm upwards.

Probe
Linear transducer 8–14 mHz or higher.

Settings
Multibeam resolution

Depth
1–2 cm

Needle Size
22 g short bevel, 50 mm insulated stimulating needle

Needling Technique, USS
It can be in-plane or out of plane. In plane, needle lateral to medial in the antecubital fossa to avoid the brachial artery. The transverse plane in either direction can be used for the block in the mid-forearm.

Optimal Needle Tip Position
Proximity to nerve, often at the "tips" of the more oval structures, ensures a visual spread around the nerve as local anaesthetic is deposited. At the level of the distal arm, ideally, the needle is once the nerve has moved away from the humerus, to avoid damage to the nerve against the bone.

Needling Technique, Nerve Stimulator
See "Midhumeral block".

Drug Choice
Surgical anaesthesia: 2-5mls of 0.5% bupivacaine or 0.75% ropivacaine.

Optimal Current if Nerve Stimulation Is Used
0.2 mA–0.5 mA

Testing Block Success
Loss of sensation (or marked dullness) over:
Little finger (fifth digit), Ulnar half of ring finger (fourth digit), and hypothenar eminence.
Motor:
Loss of finger abduction (interossei), loss of finger and thumb adduction (Froment's test).

Side Effects
Nil specific to block.

Complications Specific to the Block
Nil specific to block.

Questions

1. What are the structures surrounding the ulnar nerve at the midarm level?
2. Why should we avoid blocking the ulnar nerve at the medial epicondyle level?
3. What are the precautions to be taken during an ulnar nerve block?

Suggested Reading

1. Hazdic A. Textbook of RA copyright. McGraw-Hill Education; 2017.
2. Nicholls B, Conn D, Roberts A. The Abbott pocket guide to practical peripheral nerve blockade. Abott Laboratories Ltd.; 2003.
3. Townsley P, et al. A pocket guide to regional anaesthesia. RA-UK; 2019.
4. Ellis L. Anatomy for Anaesthetists. 9th ed. Wiley Blackwell Publishing; 2014.

Bier's Block

62

Saaman Neriman

Introduction

The Bier block is a safe, adequate, low-cost intravenous regional anaesthesia (IVRA) form. It can provide anaesthesia, analgesia, and a bloodless field to a distal limb for extremity surgery or manipulation lasting up to 1 hour.

Its success has been reported to be between 96–100%, with a low incidence of side effects.

Equipment required:
– Standard monitoring (or other National guidance).
– Resuscitation and emergency drugs available, including intralipid and methylene blue
– Airway trolley and anaesthetic machine checked.
– Trained personnel for assistance.
– IV cannula 20 g or 22 g. The alternative is a catheter over the needle for the operative side.
– IV cannula 20 g or 22 g on the non-operative side for analgesia/anxiolytic adjuncts.
– Local anaesthetics of your choice: 0.25%–2% lidocaine vs 0.5%–1% Prilocaine (see below). The LA must be preservative-free and plain.
– Syringes to draw up LA: 30–50 mls (see below).
– 2-channel tourniquet system, analogue or digital (Fig. 62.1).

S. Neriman (✉)
Charing Cross Hospital, Imperial NHS Trust, London, UK
e-mail: Saaman.neriman@nhs.net

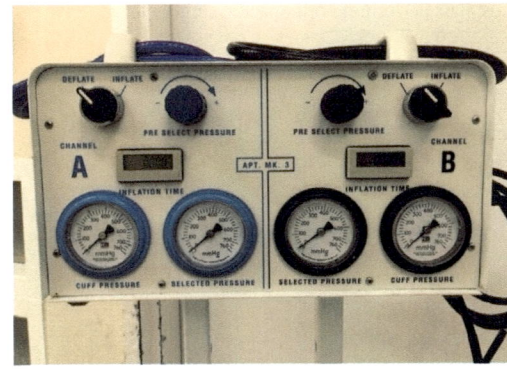

Fig. 62.1 Two-channel tourniquet system. Digital versions are available

– Elastic compression bandage
– Double pneumatic tourniquet system for upper or lower limbs (Fig. 62.2). Two single tourniquets can be used.
– Protective cotton underlayer for a tourniquet to apply over the skin (Fig. 62.3).
– Sterile skin prep.
– Sterile gloves.
– Operating table/ Arm table.
– Patient trolley.

Indications

The block can be used for upper and lower extremity surgery. Such operations/ procedures include:
– Any procedure of an extremity for up to 60 minutes which requires a still and/or bloodless field, like reduction of fractures, reduction

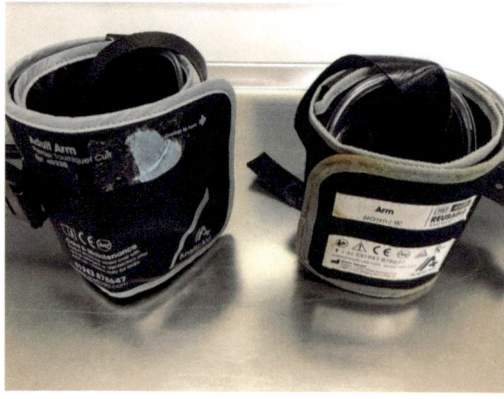

Fig. 62.2 Two-arm tourniquets- reusable and standard in hospitals performing orthopaedic surgery

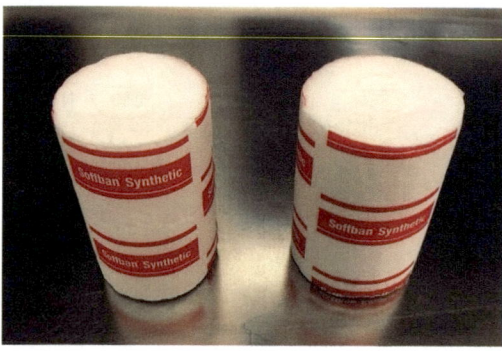

Fig. 62.3 Example of protective cotton underlayer

of dislocations, laceration repairs, removal of foreign bodies, wound debridement and/or washouts, removal of soft tissues/masses, repair to nerves, and burn debridement

- *Upper limb surgery like* peripheral surgery-ganglionectomy, carpal tunnel release, Dupuytren's contracture release and *lower limb surgery examples* like peripheral surgery-removal of plates, screws, foreign bodies, tendon grafting, accessory navicular surgery etc. may be done in IVRA.
- It can be used to assist in the treatment of Hyperhidrosis with Botulinum toxin.
- Paediatric fracture and dislocations- This may have to be used in conjunction with sedation.
- The management of pain in CRPS, Complex regional pain syndrome
- Surgery above the elbow and knee is not advisable due to suboptimal block

Contraindications:

Absolute:
- Patient refusal
- Allergy to local anaesthetics

Relative:
- Crush injuries of the limb
- Distal tibia fractures- increased risk of compartment syndrome
- Compound fractures
- Lymphoedema of the limb
- Morbidly obese patient- difficulty with tourniquet
- Cellulitis of the limb
- Local skin infections
- Vascular injury of the limb
- History of PVD in the limb
- History of AV shunts
- Severe Raynaud's disease
- Venous thrombosis
- Sickle cell anaemia
- Uncooperative patient
- Surgeries lasting >1 hr.

Technique

Preparation:

Ensuring that the equipment is checked and in working order is essential.

- Ensure the patient has been consented and appropriately marked.
- Place the patient in the semi-recumbent position.
- Obtain baseline observations—gauge systolic pressure.
- Examine the operating side for an appropriate vein. The vein to cannulate will depend on the site of surgery:

  Procedures on hand/forearm- Cannula in the dorsum of the hand.

  Procedures at the elbow- Cannula in the forearm or ACF.

  Procedures on the leg- Cannula in the foot or ankle

- Cannulate the operating and non-operating sides and secure the well with tape.
- IV fluids can be connected for hydration.
- Place a protective cotton underlayer around the upper part of the operative limb (Fig. 62.4).

Fig. 62.4 Protective underlayer cotton applied to the proximal upper limb

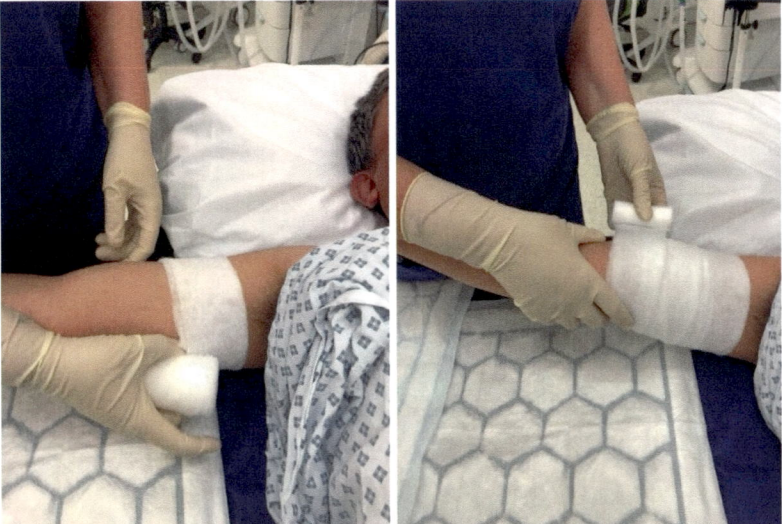

- Place the double tourniquet cuff over the underlayer. Ensure that the proximal cuff is placed higher up the arm. Two single tourniquets can also be used (Fig. 62.5).
- Elevate the operating arm to allow for passive exsanguination. This should be for 2–3 minutes (Fig. 62.6).
- Keeping the arm elevated, wrap the rubber Esmarch bandage around the fingertips up to the distal cuff in a spiral manner. This allows for further exsanguination (Fig. 62.7).
- Palpate the axillary artery on the operating side, apply pressure with fingers, and hold to occlude.
- Inflate the proximal cuff with a 50–100 mmHg pressure above the systolic pressure.
- Once inflated, remove the elastic bandage and release the pressure over the axillary artery.
- Slowly inject the desired volume of LA into the operating site (Table 62.1). Typically, 30–50 mLs for an upper arm block (Fig. 62.8). Blanching of the skin is common and expected.
- Remove the cannula from the operating side and apply a sterile pressure dressing over the entry point.
- Allow the onset of anaesthesia to ensue, typically fast within 4–5 minutes
- After 30 minutes of procedure or when the patient complains of tourniquet pain, inflate the distal cuff and deflate the proximal cuff.

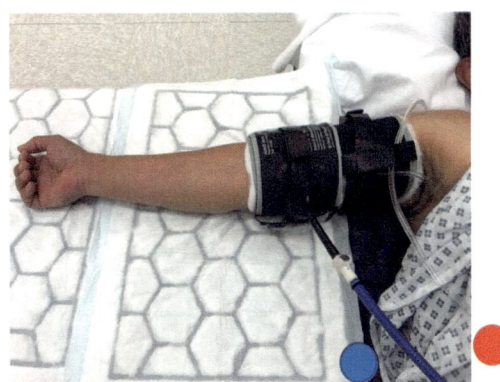

Fig. 62.5 Two single-arm tourniquets are used and connected to each system channel. A coloured dot represents each channel

This allows the surgery to continue and a resolution to the tourniquet pain.

- If the surgical time is short, one must not deflate the cuff until 30 minutes have elapsed from the injection time.
- The deflation process should follow a three-cycle deflation-inflation technique (see below).
- Deflate the cuff and immediately reinflate the cuff to 50–100 mmHg above the patient's systolic blood pressure. Observe the patient for 1 minute for any signs of local anaesthetic toxicity such as light headedness, perioral tingling, metallic taste, or central nervous system stimulation.

Fig. 62.6 Elevating the arm for passive exsanguination

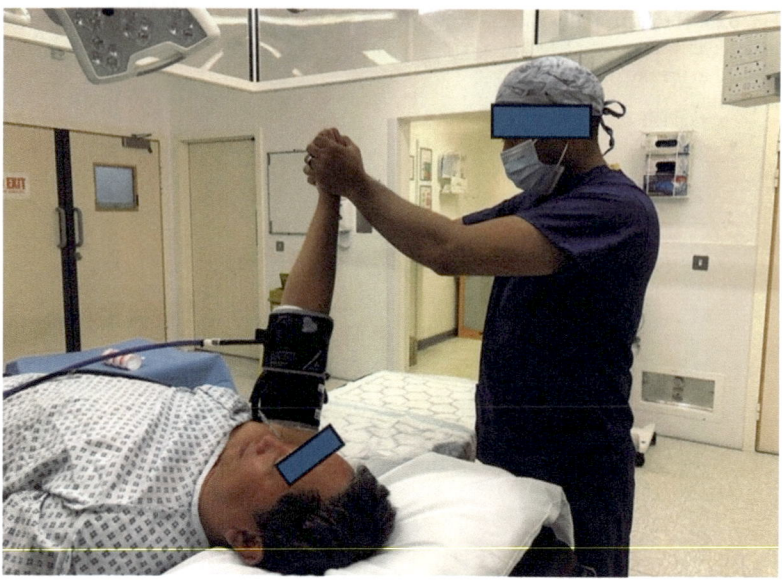

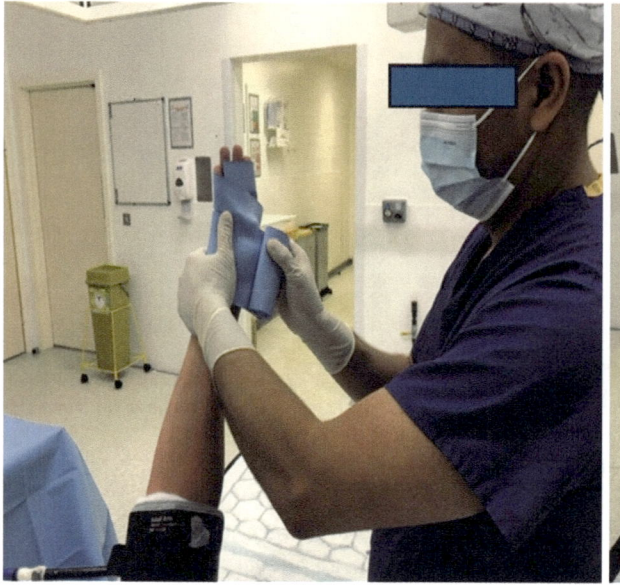

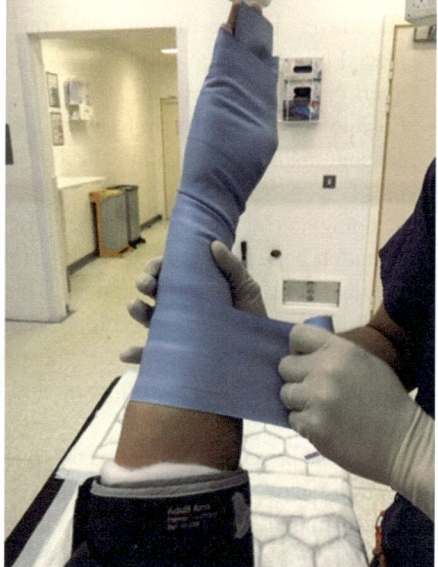

Fig. 62.7 The Esmarch bandage is wrapped in a spiral manner

- Deflate the cuff for the second time and immediately reinflate the cuff to 50–100 mmHg
  above the patient's systolic blood pressure.
  Once again, observe the patient for 1 minute
  for any adverse signs.
- Deflate the cuff for the third time and immediately reinflate the cuff to 50–100 mmHg above
  the patient's systolic blood pressure. Once
  again, observe the patient for 1 minute for any
  adverse signs.

- Finally, deflate and remove the cuff.
- After the operation, transfer the patient to a
  post-procedure recovery bay for continued
  monitoring.
- Assess the extremity for signs of venous or
  arterial insufficiency every 30 minutes.
- Peripheral nerve function will rapidly return
  following the deflation of the tourniquet.
- Continually monitor vital signs at intervals no
  more significant than every 5 minutes for the

Table 62.1 Choice of local anaesthetic (including volumes)

Drug	Lignocaine	Prilocaine
Concentration	0.25%–2%	0.5%–1%
Recommended max dose	3 mg/kg	6 mg/kg
Maximum allowed dose	200 mg	400 mg
Typical dosage for a 70 kg patient	Calculated dose: 70 × 3 = 210 mg Max dose allowed: 200 mg	Calculated dose: 70 × 6 = 420 mg Max dose allowed: 400 mg
Typical concentration and volume	40 mL of 0.5% lidocaine Dose used: 200 mg	40 mls of 0.5% Prilocaine Dose used: 200 mg

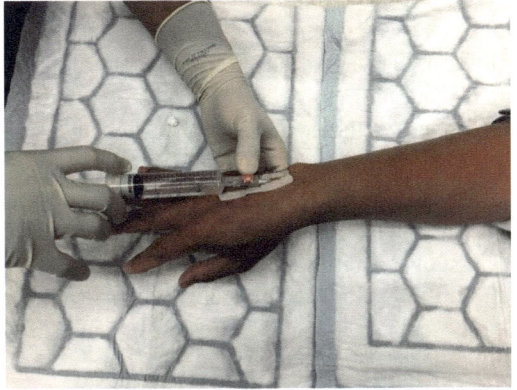

Fig. 62.8 Slow injection of dilute local anaesthetic into the cannula in the exsanguinated arm with an inflated tourniquet

first 30 minutes, as indicated by the patient's clinical status thereafter.
- Additional intravenous or intramuscular analgesics may be administered at this time if the patient is experiencing pain.

Complications/ side effects

Complications can be related to the method, equipment, or drug interactions.

- Poor exsanguination of the limb resulting in inadequate anaesthesia.
- Poor quality block: Affects lower limb more than upper limb due to LA leakage past the tourniquet.
- IV cannula failure, e.g., extravasation injury or failure of the block.
- Thrombophlebitis.
- Failure in cuff inflation.
- Failure in cuff deflation.
- Suboptimal tourniquet effect: Increased risk with lower limb and high BMI patients.

- Inadvertent deflation of the cuff.
- Cuff rupture.
- Risk of nerve damage from tourniquet use.
- Skin petechiae from tourniquet use.
- Excessive inflation pressure of the tourniquet resulting in systemic hypertension.
- Tourniquet pain: Increased risk when procedure time reaches 30 minutes.
- Paraesthesia from nerve manipulation whilst reducing fractures and/or dislocations.
- Local anaesthetic systemic toxicity.
- Side effects from adjuncts used, e.g., opioids- nausea and vomiting, pruritus, sedation.
- Methemoglobinemia.
- Compartment syndrome: Increased risk with lower limb long bone fractures.
- Crush injury: Increased risk with high inflation pressures and duration of the procedure.

Questions

1. What is methemoglobinemia?

Methemoglobinemia is an uncommon haemoglobin disorder that can potentially cause severe effects. The regular ferrous compound ($Fe2+$) is oxidised to the ferric compound ($Fe 3+$), which cannot bind to oxygen. As a result, the haemoglobin has a reduced oxygen binding capacity and a greater affinity for oxygen, resulting in a left shift of the oxygen dissociation curve.

Methaemoglobin can be produced physiologically due to the effects of nitrous oxide on haemoglobin or due to drug exposure. These include prilocaine, benzocaine, nitric oxide, phenytoin and dapsone.

When prilocaine is used, the metabolised compound ortho-toluidine is produced, which can oxidise haemoglobin. Typically, less than 1%

Table 62.2 Symptoms based on methemoglobin concentration

Methemoglobin concentration (%)	Signs and symptoms
0–3%	Asymptomatic
10–20%	Mild nonspecific symptoms: tiredness, headache. Central cyanosis described as slate-blue, saturation reading 82–85% despite supplemental oxygen and a normal paO_2, red-brown blood on arterial sampling
20–50%	Tachycardia, dyspnoea, fatigue, dizziness, headaches
>50%	Arrhythmias, ischaemia, tachypnoea, hypoxia, metabolic acidosis, CNS irritation, change of behaviour, seizures, coma
>70%	Severe hypoxia, death

accounts for methaemoglobin. The development of methemoglobinemia is more likely when 600 mg of prilocaine is reached.

2. How is methemoglobinemia present?

The presentation will depend on the amount of methaemoglobin in the blood (Table 62.2).

3. What is the treatment for methemoglobinemia (MetHb)?

The successful treatment requires prompt recognition and administration of methylene blue.

As with all anaesthetic emergencies, it is essential to call for assistance in managing the deteriorating patient.

- Provide oxygenation
- Treat adverse symptoms such as seizures and arrhythmias
- Intubate and ventilate if indicated
- IV fluid resuscitation with Dextrose 5% should be used. Helps provide NADH and NADPH
- Inject 1–2 mg/kg IV of methylene blue over 5 minutes in the non-operative side cannula.

Be aware that acutely, the patient has dyspnoea, chest pain, and haemolysis. Improvement should be seen within minutes. If the patient has failed to respond after 60 minutes, a repeated dose of methylene blue can be given.

Toxicity from methylene blue:

Doses >7 mg/kg may have significant side effects (nausea, vomiting, confusion, dyspnoea, tremulousness, diaphoresis).

Doses >> 7 mg/kg can paradoxically *worsen* MetHb.

Inform ITU and transfer patients for higher-level care.

Rebound methemoglobinemia can occur up to 18 hrs post-injection.

An alternative treatment is ascorbic acid if methylene blue is contraindicated (see below). This method is slow and requires multiple doses to reduce MetHb levels. A dose of 1.5–2 g IV infusion repeated 3–4 times is suggested.

Contraindications to methylene blue usage include G6PD patients and patients at risk of developing serotonin syndrome.

4. How does LAST present?

Please see Chap. 24.

5. What is the mechanism of action of IVRA?

Direct: The nerve endings within tissues are directly exposed to local anaesthesia. This is peripheral infiltration.

Indirect: The local anaesthetic is indirectly transported via the vasa nervorum, resulting in a conduction block.

6. Why is exsanguination so important?

Exsanguination allows for effective anaesthesia to develop in the limb. Poor exsanguination will ultimately dilute your local anaesthetic due to the presence of blood, and a suboptimal block will result.

7. Which methods of exsanguination are you aware of?

Passive: Elevating the limb for 2–3 minutes and allowing the blood to drain.

Active: Using an elastic compression bandage will allow for further exsanguination and provide the optimal condition for the success of the block.

8. By what methods does LA leak into the systemic circulation?

Direct: LA can leak past the tourniquet cuff despite appropriate inflation pressures. This can be due to poor exsanguination. If the venous pressure within the limb after injection of your LA exceeds that of the tourniquet pressure, then theoretically, LA can leak past. Lower limb procedures.

Indirect: LA enters the systemic circulation via interosseous vessels, unaffected by a tourniquet.

9. What dose of local anaesthetic would you consider if you placed the tourniquet around the proximal forearm?

Placing the tourniquet over the forearm can result in a reduction in the volume of LA used. A low volume-high concentration dose of anywhere from 8–10 mls of 2% lidocaine has been described. The benefits of a low volume-high concentration block are quicker onset of anaesthesia, more significant duration of the block, fewer rescue analgesia interventions, reduced tourniquet discomfort, less LA toxicity, and the potential to be discharged from recovery faster.

10. What volumes of LA would you require for a lower limb procedure?

Owing to the larger size of the lower limb, a greater volume of LA is required to achieve anaesthesia.

Typically, 80–100 mLs of your desired LA volumes are used.

Example:
  80 mls 0.5% prilocaine, Dose is given: 400 mg.
  Maximum dose allowed: 400 mg.

11. Which adjuncts/additives have been shown to improve your block quality/duration?

A systematic literature review identified the role of adjuncts used in IVRA. Of the studies which were included, there was substantial evidence for the use of:

(a) NSAIDS: Ketorolac showed an improved tolerance to the tourniquet during the procedure and improved postoperative analgesia. The dose at which this was observed was 0.3 mg/kg of ketorolac for an upper arm tourniquet IVRA procedure.

(b) Muscle relaxants: Atracurium, used in doses of 2–3 mg added to the LA volume, showed improved muscle relaxation, improved reduction for fractures, better operating conditions for the surgeon and improved postoperative pain scores. However, this was only observed in a small study.

Suggested Reading

1. https://rcem.ac.uk/wp-content/uploads/2021/10/Biers_block_revised_Nov_2017.pdf
2. https://www.nysora.com/techniques/intravenous-regional-anesthesia/intravenous-regional-block-upper-lower-extremity-surgery/
3. Chiao FB, Chen J, Lesser JB, Resta-Flarer F, Bennett H. Single-cuff forearm tourniquet in intravenous regional anaesthesia results in less pain and fewer sedation requirements than upper arm tourniquet. BJA. 2013;111(2):271–5. https://doi.org/10.1093/bja/aet032.
4. Kraus GP, Rondeau B, Fitzgerald BM. Bier Block. https://www.ncbi.nlm.nih.gov/books/NBK430760/
5. Arslanian B, Mehrzad R, Kramer T, Kim DC. Forearm Bier block: a new regional anaesthetic technique for upper extremity surgery. 2014;73(2):156–7. https://doi.org/10.1097/SAP.0b013e318276da4c.
6. https://resources.wfsahq.org/wp-content/uploads/uia-15-INTRAVENOUS-REGIONAL-ANAESTHESIA--BIER%E2%80%99S-BLOCK.pdf
7. Sukhani R, Garcia CJ, Munhall RJ, et al. Lidocaine disposition following intravenous regional anaesthesia with different deflation technics. Anesth Analg. 1989;68:633–7. [PubMed: 2719294]
8. Kennedy BR, Duthie AM, Parbrook GD, et al. Intravenous regional anaesthesia: an appraisal. Brit Med J. 1965;1:954–7. [PubMed: 14260623]
9. Rawal N. Analgesia for day-case surgery. Br J Anaesth. 2001;87(1). https://www.bjanaesthesia.org.uk/article/S0007-0912(17)36345-6/fulltext
10. Mabee JR, Bostwick TL, Burke MK. Iatrogenic compartment syndrome from hypertonic saline injection in Bier block. J Emerg Med. 1994;12(4):473–6.
11. Thomas C, Lumb AB. Physiology of haemoglobin. Contin Educat Anaesth Crit Care Pain. 2012;12(5):251–6. https://doi.org/10.1093/bjaceaccp/mks025.
12. The Internet book of critical care: methaemoglobinaemia. https://doi.org/10.1093/bjaceaccp/mks025
13. Iolascon A, Bianchi P. Recommendations for diagnosis and treatment of methemoglobinemia. Am J Hematol. 2021;96(12):1666–78.

Ilioinguinal/Iliohypogastric Block

63

Arunangshu Chakraborty

The ilioinguinal (II)/iliohypogastric (IH) block is a relatively simple distal branch block useful in adult and paediatric groups for surgery in the inguinal region.

Level of difficulty Basic.

Anatomy

The iliohypogastric nerve (IHN) usually originates from the L1 ventral ramus but may arise wholly or in part from the T12 ventral ramus. The ilioinguinal nerve (IIN) usually originates from the L1 ventral ramus but may receive a contribution from T12 or L2. (Fig. 63.1) Both these nerves emerge from the lateral border of the psoas and travel over quadratus lumborum and iliacus. IHN crosses obliquely behind the lower renal pole on the anterior surface of the quadratus lumborum. Above the iliac crest, it enters the posterior part of the transversus abdominis muscle (TAM) and then runs forward between TAM and the internal oblique muscle (IOM), which it supplies. It gives off a lateral cutaneous branch that pierces the internal and external oblique (EOM) muscles above the iliac crest and supplies the posterolateral gluteal skin. The IIN penetrates the transversus abdominis near the anterior part

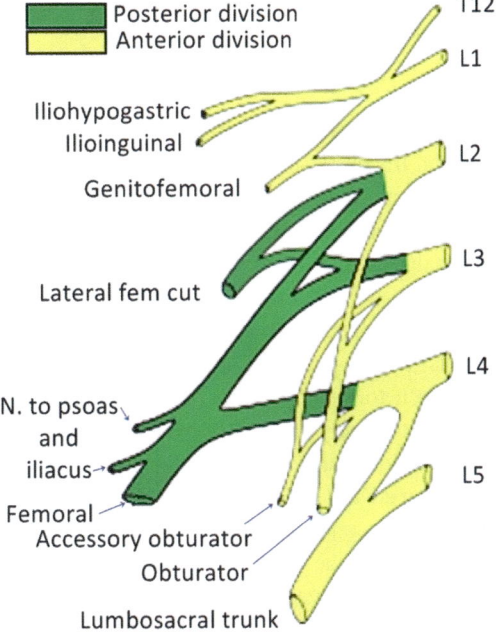

Fig. 63.1 The formation and branches of the lumbar plexus

of the iliac crest and travels between the transversus abdominis and internal oblique. It then penetrates the internal oblique and enters the inguinal canal, travels along with the spermatic cord in males (round ligament in females), and emerges through the superficial inguinal ring to supply the upper and medial thigh skin.

A. Chakraborty (✉)
Sultan Qaboos Comprehensive Cancer Care and Research Centre, Muscat, Oman

Surface anatomy
Important landmarks: anterior superior iliac spine (ASIS), Inguinal ligament.

Indications:
- Inguinal hernia repair
- Appendicectomy
- Lower abdominal surgery/Pfannensteil incisions (needs bilateral block)
- Chronic post-herniorrhaphy groin pain

Nerves blocked
Ilioinguinal & Iliohypogastric nerves (L1 dermatome).

Positioning
Supine, hip & knee extended.

Landmark-based technique
IHN and IIN blocks have been practised with landmark techniques before the advent of ultrasound for regional anaesthesia, particularly for perioperative analgesia for surgery for inguinal hernia. The needle is inserted 2 cm medial and 2 cm superior to the ASIS perpendicular to the skin. An initial loss of resistance, popularly called "pop", is felt as the needle penetrates the external oblique aponeurosis, and approximately one-half of the local anaesthetic (LA) solution is injected at this location. The needle is then advanced deeper, where a second pop is felt when the aponeurosis of the internal oblique is punctured, and the bevel of the needle lies in the fascial plane between the internal oblique and transversus abdominis. This is commonly referred to as the transversus abdominis plane (TAP) and is the region where the ilioinguinal and iliohypogastric nerves are located. The remainder of the LA is injected in this fascial plane. Careful aspiration between injections is advised as the deep circumflex iliac vessels lie in this area.

Scanning technique
The high-frequency linear probe is placed in the transverse oblique plane along the line connecting the ASIS and umbilicus; the lateral end of the probe abuts the ASIS. A nerve stimulator can be used with (dual guidance) to elicit contraction of the lower abdominal wall muscles.

Structures to identify ASIS, external oblique muscle/aponeurosis, internal oblique, transversus abdominis, II&IH nerves, deep circumflex iliac vessels (Figs. 63.2 and 63.3).

Block performance
Position/Ergonomics: Patient supine, operator on ipsilateral or contralateral side, machine facing operator.

- Probe: High-frequency linear probe (15–6 MHz, 25–38 mm)
- Settings: Nerve/MSK, Resolution, Compound imaging/Multibeam
- Depth: 1–3 cms
- Needle size: 25–50 mm B-bevel nerve block needle of 20–22 G.

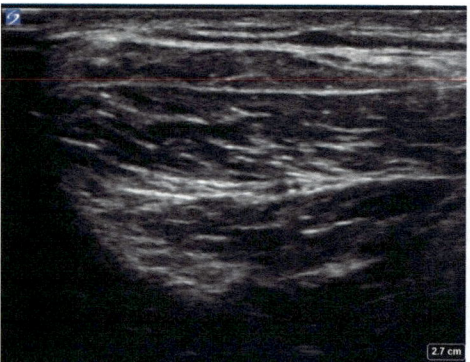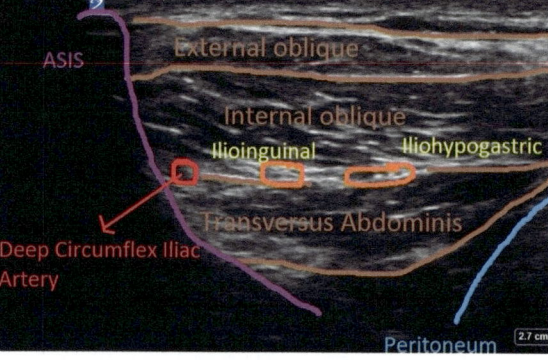

Fig. 63.2 Ultrasound image of the ilioinguinal region, with three layers of abdominal wall visible and the nerves seen in the TAP plane

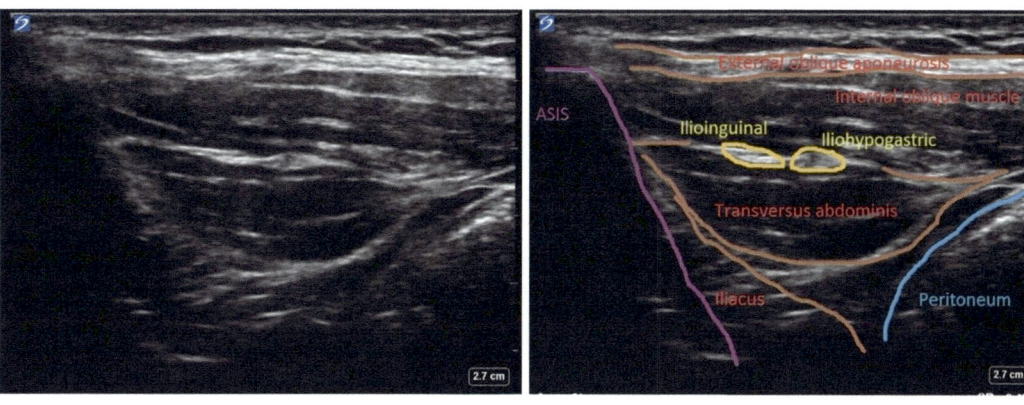

Fig. 63.3 Probe position much inferior, where the external oblique muscle is present as aponeurosis and only two muscle layers are visible

- Needling technique:
  - Transverse inplane-medial to lateral
  - Transverse- Inplane lateral to medial or
  - Transverse-out of plane caudal to cephalad
- Optimal needle tip position: Lateral to the IIN in the plane between IOM and TAM.
- Drug choice: 0.25% Bupivacaine or 0.375% Ropivacaine
- Volume: 10 mls, 5 ml per nerve
- Optimal current if NS used: <0.5 mA at 2 Hz
- Muscle responses acceptable: contraction of the lower abdominal wall muscles
- Testing block success: sensory anaesthesia to touch, pinprick, and thermal testing in the L1 dermatome
- Pearls:
  - The block can be very superficial in the paediatric population and thin patients.
  - Transverse oblique in-plane medial to lateral approach provides a safety margin due to the iliac bone; lateral to medial needling risks intraperitoneal injection/bowel injury in fragile patients.
  - Breach of the fascia iliaca can lead to femoral nerve block and quadriceps motor weakness, leading to unanticipated hospital admission or delayed discharge.
  - The block can prove to be difficult when bowel contents enter the hernial sac, risking bowel injury. Reducing the bowel

contents before the block may be prudent, or it can be performed postoperatively.
- Side effects
  - Femoral nerve block & motor weakness
- Complications
  - Vascular injection and local anaesthetic systemic toxicity (LAST)
  - Hematoma (puncture of deep circumflex vessels)
  - Bowel injury

Continuous techniques
- Indication: Postoperative analgesia for hernia surgery
- Kit: 18 G Tuhoy needle with catheter
- Regime: Infusion of bupivacaine 0.1–0.25% or ropivacaine 0.2% at the dosages of 0.1–0.2 ml/Kg

Contraindications:
- Local infection
- Allergy to LA
- Patient refusal

Suggested Reading

1. Klaassen Z, Marshall E, Tubbs RS, et al. Anatomy of the ilioinguinal and iliohypogastric nerves with observations of their spinal nerve contributions. Clin Anat. 2011;24:454–61.

2. Ndiaye A, Diop M, Ndoye JM, et al. Anatomical basis of neuropathies and damage to the ilio-inguinal nerve during repairs of groin hernias (about 100 dissections). Surg Radiol Anat. 2007;29(675):81.

3. van Schoor AN, Boon JM, Bosenberg AT, Abrahams PH, Meiring JH. Anatomical considerations of the pediatric ilioinguinal/iliohypogastric nerve block. Paediatr Anaesth. 2005;15:371–7.

4. Trainor D, Moeschler S, Pingree M, et al. Landmark-based versus ultrasound-guided ilioinguinal/iliohy-pogastric nerve blocks in the treatment of chronic postherniorrhaphy groin pain: a retrospective study. J Pain Res. 2015;8:767–70.

WALANT and Tumescent Anaesthesia

64

Shao Hong Neoh, Ashokka Balakrishnan, and Priya Tiwari-Kesavan

WALANT (Wide Awake Local Anaesthesia No Tourniquet)

Level of Difficulty Intermediate.

Background

Traditionally, hand surgery is performed under either a proximal block or general anaesthesia, which allows placement of a proximal tourniquet for a bloodless surgical field. Both techniques have disadvantages: the proximal block, especially with long-acting agents, causes prolonged motor blockade and impairs the use of the arm. General anaesthesia causes side effects like nausea, vomiting, and dizziness, which delay recovery and discharge. WALANT was subsequently developed to avoid the need for a proximal motor block, sedation, or general anaesthesia, allowing vhand surgeries to be done in an office-based setting.

S. H. Neoh (✉)
National University Health Systems,
Singapore, Singapore
e-mail: Shaohong.neoh@mohh.com.sg

A. Balakrishnan
Department of Anaesthesia, National University
Hospital, Singapore

P. Tiwari-Kesavan
NUHS
e-mail: priya_tiwari_perdit_k_t@nuhs.edu.sg

Indications

WALANT is primarily performed for hand procedures. It is ideal for patients with multiple comorbidities who are unsuitable for proximal nerve blocks due to their side effects (e.g., diaphragmatic paresis), deep sedation, or general anaesthesia. Examples of surgeries that are suitable for WALANT include:

1. Trigger Finger Release
2. Carpal Tunnel Release
3. Metacarpal Fractures
4. Dupuytren's Contracture
5. Fracture fixation of distal radius

Its contraindications are summarised in Table 64.1.

Preparation

A typical mixture used for WALANT would include 1% lignocaine with 1:100,000 epinephrine, although it is possible to use lower concentrations of epinephrine, such as 1:200,000 concentrations. Note that with this reduced concentration, the haemostatic effect is diminished. Adding epinephrine reduces the systemic absorption of lignocaine, allowing a higher dosage threshold and prolonging the duration of anaesthesia. Similar to Tumescent Anaesthesia, 8.4% sodium bicarbonate is often added to increase the pH of the mixture, facilitating a faster onset of anaesthesia and improving patient comfort during infiltration.

Table 64.1 Contraindications of WALANT block

Absolute	Relative
Lack of consent	Active infection
Lignocaine allergy	Needle phobia
Uncooperative patient	Underlying vascular disease, such as Raynaud's disease
Sickle cell disease	Coagulopathy

Safety Considerations

Dosage should be limited to 7 mg/kg of lignocaine with the administration of epinephrine to reduce the risk of local anaesthetic systemic toxicity (LAST). As the mixture contains epinephrine, there is a small risk of digital ischaemia. This rarely causes any digital necrosis but can cause post-ischaemic reperfusion pain. Injecting 1–2 mg of phentolamine in 1–2 mL of saline can help to reverse this.

Advantages

The use of WALANT allows for these hand procedures to be done in the ambulatory setting. This decreases the need for hospital admissions and reduces patients' exposure to nosocomial infections. This is also useful as it allows hand surgery in resource-poor areas.

In addition, WALANT allows the surgeon to assess the accuracy of their surgical repair. In flexor tendon repairs, for example, patients can be instructed to flex their fingers after the initial repair and adjustments can be made accordingly in the same setting. It also provides long-acting post-operative analgesia and decreases the need for opiate usage.

Techniques/Approaches

Many approaches for different types of hand surgery have been described (Fig. 64.1).

Example 1—Carpal tunnel release.

Inject 2 ml subcutaneously over the wrist crease, then 5 ml of solution beneath the deep fascia between the median and ulnar nerve, and an additional 10 ml injected deep to the incision line.

Example 2—Metacarpal fractures.

Inject 40 ml of anaesthetic solution circumferentially around the metacarpal.

Example 3—Dupuytren's contracture.

Inject 10 ml into the palm, 2 ml into the proximal phalanx, and finally 2 ml into the middle phalanx.

Example 4—Open Reduction Internal Fixation of Distal Radius.

10 mls of Subcutaneous injection at the incision site, followed by 10 mls of periosteal injection proximal to where the plate will be, and 10mls of periosteal injection at the fracture site. If there is a concurrent ulna styloid fracture, inject 10mls of periosteal injection over the ulna styloid. For a more significant surgical area such as this, it is also possible to use up to 100 mL of 0.5% lignocaine with 1:200,000 epinephrine.

Technical Pearls for WALANT

Positioning of the patient is essential in WALANT, and patient factors need to be considered. For example, patients with underlying congestive heart failure and features of dyspnoea or orthopnoea should be seated before performing the block. For younger patients, however, consider lying the patient down to prevent the occurrence of vasovagal syncope.

To improve comfort, consider using warm room temperature solutions. Inject the needle perpendicularly and use the smallest gauge possible; typically, a 27G needle is used. Inject slowly and aim to not inject into the dermis. Ensure steady needle movement and allow anaesthetic solution to take effect ahead of the needle tip before advancement. The injection technique should be to raise a forward-moving wheal of local anaesthetic rather than advancing the needle first and injecting the solution on withdrawal. Reinsert the needle only in areas that have been anaesthetized.

The clinician should allow time for local anaesthesia and the haemostatic effects of epinephrine. Typically, the block should be conducted 15–30 minutes before incision and will last up to 15 hours.

Using large volumes or tumescent anaesthesia is not uncommon, especially if coverage of a large surgical area is required. It provides the added benefit of hydro-dissection, improving surgical visibility. As a guide, it is safe to use up to 50 mL of 1% lignocaine in 1:100,000 epinephrine in an average 70 kg patient, and this is usually sufficient for most surgeries using WALANT.

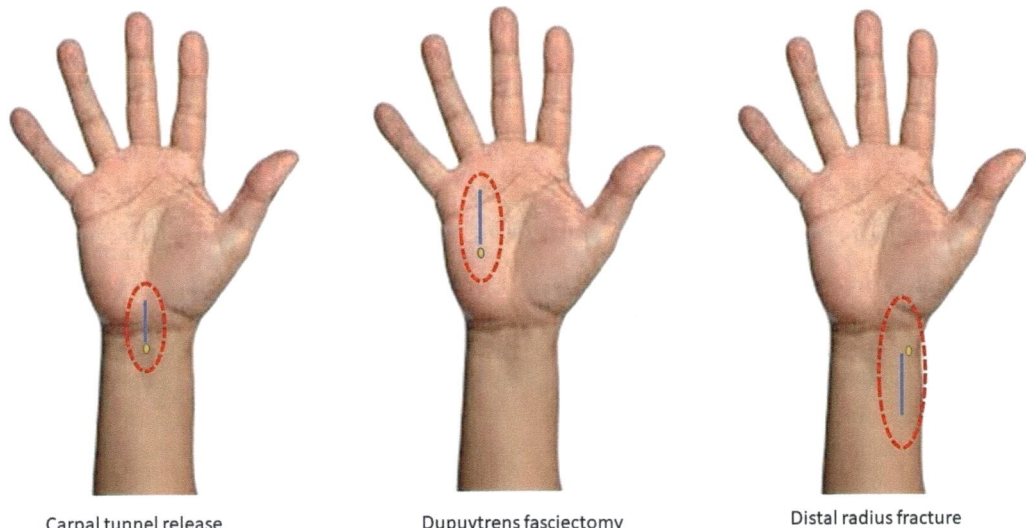

| Carpal tunnel release | Dupuytrens fasciectomy | Distal radius fracture |

Blue line- Incision site, Yellow dot- Initial needle insertion point, Red oval- zone of spread of local anaesthetic needed

Fig. 64.1 WALANT injection techniques for different hand surgeries

Tumescent Local Anaesthesia

Level of Difficulty Intermediate.

Background
Tumescent Local Anaesthesia (TLA) is a technique that was initially devised for use in liposuction but has now been adopted for use in other surgical procedures.. Tumescent, meaning 'to become swollen', describes the infiltration of relatively large volumes of highly dilute local anaesthetic into subcutaneous tissue to provide a large area of regional anaesthesia.

Indications
Initially developed by Dr. Jeffery A. Klein, TLA has revolutionized liposuction surgery, allowing the procedure to be completed with local anaesthesia alone and with minimal surgical blood loss. Its use has now been validated in other types of plastic surgeries, such as burn surgeries and breast surgeries, including breast augmentation, breast reduction, and mastectomies.

Clinicians in dermatology can also employ TLA in procedures such as laser resurfacing, blepharoplasties, facelifts, vitiligo surgery, and treatment of axillary hyperhidrosis.

TLA can also be used in vascular surgery to facilitate endovenous laser therapy (EVLT) to treat varicose veins. In contrast to its use in liposuction, TLA in EVLT involves the infiltration of tumescent solution circumferentially around the vein. This provides analgesia, heat dissipation from laser therapy, and mechanical compression of the vein to facilitate laser contact.

Other indications include surgeries such as endoscopic thyroid/parathyroid surgeries and lymph node dissection surgeries. Recent case reports also describe the use of TLA for subcutaneous implantable cardioverter-defibrillator (S-IDC) implantation as an option for patients at high risk of undergoing general anaesthesia.

Preparation
Various preparations have been described in the literature, and constituents can vary between institutions. These include:

Example 1:

- 1000 ml of lactated Ringer's solution at 21 ° C.
- 30 ml of 1% lignocaine (15 ml if large volume).
- 1 ml of 1:1000 epinephrine.

Example 2:
  Klein Solution:

- 1000 ml standard saline solution (0.9% NaCl).
- 50 ml 1% lignocaine.
- 1 ml 1:1000 epinephrine.
- 12.5 ml of 8.4% sodium bicarbonate.

Pharmacology and Safety Considerations

Lignocaine is typically the anaesthetic drug of choice, and analgesia can be provided for up to 18 hours. In the above preparation, the maximum safe dosage is estimated to be 35 mg/kg.

Use of such high quantities of lignocaine is possible because of:

- Dilute concentrations of lignocaine being used, reducing the concentration gradient and hence absorption.
- Slow infiltration of anaesthetic solution.
- Vasoconstriction of epinephrine resulting in decreased systemic absorption.
- Relative avascularity of fatty layer.
- High lipid solubility of lignocaine resulting in prolonged, slow absorption into the systemic circulation.
- Compression of vessels by infiltrate.
- Active suctioning of fat results in 7.5%–30% of the administered lignocaine being removed during the procedure.

The use of Epinephrine, while helpful in reducing systemic absorption, should be used with caution in patients with underlying hypertension, ischemic heart disease and cardiac arrhythmias. Additionally, the perivascular injection used in EVLT places patients at higher risk of systemic absorption of epinephrine and is commonly omitted for this reason. Fortunately, epinephrine is easily reversed by Phentolamine.

Sodium bicarbonate is commonly added to alkalinize the solution, increasing the amount of nonionized lignocaine, thereby increasing the speed of onset.

Advantages

The use of large volumes of TLA also confers other benefits. Fluid in the subcutaneous layer is slowly absorbed and promotes volume replacement. The use of epinephrine provides haemostasis whilst the local anaesthesia provides pain control. The solution enhances cavitation, dissipates heat, and is especially useful for ultrasound-assisted liposuction [UAL]. Finally, it is postulated that using TLA lowers infection rates as lignocaine provides concentration-dependent bacteriostatic and bactericidal activity.

Equipment

Infusion equipment is used to inject tumescent solution into the treatment area. This can be done via a syringe attached to an infusion cannula with a three-way connector. A 50-mL syringe used in this manner may be appropriate for liposuction of small areas, such as the neck. Infusions can be power-assisted for larger areas, commonly with a motorized peristaltic pump. These pumps can be adjusted for infusion speed and turned off and on manually or by foot switch. The infusion tip is usually a specially designed multi-holed infusion cannula (Fig. 64.2). Wide-bore (2–3 mm), longer stem infusion cannulas are used for filling the abdomen, thigh, and hips, while short, finer cannulas are used for areas with small fat deposits, such as the neck.

Techniques/Approaches

TLA aims to anaesthetize the superficial nerve endings in the subcutaneous layer of the skin. This is done by infiltrating the solution deep into the epidermis within the subcutaneous tissue. Anaesthetic solution is infused until the skin becomes firm and tense, giving a typical peau d'orange appearance.

The solution vasoconstricts blood vessels and allows separation of the dermis from the underlying fascia of the muscle. Liposuction can then be conducted, causing fat tunnels to collapse after the procedure.

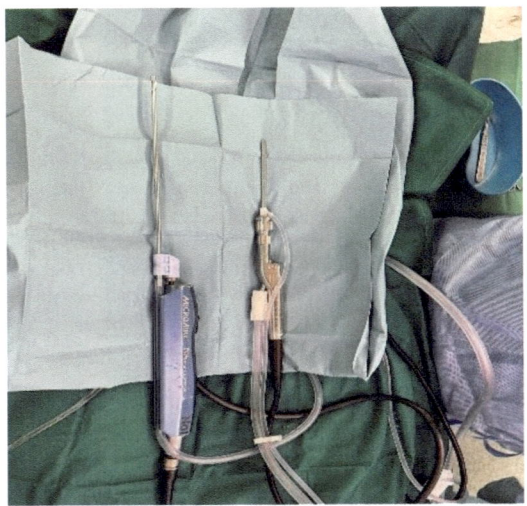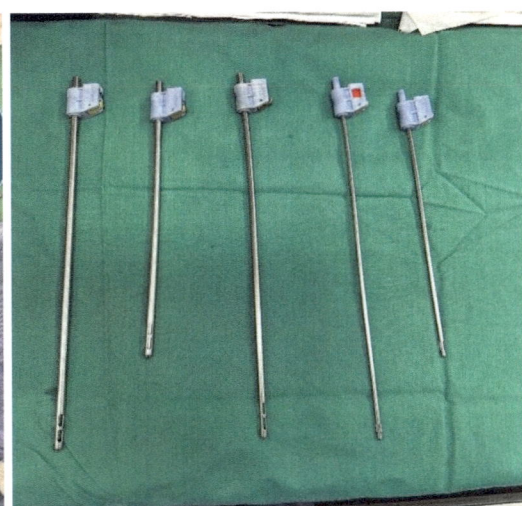

Fig. 64.2 Suctioning is then done using a power-assisted suction device such as a Microaire device, which provides a variety of suction cannulas of varying lengths and port types

Technical Pearls for Tumescent Anaesthesia in Liposuction

Tumescent solution is usually administered to the abdomen, thighs, arms and flanks before liposuction to minimise blood loss and allow fat cavitation. Small stab incisions are performed, and the cannula is inserted to allow for prefiltration and subsequently liposuction of all areas, after waiting 10 to 15 mins for adrenaline to take effect, watch for blanching and turgidity of the segment infiltrated before commencing liposuction.

Potential Issues and Solutions

The use of TLA is generally safe and effective; however, practitioners should be aware of the risks involved with the infusion of high volumes of TLA into the subcutaneous compartment.

Hypothermia is a potential problem if excessive amounts of cold solution are used. Warm saline heated to 40 degrees Celsius is commonly used to help mitigate this problem. The use of excessive volumes of tumescent anaesthesia can potentially also cause fluid overload and pulmonary edema. Clinicians should thus exercise caution when using tumescent anaesthesia in patients with a history of cardiac conditions, including heart failure.

LAST remains a valid concern for TLA. The maximum dose allowed is 7 mg/kg for lignocaine with adrenaline and 4 mg/kg without adrenaline. Care should be taken to avoid repeat LA administration for up to 12–18 hours once a patient has undergone tumescent anaesthesia. Lignocaine is metabolized via hepatic CYP3A4, and the use of lignocaine along with medications that inhibit or are metabolized by CYP3A4 enzymes can lead to toxic plasma levels. Hence, thorough screening of the patient's medical history and medications is paramount before undergoing such procedures.

Bicarbonate alkalinizes the pH of lignocaine, stabilizing the mixture to improve its onset to 3.5 mins instead of 7 mins. However, as epinephrine degrades spontaneously in neutral solutions (pH 7–7.4) with a half-life of about 10–14 days, the tumescent anaesthetic solutions should be freshly mixed on the day of surgery.

Questions

WALANT

1. Name three advantages of performing hand surgery under WALANT as compared to General Anaesthesia
2. Describe the components of a mixture to be used in WALANT

3. You decide to perform WALANT for a patient undergoing surgery for the release of his trigger finger. After the surgery, you note that his finger is pale and white. What would be your first step of management?
4. What are some of the absolute contraindications for WALANT?
5. Describe how you would administer WALANT to a patient undergoing carpal tunnel release surgery

Tumescent Anaesthesia

1. Please describe the components of tumescent anaesthesia
2. Describe your techniques for performing liposuction with tumescent anaesthesia
3. What is the maximum dose of lignocaine allowed for tumescent solution?
4. Why does the maximum dose of lignocaine in tumescent differ from systemic lignocaine administration?
5. How long should you monitor a patient for the effects of lignocaine post liposuction with tumescent solution?

Suggested Reading

1. Lalonde DH, Wong A. Dosage of local anaesthesia in wide awake hand surgery. J Hand Surg Am. 2013;38:2025–8.
2. Garmon EH, Huecker MR. Topical, local, and regional anaesthesia and anaesthetics. StatPearls [Internet]. StatPearls Publishing; Treasure Island. 2021.
3. Lalonde D, Bell M, Benoit P, Sparkes G, Denkler K, Chang P. A multicenter prospective study of 3,110 consecutive cases of elective epinephrine use in the fingers and hand. J Hand Surg. 2005;30:1061–7.
4. Lalonde DH. Latest advances in wide awake hand surgery. Hand Clin. 2019;35:1–6.
5. Uttamani RR, Venkataram A, Venkataram J, Mysore V. Tumescent anesthesia for Dermatosurgical procedures other than liposuction. J Cutan Aesthet Surg. 2020;2020(13):275–82.
6. Gunes T, Altin F, Kutas B, Aydin S, Erkoc K, Eygi B, et al. Less painful tumescent solution for patients undergoing endovenous laser ablation of the saphenous vein. Ann Vasc Surg. 2015;29:1123–7.
7. Romero J, Diaz JC, Alviz I, Briceno D, Zhang X, Palma E, et al. Tumescent local anesthesia for subcutaneous implantable cardioverter-defibrillator implantation: an alternative for general anesthesia. Heart Rhythm Case Rep. 2021;7:286–91.
8. Afolabi O, Murphy A, Chung B, Lalonde DH. The effect of buffering on pain and duration of local anesthetic in the face: a double-blind, randomized controlled trial. Can J Plast Surg. 2013;21:209–12.

Chronic Postsurgical Pain

65

Prateek Maurya, Nishkarsh Gupta, and Anju Gupta

Case History

A 65-year-old male underwent an uncomplicated total knee replacement under spinal anaesthesia. The postoperative course was quite stormy; the patient had severe pain after regression of spinal anesthesia and required a PCA with morphine. The pain was very difficult to control, and the patient, on discharge, still had moderate pain. The patient came back for manipulation under GA because of stiffness post-surgery. The patient had aggravation of severe pain and required a femoral block to control pain this time. One year down the line, the patient still has persistent pain and has been referred to the pain specialist for further management.

1. What is the definition of chronic post-surgical pain (CPSP) ?

Chronic postsurgical pain (CPSP) or persistent post-surgical pain (PPP) is defined as pain that develops or increases in intensity after a surgical procedure or tissue injury, persists beyond the healing process (at least 3 months after the surgery or trauma), and is localized to the surgical

area, the innervation area of a nerve in that area, or related to a dermatome or Head's zone.

Key aspects of the definition include:

- Pain development: Pain emerges or intensifies following a surgical procedure or tissue injury.
- Duration: Pain persists for at least 3 months post-surgery or injury, exceeding the standard healing period.
- Location: Pain is typically localized to the surgical site, the distribution of a nerve in the surgical field, or a dermatome associated with the affected area.
- Exclusion of other causes: It's essential to rule out other potential pain sources like pre-existing conditions, infections, or malignancies.
- Neuropathic characteristics: CPSP can exhibit features of neuropathic pain.

2. What is the incidence of CPSP?

The incidence of chronic postsurgical pain (CPSP) varies, with the median incidence of chronic pain reported as **20%–30%** at 6–12 months post-surgery. However, reported incidences differ significantly, ranging from **5% to 85%**. This wide variability is attributed primarily to methodological differences, including variations in data collection methods and inconsistent definitions of CPSP.

Even minor surgical interventions are linked to the risk of developing CPSP. Recent data from

P. Maurya (✉) · N. Gupta
Onco-Anesthesia and Palliative Medicine, All India Institute of Medical Sciences, New Delhi, India

A. Gupta
Anesthesiology Pain and Critical Care, All India Institute of Medical Sciences, New Delhi, India

S. Phillips et al. (eds.), *Regional Anaesthesia*, https://doi.org/10.1007/978-3-032-05165-3_65

ambulatory surgical settings indicate that more than one in ten patients develop CPSP, with 93% of these patients having no pain before surgery. Severe CPSP (a score > 5 on the Numeric Rating Scale) affects 2%–10% of adults undergoing surgery in the UK.

3. What are the consequences of CPSP?

Chronic postsurgical pain (CPSP) has significant consequences for postoperative recovery, quality of life, and economic and healthcare burdens.

- Impact on Quality of Life: Patients with neuropathic CPSP report more intense pain, more significant limitations in activities of daily life, and reduced quality of life. CPSP is now recognised as a global measure of the impact of pain on the quality of life and considers pain severity encompassing pain intensity, pain-related distress, and pain-related functional interference.
- Healthcare burden: CPSP results in significant economic and healthcare burdens.
- Postsurgical Rehabilitation: CPSP has a debilitating impact on postsurgical rehabilitation.

4. What type of surgeries are more common?

Chronic postsurgical pain (CPSP) incidence varies depending on the type of surgery, with reported incidences ranging from 5% to 85%.

Surgeries with relatively high incidences of CPSP include:

- Amputation (30%–85%)
- Thoracotomy (5%–71%)
- Craniotomy (7%–65%)
- Inguinal herniotomy (5%–63%)
- Mastectomy (11%–57%)
- Caesarean section (6%–55%)
- Sternotomy (7%–50%)
- Knee arthroplasty (13%–44%)

Other surgeries where CPSP can occur, though potentially at lower rates, include:

- Cholecystectomy (3%–56%)
- Abdominal surgery (17%–21%)
- Hip arthroplasty (7%–23%)
- Dental surgery (5%–13%)
- Coronary bypass (30–50%)
- Melanoma resection (9%)
- Vasectomy (0%–37%)

It is worth noting that methodological differences in data collection and variable definitions of CPSP contribute to the wide variability in reported incidence.

5. What are the risk factors for the development of CPSP?

These risk factors can occur before, during, and after surgery. The risk factors can be broadly identified by temporal characteristics in the pre-, peri-, and post-operative periods and cover six general domains: genetic, demographic, psychosocial, pain, clinical, and surgical factors. Prediction models can be applied clinically for risk stratification and tailoring appropriate treatments for patients most at risk of developing CPSP.

Risk factors include:

- **Surgical Factors**:
  - **Type of surgery:** The type of surgery is predictive of CPSP. Procedures such as thoracotomy, amputation, and mastectomy are associated with a higher incidence.
  - **Extent and duration of surgery**. Surgeries lasting longer than 3 hours led to increased pain and poor functional outcomes.
  - **Surgical technique:** Minimally invasive surgery does not always reduce the risk of CPSP. For example, a laparoscopic approach can reduce the risk in certain types of surgery but not others.
  - **Nerve damage**. Nerves risk injury from partial or complete transection, stretching, crushing, electrical damage, entrapment, or compression during surgery.
  - **Postoperative complications**, reoperation, and infection are additional surgery- and disease-related risk factors for CPSP.

- **Patient-Related Factors**:
  - **Pre-existing pain.** Patients with preoperative chronic pain, particularly at the surgical site, are at increased risk of developing CPSP. Pre-existing chronic painful conditions (e.g, fibromyalgia, migraine, low back pain) increase the risk of CPSP.
  - Younger age (adult) is associated with increased risk. Older patients tend to have a lower risk of developing CPSP than younger patients.
  - **Sex** Female sex is associated with increased risk.
  - **BMI** High BMI is associated with increased risk.
  - **Genetics** Pain susceptibility is known to be influenced by several genes, and the genetic basis of the individual physiological response to injury and pain management in post-operative patients.
- **Psychosocial Factors:**
  - Psychological distress, anxiety, catastrophising, reduced ability to cope with pain, depression, and hypervigilance increase the risk of CPSP. State anxiety is the primary psychological risk factor for CPSP.
- **Anaesthesia-Related Factors:**
  - **Opioid use:** Long-term consumption can lead to tolerance, addiction, and opioid-induced hyperalgesia. Pre-operative opioid consumption is a risk factor for CPSP. Intraoperative remifentanil dosage is correlated with increased incidence of CPSP up to 1 year after cardiac surgery.
- **Postoperative Pain**:
  - **Severity of acute postoperative pain.** The severity of acute postoperative pain is a consistent predictor of CPSP.
  - **Duration of intense pain.** The duration of intense pain and pain trajectories are essential. Postoperative pain of neuropathic-like symptoms within the first days after surgery is strongly associated with neuropathic CPSP.

6. What is the mechanism of development of CPSP?

The development of CPSP involves complex mechanisms, including peripheral and central sensitization, but translational research is sparse, and findings are often inconsistent.

Key aspects of the mechanisms of CPSP include:

- **Peripheral Sensitisation**:
  - Nerve damage is associated with both the incidence and severity of CPSP. Many CPSP syndromes may arise from neural trauma, whether from crush, stretch, transection, hypoxia, or additional mechanisms. Beginning in the periphery, neuromas are one source of pain from damaged nerves.
  - **Immune Response** Molecules associated with the innate immune system, including cytokines, arachidonic acid metabolites, and complement system fragments, are generated in large quantities in surgical wounds and traumatised tissues. The inflammatory and immune response to axonal and tissue damage, including the release of neurotransmitters peripherally, leads to glial activation, ectopic neural activity, and altered activity in the dorsal horn.
  - **Peripheral Nerve Hyperexcitability** Damaged or adjacent C- and Aδ-fibers demonstrate hyperexcitability and ectopic firing due to alterations in sodium, potassium, and calcium ion channels.
- **Central Sensitisation**:
  - **Neuroplasticity**: Central sensitisation is a form of long-term adaptive neuroplasticity that amplifies central pain pathways.
  - **Neuroinflammation:** Activation of microglia and astrocytes has been demonstrated using the incisional pain model and bone fracture pain models. A large body of laboratory research supports the role of neuroinflammation in pain after nerve injury, which can occur during surgery.
  - **Changes in the brain.** There are also changes in the supraspinal processing including brain network connectivity and changes in endogenous, descending pain modulation.

- **Genetic Factors:**
  - Single-nucleotide polymorphisms (SNPs) and epigenetic changes can affect various inflammatory and stress response functions.

As a consequence of the central sensitisation processes, patients developing CPSP often report clinical symptoms such as hyperalgesia, allodynia, and dysaesthesia. Hyperalgesia detected early after surgery might predict prolonged, chronic neuropathic pain after surgery.

7. What are the evidence-based methods for the prevention of CPSP?

It is important to note that there are limitations in the evidence base, including that most clinical trials report CPSP as a secondary outcome. The definition of CPSP has evolved, and different time points and measurement instruments are used; therefore, it is difficult to synthesize the data.

Preventive strategies for CPSP include regional anaesthesia, pharmacological interventions, optimising the surgical approach, and non-pharmacological interventions. The data suggest that the patient cohorts most likely to benefit from regional anesthesia are those having epidurals for thoracotomy, wound infiltration for significant breast surgery, and cesarean delivery, and there is emerging evidence supporting SAP or pectoserratus/interpectoral plane blocks in breast surgery.

Key strategies include:

- **Regional Anaesthesia**: Perioperative regional anaesthesia has been shown to reduce the risk of CPSP in most types of surgery studied. By blocking nociceptive input to the central nervous system, central sensitisation processes can be reduced if not prevented.
  - **Epidural Analgesia**: May reduce the incidence of CPSP in patients undergoing thoracotomy. Following open thoracotomy, epidural analgesia halves the odds of CPSP at 3–18 months.
  - **Thoracic Paravertebral Block (TPVB)**: TPVB block has a more favourable safety profile than epidural analgesia. However,

in thoracic surgery, TPVB is not associated with a reduced incidence of CPSP. In breast surgery, evidence is increasingly demonstrating that TPVB has little benefit in reducing the incidence of CPSP.
  - **Fascial Plane Blocks**: Limited data show that the fascial plane block contributes to a reliable reduction in CPSP, but some approaches may have more benefits than others.
    - **Serratus Anterior Plane (SAP) Block**: In patients receiving it for analgesia in mastectomy, one randomized trial reported a reduced incidence of CPSP at 3 and 6 months and a reduced severity.
    - **Interpectoral/Pectoralis Plane Blocks**: One trial reported that the interpectoral/pectoserratus plane block substantially reduced the incidence of moderate-to-severe CPSP at 6 months compared with the SAP block.
  - **Peripheral Nerve Blocks**: Preoperative sciatic nerve block does not reduce the incidence of phantom limb pain, although pain outcomes at 4 weeks might be improved.
  - **Wound Infiltration**: Meta-analyses have demonstrated that wound infiltration and continuous infusions can reduce the incidence of CPSP following breast cancer surgery and cesarean delivery, but there was insufficient evidence in other settings.
- **Pharmacological Interventions**:
  - **Multimodal Analgesia**: Using multimodal analgesia during the perioperative phase has also prevented CPSP.
  - **Ketamine**: Perioperative ketamine may reduce opioid consumption and acute postoperative pain.
  - **Gabapentinoids**: Perioperative use of gabapentinoids does not reduce the incidence of CPSP.
  - **I.V. Lidocaine**: Lidocaine i.v.... for 24 h or less potentially helps to reduce CPSP in patients undergoing breast surgery.
  - **NSAIDs**: A recent meta-analysis has reported positive effects in the prevention of CPSP.

- **Optimising Surgical Approach**:
  - Minimizing tissue damage, including damage to nerves, during surgery.
  - Performing less extensive surgery may reduce the incidence of CPSP for some interventions.
  - Avoiding damage to local nerves, minimizing the duration of surgery, choosing a minimally invasive procedure, and avoiding extensive surgery where possible.
- **Non-pharmacological intervention and transitional pain services**
  - A multidisciplinary approach might be far more effective, including non-pharmaceutical therapies such as physiotherapy and psychological support.
  - Transitional pain services aim to close the gap between acute postoperative pain management and pain management after discharge from the hospital.

8. How to manage CPSP?

Questions

Chronic postsurgical pain (CPSP) management includes a range of strategies, including pharmacotherapies, nerve blocks, and other interventional and non-pharmacological approaches. An individualised patient-centred approach is essential in the prevention and treatment of CPSP.

Key elements in the management of CPSP are:

1. **Identify the aetiology and type of pain**: exclude recurrent malignancy in the case of cancer surgery, or to exclude other postoperative complications such as infection.
2. **Pharmacotherapies** Current pharmacotherapies for the management of CPSP include topical local anaesthetics, non-steroidal anti-inflammatory drugs (NSAIDs), paracetamol, weak opioids (codeine or tramadol), and adjuvant analgesics such as gabapentin and pregabalin. Strong opioid use is to be avoided to reduce the risk of dependency, which highlights the need for novel analgesics.
3. **Nerve blocks**: For patients whose pain levels are not responsive to pharmacotherapy, interventions such as nerve blocks, nerve ablation, and neuromodulation can also be used.
   - (a) Axillary brachial plexus blocks for complex regional pain syndrome type I (CRPS I) of the upper limb, Epidural analgesia, and Ilioinguinal block have all been used successfully for various CPSP
   - (b) Botulinum toxin injections injected into painful areas of chronic post-thoracotomy pain can provide significant pain relief, as well as the abdominal wall after laparoscopic ventral hernia repair.
4. **Neuromodulation** Spinal cord stimulation is a valuable method to treat neuropathic pain.
5. **Other interventional methods, such as** Radiofrequency ablation of the dorsal root ganglion (DRG) or dorsal root entry zone (DREZ), show potential for the treatment of chronic ilioinguinal pain following inguinal hernia repair as well as for chronic post-thoracotomy pain.
6. **Surgical resection** may be appropriate in the case of neuroma formation.
7. **Physical therapies**, including massage, physiotherapy, and acupuncture, may be helpful.
8. **Psychological interventions, such as** Cognitive behavioural therapy, may help manage chronic pain.
9. **Multidisciplinary approach** Given the complexity of CPSP, an individualized patient-centred approach is essential in its prevention and treatment.

Suggested Reading

1. Fuller AM, Bharde S, Sikandar S. The mechanisms and management of persistent postsurgical pain. Front Pain Res. 2023;4:1154597.
2. Searle RD, Simpson KH. Chronic post-surgical pain. Contin Educ Anaesth Crit Care Pain. 2010;10(1):12–4.
3. Rosenberger DC, et al. Chronic post-surgical pain – update on incidence, risk factors and preventive treatment options. BJA Educ. 2022;22(5):190–6.
4. Elsharkawy H, Clark JD, El-Boghdadly K. Evidence for regional anesthesia in preventing chronic postsurgical pain. Reg Anesth Pain Med. 2025;50:153–9.

Acute Compartment Syndrome

Anju Gupta, Nishkarsh Gupta, and Prateek Maurya

Scenario

A 25-year-old male, with a history of a fall from a motorbike, sustains a closed fracture of his left tibia and fibula. He undergoes intramedullary nailing of the tibia in the trauma list under a general anaesthetic. Intraoperatively, a popliteal block was performed with 20 mls 0.5% Bupivacaine. Twelve hours after the procedure, he develops severe pain and a tense calf.

1. **What is the most probable diagnosis?**

   Acute compartment syndrome of the lower limb.

2. **What is the definition of acute compartment syndrome?**

   Acute compartment syndrome (ACS) is when increased pressure within a closed compartment compromises the circulation and function of the tissues within that space. It is a serious condition that can threaten a limb and, in rare cases, a life, and it can cause significant disability if it is not treated early.

3. **What are the cardinal signs and symptoms of compartment syndrome?**

The **cardinal symptom of compartment syndrome** is **severe pain** over the affected compartment, often disproportionate to the apparent injury. This pain is typically aggravated by passive stretching of the muscles involved.

Further signs and symptoms include:

- **Paraesthesia** is considered characteristic, especially a loss of two-point discrimination in the distribution of the nerves traversing the compartment.
- **Weakness or paralysis** of the limb is a late sign.
- The affected compartment may present with **tense and tender swelling**, along with dysfunction of the nerves traversing it.
- **Pulselessness** is uncommon and suggests a late stage, as extensive muscle and nerve injury typically occurs by the time compartment pressures rise enough to occlude the traversing arteries.

It is important to note that not all of these signs are required to make a diagnosis, and the clinical findings can change as the syndrome progresses. Also, many of the above conclusions may not be present until late in the disease process when damage is irreversible. **Pain can be an unreliable symptom**, as it is subjective and variable and may be absent in an established compartment syndrome. ACS can present without pain in up to 10% of patients.

A. Gupta
Anesthesiology Pain and Critical Care, All India Institute of Medical Sciences, New Delhi, India

N. Gupta · P. Maurya (✉)
Onco-Anesthesia and Palliative Medicine, All India Institute of Medical Sciences, New Delhi, India

© The Author(s), under exclusive license to Springer Nature Switzerland AG 2026
S. Phillips et al. (eds.), *Regional Anaesthesia*, https://doi.org/10.1007/978-3-032-05165-3_66

4. What are the differential diagnoses of compartment syndrome?
   a. Deep venous thrombosis
   b. Acute arterial insufficiency
   c. Cellulitis
   d. Failed regional anaesthesia (kink, occlusion, displacement of regional anaesthesia catheter)
5. How is compartment syndrome diagnosed?

Compartment syndrome is **usually diagnosed clinically**, although compartmental pressure monitoring is recommended for use in high-risk patients as an adjunct. A high index of suspicion is needed, and repeated assessment and observation are required. Not all signs are necessary for the diagnosis, and the clinical findings can change as the syndrome progresses. Diagnosis can be incredibly challenging in children and patients with neurological compromise or altered mental status.

In addition to the above clinical signs/symptoms, compartment pressure monitoring and other imaging modalities can be used.

- **Compartmental pressure monitoring:**
  - Normal pressure in the muscle compartments is <10–12 mm Hg.
  - Compartmental pressure monitoring can be performed using a pressure transducer attached to a needle or cannula, which is placed into the suspect compartment and the transducer zeroed to the level of the needle.
  - All compartments in a limb suspected of having CS should be measured.
  - It has been recommended that fasciotomy is required if the compartmental perfusion pressure is ≤30 mm Hg.
  - Muscle compartment pressures have also been advocated, with fasciotomy recommended if the compartment pressure is >30 mm Hg.

Other investigations, such as near-infrared spectroscopy, infrared imaging, ultrasound, and MRI, show promise in monitoring for compartmental ischaemia. Still, these methods are not yet widely available and all have limitations. Serum creatine phosphokinase or myoglobinuria has been used to indicate CS as it reflects muscle necrosis. Still, it is not helpful for early diagnosis and may reflect muscle damage from one or more sites around the body.

6. What are the pathophysiological mechanisms of compartment syndrome?

The **pathophysiology of acute compartment syndrome** is complex and involves a cascade of events triggered by various traumatic and non-traumatic causes, ultimately leading to tissue ischaemia and potential necrosis.

- **Initiating Factors**: tissue injury, which starts the process of tissue ischaemia and reperfusion. These causes can include fractures, soft tissue injuries, crush injuries, burns, and surgical procedures.
- **Microvascular Changes** Precapillary vasodilation in the arteriole system, collapsing venules, and increased permeability of the capillary bed are the predominant microvascular mechanisms. These changes increase net filtration, leading to elevated interstitial pressure within the affected compartment.
- **Increased Intracompartmental Pressure** After direct injury, ischaemia-reperfusion, or fluid extravasation, the pressure within these compartments rises, reducing perfusion and leading to local ischaemia of muscles and nerves. The ischaemia results in tissue membrane damage and leakage of fluid through capillary and muscle membranes, with a subsequent increase in tissue pressure.
- **Reduced Tissue Perfusion.** As interstitial pressure increases, sufficient perfusion to tissues decreases, resulting in tissue hypoxemia. This can be measured as critical tissue delta pressure (diastolic blood pressure minus compartment pressure) with a threshold of 30 mm Hg, which is widely accepted as an indication for fasciotomy.
- **Cellular Damage** Hypoxia, oxidant stress, and local hypoglycaemia cause cell oedema. The cellular osmotic balance is disturbed due to a deficiency of adenosine triphosphate (ATP) and shutdown of the sodium-potassium ATPase channels, caus-

ing an influx of chloride ions, cell swelling, and cell necrosis. Damaged membranes continue to leak, increasing oedema formation and pressure in the enclosed compartment.

- **Reperfusion Injury** Reperfusion injury is the next pathophysiological step of compartment syndrome, involving the production of oxygen radicals, lipid peroxidation, and calcium influx, which disturbs intracellular homeostasis. This leads to hyperkalaemia and acidosis, potentially facilitating systemic organ failure.
- **Venous Obstruction:** Raised tissue pressure can obstruct venous outflow and increase venous pressure. The consequent increase in capillary pressure induces a vicious cycle of increased fluid transudation, more significant tissue swelling, and a rise in intra-compartmental pressure. Eventually, as intra-compartmental pressure approaches capillary pressure, microcirculatory perfusion ceases.
- **Ischaemia-Reperfusion Cycle** The underlying pathophysiology of acute compartment syndrome is an ischaemia–reperfusion–ischaemia cycle. Ischaemia can be precipitated by remote perfusion failure or increased resistance to flow within the compartment. The damaged membrane leaks with arterial reperfusion, increasing oedema formation and pressure in the closed compartment.
- **Irreversible Damage**: If the pressure is not relieved within a few hours of onset, irreversible changes will occur with muscle necrosis, contracture, and nerve and vessel damage. The time required to develop irreversible injury to nerves and muscle varies depending on the site. Still, within the leg, it may occur as early as four hours after the onset of injury.

7. **How is acute compartment syndrome managed?**

Acute compartment syndrome (ACS) requires **urgent treatment**, with **surgical decompres-**

sion being the primary and most reliable method of therapy.

The goals of management are to alleviate tissue pressure, restore blood flow, and minimise tissue damage and related functional loss.

Key steps in the management of ACS:

- **Release external pressure:** While arranging surgery, any constricting bandages, dressings, or casts encircling the limb should be removed to release external pressure.
- **Limb positioning:** The limb should be maintained at the level of the heart, avoiding elevation, as this may further decrease perfusion below critical levels.
- **Surgical decompression:** Urgent decompression is required, and resuscitation should occur during the procedure rather than delaying it.
  - **Open fasciotomy** involves incising both skin and fascia, is the most dependable method for achieving adequate compartment decompression.
- **Management of systemic effects.** The patient may develop systemic effects of massive rhabdomyolysis, including hyperkalaemia, myoglobinuria, acute renal failure, and a systemic inflammatory response syndrome with cardiovascular and respiratory failure. In such cases, early amputation may be life-saving.
- **Adjunctive therapies**
  - **Hyperbaric oxygen therapy** shows promise as an adjunct to fasciotomy or when immediate surgical treatment is not possible. However, it requires further evaluation and is seldom practicable locally.
  - **Mannitol** may reduce the incidence of CS after revascularisation by acting as a free-radical scavenger and reducing oedema. While it may be beneficial, more human studies are required.
  - In phlegmasia caerula dolens (venous gangrene), early aggressive limb elevation is essential, along with anticoagulation.

8. What are the consequences of untreated compartment syndrome?

If compartment syndrome is left untreated, it can lead to significant functional morbidity for the patient due to permanent nerve injury, poor muscle function, and ischaemic contractures. Limbs with extensive muscle infarction may ultimately require amputation. Delays in recognition and surgical management are a frequent cause of litigation.

Some of the consequences of untreated compartment syndrome are:

- **Nerve damage:** Irreversible changes to functional outcomes, such as axonotmesis of peripheral nerves, can occur after a maximum time of 6 hours of persistent anaerobic conditions.
- **Muscle damage:** Muscle necrosis and contracture can occur, potentially leading to poor muscle function. Significant muscle necrosis can occur after 8 hours with a compartmental pressure of 30 mm Hg.
- **Amputation:** In cases with extensive muscle infarction, the affected limb may require amputation.
- **Systemic effects:** The patient may develop systemic effects of massive rhabdomyolysis, including hyperkalaemia, myoglobinuria, acute renal failure, and a systemic inflammatory response syndrome with cardiovascular and respiratory failure.
- **Increased risk of litigation:** Perceived delays in recognition and surgical management frequently cause litigation. Defence is always successful when a fasciotomy is performed within 8 h of the first presenting symptom.

9. What are the controversies surrounding regional anaesthesia in compartment syndrome?

The central concern revolves around whether regional anaesthesia may **delay the diagnosis of ACS**.

Key points of contention include:

- **Masking of pain**: A primary concern is that regional anaesthesia, by blocking sensory nerves, could mask the early pain associated with ACS, leading to a delay in diagnosis and treatment. Pain is often described as the cardinal symptom of compartment syndrome, but many consider it unreliable. However, some sources suggest that breakthrough pain may still occur despite regional anaesthesia, and that ischaemic pain may not be masked by regional anaesthesia.
- **Diagnostic challenges**: Diagnosis can be especially challenging in children and patients with neurological compromise or altered mental status.
- **Impact on clinical assessment**: Dense local anaesthetic blocks can influence in the evaluation of pain and movement, making the diagnosis of compartment syndrome difficult without invasive pressure monitoring.
- **False positives**: Clinical findings of compartment syndrome were more likely to be present in patients who do not have compartment syndrome than in those who do.
- **Type of regional anaesthesia**: The type of regional anaesthesia may influence the potential for delayed diagnosis. While most publications report on the use of peripheral nerve blocks and their possible delay in the diagnosis of compartment syndrome, neuraxial anaesthesia (ie, epidural) has been associated with masking acute compartment syndrome in more reported cases.
- **Concentration of local anaesthetic**: The concentration of local anaesthetic used for nerve blocks has been identified as a factor in the timely detection of compartment syndrome. Using blocks with dilute concentrations of local anaesthetic is recommended in high-risk scenarios.
- **Conflicting perspectives**: There is a divergence in opinions between surgeons and anaesthesiologists. Orthopaedic surgeons mainly report cases of delayed diagnosis of compartment syndrome when regional anaesthesia was performed. In contrast, anaesthesiologists primarily describe the

harmless use of regional anaesthesia in the context of compartment syndrome.

- **Lack of high-quality evidence**: The available data are mainly from case reports and case series, which are considered low-quality evidence with a high risk of bias. No randomised controlled studies dedicated to this topic were found.
- **Alternative analgesic methods**: Every single analgesic method can be associated with the delay in ACS diagnosis if pain is the sole diagnostic criterion. As opioids (PCA) can lead to even higher incidence of delay compared to regional anaesthesia, and it is highly unethical not to treat the pain, the complex management of the whole patient at risk of ACS appears to be more important than the analgesic method alone.

Despite these concerns, some sources suggest that regional anaesthesia may not necessarily delay the diagnosis of compartment syndrome if certain precautions are taken:

- **Careful monitoring**: Frequent clinical evaluation and breakthrough pain, despite a functional regional anaesthesia, in combination with intracompartment pressure measurement, remains the keystone of recommended management for patients at risk of ACS.
- **Dilute local anaesthetics**: Low concentrations of local anaesthetics can facilitate the motor function of the limb and allow breakthrough pain detection. The optimal concentration of ropivacaine for epidural analgesia and avoidance of motor block is 0.2%.
- **Ultrasound guidance**: Ultrasound guidance for regional blockade and catheter insertion can lead to a reduction in the dose of local anaesthetics, which is strongly recommended.
- **Vigilance**: All reported severe consequences of compartment syndrome in the presence of peripheral nerve blocks would have easily been detected by adequate vigilance.
- Some sources advocate that because regional blockades can increase the blood flow through partial sympathetic blockades without blocking the warning signs of ACS, the implementation of regional anaesthesia in patients at risk of ACS should be encouraged.

Questions

1. What are the other aetiologies for compartment syndrome?
2. What other medical conditions can mask compartment syndrome?
3. Where else can compartment syndrome present?
4. What are the compartments of the upper limb?
5. What are the compartments of the lower limb?

Suggested Reading

1. Farrow C, Bodenham A, Troxler M. Acute limb compartment syndromes. Contin Educ Anaesth Crit Care Pain. 2011;11(1):24–8.
2. Mar GJ, Barrington MJ, McGuirk BR. Acute compartment syndrome of the lower limb and the effect of postoperative analgesia on diagnosis. Br J Anaesth. 2009;102(1):3–11.
3. Marhofer P, Halm J, Feigl GC, Schepers T, Hollmann MW. Regional anesthesia and compartment syndrome. Anesth Analg. 2021;133(5):1348–52.

Failed Spinal Anaesthesia

67

Nishkarsh Gupta, Mageshwaran Sivashanmugavel, and Kiran Koneti

Scenario

35-year-old patient, scheduled for an elective ACL reconstruction, requests a spinal anaesthetic due to severe postoperative nausea and vomiting from a previous general anaesthesia. You performed a spinal anaesthetic with 2.5 mls of 0.5% Hyperbaric Bupivacaine; there was aspiration of CSF at the start of the procedure, but not at the end. Ten minutes later, the patient can still move the leg, but there is a sensory block up to the level of the knee bilaterally and the sacral segments. Further 100 minutes later, there is very little increase in the block height. How will you proceed?

1. How would you define a failed spinal anaesthesia?

A failed spinal anaesthesia can be defined as when a spinal anaesthetic has been attempted, but satisfactory conditions for proceeding with surgery have not been obtained, which may be

- The total absence of any neuraxial block.
- The development of a partial block that is of insufficient height, duration, or quality and is inadequate for the proposed surgery

Additionally, the definition of failure has been questioned, especially when considering the patient's experience. Analgesic supplementation or intraoperative conversion to general anaesthesia may underestimate the incidence of intraoperative pain.

2. What is the incidence of failure with spinal anaesthesia?

The incidence of failure with spinal anaesthesia varies, but most experienced practitioners consider it to be shallow, perhaps less than **1%**. However, some reports indicate higher failure rates. A retrospective review of more than 5300 spinal anaesthetics for caesarean delivery found a spinal anaesthesia failure rate of **2.1%**.

N. Gupta
Onco-Anesthesia and Palliative Medicine, All India Institute of Medical Sciences, New Delhi, India

M. Sivashanmugavel
Department of Anaesthesia, Frimley Park Hospital, Camberley, UK

K. Koneti (✉)
Department of Anaesthesia, Sunderland Royal Hospital, Sunderland, UK

© The Author(s), under exclusive license to Springer Nature Switzerland AG 2026
S. Phillips et al. (eds.), *Regional Anaesthesia*, https://doi.org/10.1007/978-3-032-05165-3_67

3. Enlist the mechanisms of failed spinal anaesthesia

The mechanisms of failed spinal anaesthesia can be distilled into five distinct phases:

- **Unsuccessful lumbar puncture**.
- **Solution injection errors**.
- **Inadequate intrathecal spread**.
- **Drug failure**.
- **Failure of subsequent management**.

Within these phases, failure can arise from several specific issues:

Unsuccessful Lumbar Puncture
- Inability to access the subarachnoid space due to incorrect needling technique, poor patient positioning, anatomical abnormality, or equipment-related factors.
- Manufacturing problems resulting in a needle with a blocked lumen, or obstruction of the lumen by clot or tissue, are more likely. Failure to obtain CSF flow despite an successful needle placement(s) should raise the suspicion of needle blockage and prompt needle withdrawal and "flush test" to assure patency.
- Rarely, the flow of a clear fluid of non-cerebrospinal origin through the spinal needle may mimic a successful lumbar puncture without this having occurred.

Solution Injection Errors
- To ensure a block suitable for surgery, a proper dose of local anaesthetic must be calculated, prepared, and delivered to the site of action.
- Leakage may occur at the Luer connection between needle and syringe or from a deficiency at the joint between needle hub and shaft.
- Accidental movement of the needle. If the needle tip is misplaced such that the arachnoid mater acts as the flap valve, local anaesthetic will spread into the subdural space.

Inadequate Intrathecal Spread
Even when the entire volume of injectate is successfully delivered to the intrathecal space, the spread of solution within the CSF can be somewhat unpredictable.

- Dispersion of injectate within the CSF is dictated by the complex interaction between
  - The anatomy of the spinal canal,
  - The physical properties of the solution
  - gravity
  - Density of the injected solution relative to the CSF
- To achieve a uniform symmetrical block, the local anaesthetic should diffuse freely within CSF, without anatomical barriers.

Drug Failure
- A faulty drug batch, ineffective drug, or degradation could be potential causes.
- Wrong drug, drug identity error
- The common practice of utilizing adjuvants to local anaesthetics in spinal injections necessitates mixing solutions, introducing the possibility of a chemical reaction, incompatibility, and potentially reducing efficacy.
- Several cases of failed spinal anaesthesia have been attributed to local anaesthetic resistance.

Failure of Subsequent Management
- The patient may perceive unblocked sensations of movement, pressure, or traction experienced intraoperatively to be painful or uncomfortable experiences. Even for the most composed patients, lying supine in the operating theatre completely awake while undergoing an operative procedure may be an unnatural and anxiety-provoking experience.

4. Enlist causes where fluid flow is not CSF, or a pseudo-successful spinal anaesthesia?
In rare instances, the flow of a clear fluid of non-cerebrospinal origin through the spinal needle may mimic a successful lumbar puncture without this having occurred. There are a few scenarios in which this may happen:

- **"Topping up" a lumbar epidural** in obstetric practice for a caesarean section may result in a reservoir of local anaesthetic in the epidural space. This may be mistaken for CSF at subsequent spinal injection.
- An **epidural spread of injectate** has also been reported following lumbar plexus block. This may be mistaken for CSF at subsequent spinal injection.
- Another potential source of fluid mimicking CSF is the presence of a **congenital arachnoid cyst**. Tarlov cysts are meningeal dilatations of the posterior spinal nerve root, reportedly present in 4.5%–9% of the population. Such a cyst could result in CSF flow through the needle, but anaesthetic injected may fail to result in anaesthesia.

5. How do you manage a failed spinal block?
Managing a failed spinal anaesthetic depends on the time of detection and the nature of the failure.

General strategies for managing an inadequate spinal anaesthetic:

- Closely monitor the patient for the expected signs of neuraxial block, like sympathetic block, drop in blood pressure, and motor blockade
- Note that lack of autonomic response or slower-than-expected motor or sensory block development should alert the clinician to inadequate or failed spinal anaesthesia potential.
- Allow sufficient time because the development of anaesthesia can be more gradual in some patients before assuming failure. If 15 minutes have lapsed since intrathecal injection and the spinal block does not follow a typical onset pattern, the spinal anaesthetic will likely be inadequate for surgery and additional anaesthetic interventions will be required.

Specific management strategies based on the clinical presentation of the failed block:

- **No block**: If there is no appreciable block at 15–20 minutes, the most logical step is to repeat the injection, taking steps to eliminate the proposed cause of the previous failure.
  - *Suggested management:* Repeat injection (with caution) or administer general anaesthesia. If the spinal injection is repeated, sufficient time (20 minutes) must be allowed to pass to ensure that there is truly no block developing. If a second injection is performed after a successful but slowly developing first procedure, a "total spinal" may result.
- **Spinal block of insufficient height**: Manipulating posture and utilising gravity may overcome these difficulties.
  - *Possible causes:* Local anaesthetic has been lost during injection (e.g., leakage at needle-syringe connection), lumbar puncture was in too low a lumbar interspace, or an anatomical barrier is preventing diffusion of anaesthetic.
  - *Suggested management:* If a hyperbaric formulation was used, the patient should be placed in the Trendelenburg position with the hips and knees flexed. This will flatten the lumbar lordosis, allowing injectate to travel cephalad. Change in position after injection of isobaric bupivacaine is unlikely to be successful. Consider intravenous analgesia or sedation.
- **Unilateral block**: Encourage bilateral spread of the block by moving the patient so that the unblocked side is downward. A unilateral block should be sufficient for ipsilateral lower limb surgery, but the surgeon must be warned that the other limb is not anaesthetised.
  - *Possible causes:* Patient position or anatomical barrier formed by the longitudinal ligaments to prevent spread.
  - *Suggested management:* Postural manoeuvres or proceed with care (if correct side blocked).
- **Patchy block**: Additional sedation and opiate analgesia may prove successful, mainly if anxiety is a prominent factor. Alternatively, conversion to general anaesthesia may be required.
  - *Possible causes:* This describes a block that appears to have spread adequately but is of

inconsistent quality with variable sensory and motor block. There are multiple potential explanations, but the most common is administering an insufficient dose of anaesthetic drug, either due to underdosing or the solution not reaching the target.

– *Suggested management:* Repeat injection (with caution), intravenous analgesia/sedation, or general anaesthesia.

- **Inadequate duration**: The only realistic solutions are additional intravenous analgesia, sedation, or general anaesthesia.
  – *Possible causes:* Delivery of an insufficient dose of local anaesthetic, a "syringe swap" by which a short-acting agent such as lidocaine is injected instead of the intended bupivacaine, or the procedure may have lasted longer than anticipated.
  – *Suggested management:* Intravenous analgesia/sedation or general anaesthesia.

Additional considerations for management

- Judicious use of analgesia and sedation-Intravenous infusions of propofol and remifentanil can be used at low concentrations to good effect.
- Repeating subarachnoidal injection should not be done routinely unless the previous injection is a complete failure.
  – High concentrations of local anaesthetic intrathecally can be neurotoxic (especially with anatomic barriers)
  – unpredictable extensive cephalad spread with the potential for cardiovascular instability, respiratory embarrassment, or total spinal anaesthesia.
  – If block failure is secondary to anatomical factors, repeat injection is unlikely.
  – Risk of direct needle trauma to neural tissues is increased (patients may not have pain or paresthesia)

Postoperative Management

- At the postoperative visit, the patient should be offered an apology and given a complete explanation, a written summary of events, and fully documented in medical records to inform future anaesthetic procedures.
- Rarely, unusual patterns of failure may signal the presence of severe pathology within the vertebral canal, and if there are other signs or symptoms, then a neurology consultation is advised. If a patient has experienced failure of spinal anaesthesia on more than one occasion, MRI of the spine may be used to exclude or delineate abnormal anatomy.
- Suppose the procedure has been routine and straightforward. In that case, concerns can arise that the current supply of local anaesthetic is defective, especially if two or more such failures occur in the same hospital within a short period.

(Also check failed spinal anaesthesia in Caesarean section)

Questions

1. How will you manage a unilateral block?
2. How will you manage a block that has inadequate height?
3. What are the problems due to repeating a spinal block?
4. What is the role of ultrasound in reducing spinal failure?
5. What needle design factors can reduce the failure of spinal anaesthesia?

Suggested Reading

1. Fettes PDW, et al. Failed spinal anaesthesia: mechanisms, management, and prevention. Br J Anaesth. 2009;102(6):739–48.
2. Bekele Z, Jisha H. Type, management, and associated factors of failed spinal anesthesia in cesarean section. Prospective cohort study. Ann Med Surg. 2022;77:103616.
3. Demilie AE, Denu ZA, Bizuneh YB, et al. Incidence and factors associated with failed spinal anaesthesia among patients undergoing surgery: a multi-center prospective observational study. BMC Anesthesiol. 2024;24:129.
4. Girard T, Savoldelli GL. Failed spinal anesthesia for cesarean delivery: prevention, identification, and management. Curr Opin Anaesthesiol. 2024;37(3):207–12.

Recognition and Management of Accidental Intrathecal Catheter

68

Suresh Jeyaraj, Anju Gupta, and Nixon Thirumaran

Scenario

A 24-year-old labouring primipara requests an epidural catheter placement for pain relief. As a trainee anaesthetist, you are called in to do the procedure. While you are performing the procedure, the patient accidentally moves abruptly, and you encounter a dural puncture, you decide to thread the catheter intrathecally. How will you manage labour?

1. What is the incidence of inadvertent dural puncture in obstetrics?

The incidence of inadvertent dural puncture during attempted epidural analgesia in obstetric patients ranges from **0.4% to 1.5%**.

Factors that may influence the rate of inadvertent dural puncture include:

- **Cervical dilatation:** A greater degree of cervical dilatation at the time of epidural insertion was positively associated with an increased risk of inadvertent dural puncture.

- **Operator experience.** Inadvertent dural puncture rates are higher for low-case volume specialists and anaesthetists in training, particularly those who are novices.

- **Time of day.** The relative risk of inadvertent dural puncture may be higher at night due to fatigue, sleep deprivation, and fewer, less experienced anaesthesia providers working out-of-hours.

2. How is inadvertent dural puncture recognised?

Inadvertent dural puncture is most frequently recognised by **persistent leak of CSF from an epidural needle**.

Several techniques have been suggested to distinguish CSF from saline:

- Testing for protein or glucose.
- Temperature, pH.
- Changes in turbidity when mixed with thiopental.

One study found that the **glucose test was most accurate at 97%**, compared with 91% for pH, 84% for temperature, and 50% when using thiopental.

It has been estimated that around a third of inadvertent dural punctures are unrecognised. Dural puncture may only be spotted following catheter insertion. If an epidural dose of local anaesthetic is injected into the subarachnoid space, a **higher and denser than expected neur-**

S. Jeyaraj (✉)
Anaesthetic Department, Frimley Park Foundation Trust NHS Hospital, Frimley, Surrey, UK

A. Gupta
Anesthesiology Pain and Critical Care, All India Institute of Medical Sciences, New Delhi, India

N. Thirumaran
Department of Anaesthesia, Frimley Park Hospital, Camberley, UK

axial block is likely. Catheter aspiration is used widely to detect an intrathecal catheter. Studies suggest that direct intrathecal injection after negative aspiration through needle or catheter is rare, estimated to be between 1 in 1750 (0.06%) and 1 in 126,000 (0.0008%).

3. What are the risks of an intrathecal catheter?

The use of intrathecal catheters carries several risks, including:

- Mismanagement of the intrathecal catheter can lead to
  - increased motor block,
  - drug error (wrong drug injected or epidural dose of local anaesthetic administered)
  - high spinal or total spinal anaesthesia, hypotension, respiratory depression, cardiac arrest
  - Fetal bradycardia.
- Potential for damage to the spinal cord, cerebrospinal fluid-cutaneous fistula.
- Central neuraxial infection is a concern with intrathecal catheter use as the dura is breached and the catheter is placed within the CSF adjacent to nerve roots and meninges, which can act as a conduit for infection.
- Catheter failure: Intrathecal catheter failure after inadvertent dural puncture is comparable with epidural failure.
- Inadequate analgesia. Inadequate spread of local anaesthetic within the CSF, low flow rates of intrathecal infusion, the use of single-orifice catheters, and inconsistency in maintenance labour analgesia regimens between patients.
- Catheter migration and dislodgement.

To reduce risks, institutions should have clear guidelines for intrathecal catheter use, including labour analgesia protocols, management of top-ups for operative delivery, and management of breakthrough pain.

4. What are the benefits of an intrathecal catheter?

Intrathecal catheters (ITCs) offer several benefits when used following an accidental dural puncture, including providing analgesia and anaesthesia.

Primary Advantages:

- Rapid pain relief
- Avoidance of repeat dural puncture, placing an ITC after many unsuccessful attempts, avoids repeated accidental dural punctures, or the inability to identify the epidural or intrathecal space again.
- Flexibility for operative delivery: Intrathecal catheters facilitate rapid extension of a block for operative delivery while eliminating the requirement for a large epidural top-up in the presence of a breach in the dura, especially in patients with non-reassuring fetal tracings.
- May decrease post-dural puncture headache (PDPH). Purported advantages of inserting an intrathecal catheter after an accidental dural puncture are the reduced incidence of post-dural puncture headache and the decreased need for an epidural blood patch.
- Comparable effectiveness . Most studies have indicated satisfactory labour analgesia with intrathecal catheters. A recent meta-analysis showed no significant difference between intrathecal catheter insertion and re-siting the epidural.
- Reduced pain. A retrospective study found that women with accidental dural puncture managed by intrathecal catheter insertion had less pain throughout labour compared with women managed by re-siting the epidural.

5. When may you consider an intrathecal catheter?
   - In maternity units that are familiar with ITC.
   - Difficult to position the patient, very difficult to insert (high BMI, or spine abnormalities), severe pain, and unable to be still for siting catheter, nearing delivery, labouring patient.
   - Nonreassuring fetal trace, where operative intervention is highly likely

6. What are the benefits of resiting an epidural catheter
   - Technique is familiar, maternity units can manage an epidural catheter safely
   - Option to administer prophylactic blood patch.
7. What are the safety aspects and practices when managing an intrathecal catheter?

Key Safety Practices:
- **Aseptic Technique:** during insertion and subsequent top-ups
- **Clear Identification and Labelling:**
  - Label the catheter, infusion tubing, and infusion pump clearly to avoid inadvertent epidural dosing.
- **Communication and Handovers:**
  - The multidisciplinary team must be aware of the intrathecal catheter through verbal and written communication, including at every handover. An alert must be placed on multidisciplinary handover boards and a notice on the door of the patient's room
  - Insertion of an intrathecal catheter should be clearly documented and highlighted in the patient's record.
- **Medication Management:**
  - All intrathecal medications must be preservative-free and given through a filter connected to the catheter.
  - Account for the dead space of the intrathecal catheter and filter.
  - Medications should be drawn up through filtered needles and given through a filter connected to the catheter to reduce the risk of contamination and particulate injection.
  - Avoid frequent catheter disconnections and reconnections.
- **Closed-Loop Infusion Systems:** To minimise the risks of infection, accidental overdose, and drug errors, consideration may be given to using closed-loop infusion systems for intrathecal analgesia. Boluses for breakthrough pain should be administered through the pump whenever possible.

- **Qualified Personnel:**
  - Only anaesthetists should administer top-ups through an intrathecal catheter, and connect, disconnect, or reconnect the catheter and tubing.
  - Anaesthetists must be aware of the risk of high- or total-spinal anaesthesia when topping-up an intrathecal catheter.
  - Appropriate fluid loading and vasoconstrictor use should be used when topping up an intrathecal catheter for operative delivery.
- **Monitoring:** Maternal blood pressure should be checked every 5 minutes for 15 minutes following the first dose, and after every subsequent bolus given via an intrathecal catheter. Sensory and motor block should be checked every hour during intrathecal catheter analgesia. Fetal heart rate should be continuously monitored during intrathecal analgesia. Full AAGBI monitoring, including Non-invasive blood pressure, ECG, and oxygen saturations, should be monitored throughout intrathecal anaesthesia.
- **Institutional Guidelines:.** These should highlight key risks, monitoring protocol, and other safety measures.
- **Removal of Catheter:** Remove it at the earliest opportunity following delivery. An intrathecal catheter should be removed if an accidental and unwitnessed disconnection between the catheter and bacterial filter occurs.
8. What are the usual intrathecal dosage regimes for labour analgesia?
General recommendations: Qualified personnel, aseptic technique, dilute local anaesthetic with opioids in titrated aliquots, minimise disconnections, minimise ambulation (due to risk of motor weakness and falls), frequent monitoring (Heart rate, NIBP, sensory & motor levels, Fetal heart rate) (Table 68.1).
9. What are the usual intrathecal dosage regimes for surgical anaesthesia? (Table 68.2)

Table 68.1 Intrathecal doses for labor analgesia

Dosing technique	Medication
Initial	Bupivacaine 1.25–2.5 mg or ropivacaine 2–5 mg and fentanyl 12.5–25 μg or sufentanil 2–7 μg.
Infusion only	Bupivacaine 0.05–0.125% + fentanyl 2–5 mcg/ml. Basal: 0.5–3 ml/h Ropivacaine 0.1–0.2% and fentanyl 2–2.5 μg/ml or sufentanil 0.75–1 μg/ml at a rate of 1–3 ml/h
Patient-controlled Intrathecal analgesia	Bupivacaine 0.125% + fentanyl 2 mcg/ml Basal: 1–2 ml/hr. Bolus: 1 ml Lockout: 20–30 min
Top ups	Bupivacaine 0.25% 0.5–1 ml (1.25–2.5 mg) with or without fentanyl 15–20 mg Ropivacaine 2–5 mg and fentanyl 12.5–25 μg or sufentanil 2–7 μg.

Table 68.2 Intrathecal dose regimens for surgical anesthesia

Dosing technique	Medication
Initial	Fentanyl 15–20 mg Morphine 0.05–0.3 mg Bupivacaine plain or hyperbaric 0.5%, 1 ml (5 mg) initial dose, and then titrate to the desired level with additional 0.5 ml (2.5 mg) boluses
Subsequent intraoperative dosing	Titrate to desired level with additional 0.5 ml (2.5 mg) boluses of bupivacaine plain or hyperbaric 0.5%

Questions

1. What are the Association of Anaesthesia recommendations for managing pain and distress during caesarean section and their grade/strength of evidence

2. What length of intrathecal catheter should be left in the intrathecal space?

3. Why may an intrathecal catheter fail?

4. Which technique provides better analgesia and maternal satisfaction, epidural or intrathecal catheters?

5. What is the incidence of high and total spinal incidence in Obstetric neuraxial anaesthesia, and when is it most common?

6. When is an accidental overdose via an intrathecal catheter likely to happen, and how can this be mitigated?

7. What are the signs and symptoms of a high spinal & and a total spinal?

Suggested Reading

1. Heesen M, et al. Intrathecal catheterisation after observed accidental dural puncture in labouring women: update of a meta-analysis and a trial-sequential analysis. Int J Obstet Anesth. 2020;41:71–82.
2. Newman MJ, Cyna AM, Middleton P. Epidural catheter replacement and intrathecal catheter techniques for preventing post-dural puncture headache following an inadvertent dural puncture in labour. Cochrane Database Syst Rev. 2018;2018(7)
3. Orbach-Zinger S, Jadon A, Lucas DN, et al. Intrathecal catheter use after accidental dural puncture in obstetric patients: literature review and clinical management recommendations. Anaesthesia. 2021;76(8):1111–21.
4. Griffiths SK, Russell R, Broom MA, Devroe S, Van de Velde M, Lucas DN. Intrathecal catheter placement after inadvertent dural puncture in the obstetric population: management for labour and operative delivery. Guidelines from the Obstetric Anaesthetists' Association. Anaesthesia. 2024;79(12):1348–68.

Management of Pain During Caesarean Section

69

Venkatesh Kempulraj, Suresh Jeyaraj, and Anju Gupta

Scenario

21-year-old female, first pregnancy, undergoing elective caesarean section for breech. You perform an uneventful spinal anaesthetic with 2.4mls of 0.5% Bupivacaine heavy. The patient has developed motor block in the legs and does not feel cold sensation up to T12 dermatome. You wait for another 5 minutes and decide to proceed with surgery. The patient complains of pain 15 minutes after surgery, and the child hasn't been delivered. How will you manage?

1. What are the consequences for this lady who experiences pain during a caesarean section?

A woman who experiences pain during a caesarean section under neuraxial anaesthesia is at risk of adverse psychological sequelae. Litigation arising from pain during caesarean section under neuraxial anaesthesia is the most common successful medicolegal claim against obstetric anaesthetists. Subjective birth experience is the strongest predictor of postnatal trauma.

2. What Is the Failure Rate of Neuraxial Anaesthesia?

The incidence of inadequate neuraxial anaesthesia for caesarean section varies based on the definition of "failure", the neuraxial technique used, and the urgency of the caesarean section. "Failure" can refer to completely failed blocks, partial blocks (e.g., unilateral or inadequate height), the use of adjuvants, or the requirement for conversion to general anaesthesia.

Spinal anaesthesia typically has a quicker onset, fewer complications, and lower intraoperative supplementation rates than epidural anaesthesia.

Based on the literature, the rate of failure to achieve a pain-free operation is:

- 6% with spinal anaesthesia
- 24% with epidural top-up
- 18% with combined spinal-epidural

3. What are the risk factors for inadequate neuraxial block?

Risk factors for inadequate neuraxial block depend on the definition of failure used.

V. Kempulraj (✉)
Department of Anaesthesia, Rajiv Gandhi Government General Hospital, Chennai, Tamil Nadu, India

S. Jeyaraj
Anaesthetic Department, Frimley Park Foundation Trust NHS Hospital, Frimley, Surrey, UK

A. Gupta
Anesthesiology Pain and Critical Care, All India Institute of Medical Sciences, New Delhi, India

Factors associated with pre-operative failure include:

- Operative urgency
- Increased BMI
- Women having their first caesarean section
- Indications for caesarean section include acute fetal distress or a maternal medical condition

For intra-operative failure, the following are significant risk factors:

- Inadequacy of pre-operative anaesthetic block
- Duration of surgery
- Technique: When spinal anaesthesia was used, the use of a spinal opioid was associated with less pre-operative failure. When a labour epidural was extended for caesarean section, lower epidural top-up volume was associated with less pre-operative failure, and use of adrenaline was associated with both reduced pre-operative and intra-operative failure.

Risk factors for failed conversion of labour epidural analgesia to caesarean section anaesthesia include:

- Greater urgency of caesarean section
- An increased number of clinician-administered boluses during labour
- Provision of anaesthetic care by a non-obstetric anaesthetist

4. What is an adequate level of block for a caesarean section?

The level required for a lower transverse abdominal skin incision for caesarean section is the T10 dermatome. The uterus receives sympathetic innervation from the inferior hypogastric plexus (T10–L1) and parasympathetic fibres from pelvic splanchnic nerves (S2–S4). However, because several visceral organs send sympathetic afferent impulses to the thoracic spinal cord (T4–L2), a block height to higher thoracic dermatomes is required. In the study by Russell et al., no woman with an anaesthetic level that remained above T5 experienced intra-operative pain. This suggests that loss of touch sensation up to and including T5 is required to minimise the risk of pain during caesarean section.

5. How can we test the adequacy of the level of spinal anaesthesia?

A multimodal approach incorporating sensory, motor, and autonomic block assessments is used to test the adequacy of spinal anesthesia.

Sensory Block Assessment:

- **Light touch** should be the primary testing modality, aiming for a block to sensation at the T5 level or higher. The T5 dermatome is considered an acceptable block height for caesarean section. A second, confirmatory sensory modality should be used if the block level is in doubt.
- Identify the block level at which sensation is first felt when moving from blocked to unblocked dermatomes bilaterally between the mid-axillary and mid-clavicular lines.
- Test the lower limit of the block and the upper limit, using the back of the leg if necessary to avoid spraying near the genital area.
- Allow sufficient time, avoiding rapid movement along dermatomes.

Motor Block Assessment:

- Use straight leg raising as a simple and reproducible test for motor block of L1-L4. An effective block is indicated by the inability to raise the straight leg against gravity bilaterally.
- If the mother can perform a straight leg raise, no matter how high the loss of sensation, the block is unlikely to be suitable for anaesthesia for caesarean section.
- Complete motor block of S1 (plantar-flexion) is a characteristic of spinal anaesthesia but unusual with an epidural.
- Normal ankle motor function during epidural anaesthesia may indicate absent or inadequate sacral anaesthesia, which will likely result in pain during surgery.

Autonomic Block Assessment:

- Although not objectively proven part of routine practice, sympathetic block can be a helpful adjunct to sensory and motor testing to confirm bilateral spread.
- A sympathetic block of the feet does not develop until a well-defined sensory block to T10 exists.
- Assess by feeling the temperature on the underside of the toes bilaterally. Differences in foot temperature or the dampness of the feet indicate an asymmetrical or unilateral block.

The assessment of the neuraxial block should be comprehensively and accurately documented, including the precise modalities used, the testing time, and, when applicable, the pre-operative block height. Documenting the height of the sensory block using a dermatome map may be the most reproducible method.

6. What are the key aspects of communication with the patient?

Communication with the patient during neuraxial anaesthesia for caesarean section involves establishing rapport, providing information, and ensuring the woman feels heard and understood.
  - Establishing rapport is vital to improving the assessment of the block.
  - Responding to verbal and non-verbal cues.
  - Using appropriate language- be wary of language & cultural differences
  - Confirming understanding.
  - Demonstrating empathy & active listening.
  - Providing verbal facilitation and non-verbal encouragement.
  - Legitimising the woman's concerns.
  - Avoid leading questions; questions should be open and neutral.
  - Acknowledging distress: Acknowledge any complaint of pain or distress.
  - Ensuring follow-up: Ensure that everyone caring for the woman before and following discharge is aware of intra-operative events.

7. How to manage pain and distress during caesarean section under neuraxial anaesthesia?

Management of pain and distress depends on
  - The urgency of the situation,
  - The stage of the procedure, and
  - The neuraxial technique used

The patient is the primary source of information regarding the block's effectiveness and should be carefully listened to. Inadequate or delayed management, rather than the block's failure, can cause the most distress.

The following steps should be taken when managing pain and distress:

- Acknowledge the patient's distress and inform the operating theatre team.
- Ask the surgeon to stop surgery as soon as it is safe to do so. If the pain is severe and the lives of the woman and baby are not in danger, surgery should be immediately halted, except between uterine incision and delivery. At this stage, the obstetrician should be asked to achieve delivery as quickly as possible.
- Reassure the woman (and her partner) that the pain will be managed.
- If pain occurs early on, especially before delivery, analgesic adjuvants are unlikely to be fully effective. If the urgency of surgery permits,
  - consider a second neuraxial technique (in the case of spinal anaesthesia)
  - extending the neuraxial technique (in the case of combined spinal–epidural or epidural extension anaesthesia).
  - If there is an indwelling epidural catheter and time, additional top-ups could be considered, with alkalinised lidocaine with adrenaline likely to achieve the most rapid effect. Do not allow surgery to restart without re-checking the block.
  - Nitrous oxide and oxygen alone are unlikely to be sufficient. Consider repeated boluses of fast-acting opioids (fentanyl 25–50 mcg, alfentanil 250–500 mcg) or ketamine (10 mg boluses) if the woman chooses to continue with neuraxial anaesthesia. Do not treat pain with anxiolytics.

- Recheck the block and ensure the patient is pain-free before surgery is allowed to restart
- Ask the surgeon to minimise surgical stimuli, for example, exteriorisation of the uterus is not recommended.
- If these options are not possible, general anaesthesia should be recommended.

8. What are the key aspects of documentation that reduce medicolegal claims?
   - Make a detailed record of events on the anaesthetic chart, including what treatment was offered, the patient's response, and any recommendation of general anaesthesia.
   - Provide general anaesthesia if other strategies have failed and the woman requests it; do not persist with the neuraxial technique.
   - Postoperatively, explain the possible reasons for intraoperative pain and address any questions or concerns as fully as possible.
   - Ensure follow-up to minimise the development of long-term psychological sequelae.

9. What are the key recommendations?
   1. Informed consent for anaesthesia for caesarean section requires an explanation of neuraxial techniques and general anaesthesia.
   2. For neuraxial techniques, discuss the planned level of block and how it will be tested, the sensations that should be expected with an effective block, the possibility of pain, and the potential ways of treating it, including general anaesthesia.
   3. For non-elective caesarean section, the discussion should include any potential fetal risks arising from the time taken to deliver, the possible modes of anaesthesia.
   4. Use a recognised technique for neuraxial block for caesarean delivery with suffi-

cient doses of local anaesthetic and opioids.

5. Light touch is the primary testing modality, aiming for a block sensation of T5 or higher. A second, confirmatory sensory modality should be used if the block level is in doubt. Identify the block level at which sensation is first felt when moving from blocked to unblocked dermatomes bilaterally between the mid-axillary and midclavicular lines.

6. Test the lower limit of the block and the upper limit, using the back of the leg if necessary to avoid spraying near the genital area.

7. In addition, straight leg raising can be used as a simple and reproducible test for motor blocks. An effective block is indicated by the inability to raise the straight leg against gravity bilaterally.

8. Acknowledge any complaint of pain or distress and ask the surgeon to stop if safe, then use intravenous fast-acting opioids or ketamine in the first instance.

9. A request for general anaesthesia should be honoured if possible. It is good practice for the anaesthetist to recommend general anaesthesia if adequate analgesia is unlikely to be achieved using other methods.

10. Any patient who feels pain during a caesarean section should be followed up before they leave the hospital by a senior anaesthetist, who should also contact the patient's general practitioner.

Suggested Reading

1. Kinsella SM. A prospective audit of regional anaesthesia failure in 5080 caesarean sections. Anaesthesia. 2008;63:822–32.
2. Russell IF. Levels of anaesthesia and intraoperative pain at caesarean section under regional block. Int J Obstet Anesth. 1995;4:71–7.
3. Plaat F, Stanford SER, Lucas DN, et al. Prevention and management of intra-operative pain during caesarean section under neuraxial anaesthesia: a technical and interpersonal approach. Anaesthesia. 2022;77(5):588–97.

Rebound Pain After Peripheral Nerve Blocks

70

Roche John Alexis Martin, Nishkarsh Gupta, and Kiran Koneti

Scenario

28-year-old male, received an interscalene nerve block with 10mls 0.5% Bupivacaine for an arthroscopic rotator cuff repair. He was very comfortable postoperatively, had a numb arm, was given standard analgesics, postoperative instructions, and was discharged. Twenty-four hours later, he was readmitted to the hospital with severe postoperative pain and required a PCA with opioids.

1. What is the definition of rebound pain?

Rebound pain is an acute increase in pain severity after a peripheral nerve block (PNB) has receded, typically manifesting within 24 hours after the block was performed. The common characteristics: severe pain related to regional anaesthesia, which occurs after the resolution of the sensory peripheral nerve block (PNB) in the first 12–24 hours after performing the PBN, with a duration of around 2 hours, and does not respond to intravenous opioid administration.

R. J. A. Martin
Department of Anaesthesia, Basingstoke Hospital, Hampshire Hospital NHS Trust, Basingstoke, UK

N. Gupta
Onco-Anesthesia and Palliative Medicine, All India Institute of Medical Sciences, New Delhi, India

K. Koneti (✉)
Department of Anaesthesia, Sunderland Royal Hospital, Sunderland, UK

- Patients describe RP mainly as an intense burning or aching pain.
- Rebound pain is defined as the transition from well-controlled pain (Numerical Rating Scale [NRS] $\leq$ 3) while the block is working to severe pain (NRS $\geq$ 7) within 24 hours of block performance.
- The rebound pain score is calculated by subtracting the pain score recorded within the first 12 hours after the PNB wears off from the lowest pain score reported within the initial 12 hours after the block was administered.

2. What is the incidence of rebound pain?
The incidence of rebound pain can vary. The incidence of RP could reach around 40% of patients for ambulatory surgery. The incidence differs after discharge following inpatient care, and it is 12–13% for severe-to-extreme pain. This may be due to abnormal spontaneous C-fiber hyperactivity and nociceptor hyper-excitability without mechanical nerve lesions.

3. What is the mechanism for the development of rebound pain?

Rebound pain refers to surgical pain of a mechanical nature that intensifies after the resolution of PNB, due to unimpeded nociceptive signals. The mechanism of rebound pain (RP), which is described as an intense burning pain, has more of a **neuropathic mechanism than a nociceptive component after nerve block**. In neuropathic

© The Author(s), under exclusive license to Springer Nature Switzerland AG 2026
S. Phillips et al. (eds.), *Regional Anaesthesia*, https://doi.org/10.1007/978-3-032-05165-3_70

pain, ongoing burning pain is caused by abnormal spontaneous C-fiber activity and hyperexcitability of nociceptors **without mechanical nerve lesions**.

4. What are the risk factors for the development of rebound pain?

Risk factors for the development of rebound pain include patient-related, surgical, and anaesthesia-related factors.

Specific risk factors:

- Younger age: age < 60.
- Female gender.
- Bone surgery. Rebound pain was 6.5 times more likely to occur after bone surgery compared to soft tissue surgery.
- Absence of intraoperative intravenous dexamethasone.
- Pre-existing preoperative pain.
- Single-injection techniques.
- Type of surgery. Upper and lower limb surgery, such as shoulder surgery performed under brachial plexus block, and ankle fracture surgery under popliteal sciatic nerve block, are significant risk factors for rebound pain.
- Patients' cognitive functioning and anticipation of postoperative pain.

5. What are the consequences of rebound pain?

Rebound pain has significant consequences for patients and can impact their overall recovery and well-being. Despite the early benefits of PNBs, rebound pain presents a challenge in perioperative care.

The adverse consequences include:

- Patient discomfort and impaired sleep:
- Increased risk of chronic pain: Orthopaedic surgery carries an almost three-fold increased risk of developing moderate to severe chronic pain compared with all other types of surgery at one year.
- Reduced quality of life: Evidence suggests that complex regional pain syndrome in adults can result from the childhood onset of the condition.
- Undermines pain management efforts
- Increased healthcare utilisation: Poorly managed postoperative pain can lead to

adverse outcomes, such as impaired quality of recovery, dependency on opioids, persistent postsurgical pain, and elevated medical expenses.

- Negative impact on patient satisfaction
- Failure to return to daily activities
- Unpleasant experience for ambulatory surgery.

6. What are the strategies to manage rebound pain?

Strategies to manage rebound pain include both preventative and active management techniques. A multimodal approach, started before the peripheral nerve block (PNB resolution), is typically recommended.

Key strategies include:

- **Pre-operative education**: Informing patients about the possibility of severe but transient pain at the resolution of PNBs is crucial. Patients should be warned about the limits of regional anaesthesia and instructed to take rescue analgesic medication before discharge, somewhat earlier than later. "Acknowledging 'rebound pain' after the use of regional anaesthesia associated with patient counselling regarding early narcotic administration may allow patients to have more effective postoperative pain control".
- **Preoperative evaluation of anxiety**: Evaluate the anxiety score and catastrophising tendencies because both scores significantly correlate with postoperative pain scores.
- **Preemptive analgesia:** Preoperative analgesia can function as preemptive or preventive analgesia to diminish peripheral and central sensitisation.
- **Perioperative and postoperative multimodal analgesia**: Combining PNB with systemic multimodal analgesia improves postoperative pain and related outcomes. Multimodal analgesia addresses peripheral sensitisation and other physiological responses mediated by the humoral inflammatory response to surgery, which are unaffected by the PNB. Different classes

of analgesics could be combined: paracetamol, non-steroidal anti-inflammatory drugs/COX-2 inhibitors, and oral opioids. The administration of the multimodal analgesia before the sensory block resolution could lower the intensity and severity of RP.

- **Continuous catheter PNB techniques**: Increasing the sensory block allows more time for healing, decreases the inflammatory process, and impacts the incidence of RP. Although this strategy has advantages, it is not the first option for the patient in ambulatory surgery because it is time-consuming, can be performed by highly skilled personnel, and has a failure rate.

- **Local anaesthetic adjuvants in single-injection PNB**: Using adjuvants can prolong the duration of the sensory bloc; clonidine, buprenorphine, dexamethasone, and dexmedetomidine have been used. Dexamethasone is a promising adjuvant because it is cheap and easy to find, but the perineural use is off-label. Dexamethasone (perineural more so than intravenous) can prolong the analgesic benefit of PNB. Liposomal bupivacaine could be an effective strategy to prolong the duration of analgesia (up to 72 h) with single-injection PNB. Still, current evidence fails to support its routine use.

- **Perineural or intravenous dexamethasone:** Meta-analyses suggest that both perineural and intravenous dexamethasone have comparable effects on the duration of block, 24-hour pain scores, and postoperative opioid consumption. Dexamethasone, when administered perineurally, may extend the duration of PNB compared to intravenous administration. Administering dexamethasone at doses below 0.1 mg/kg can effectively alleviate postoperative pain.

- **Early administration of analgesics:** Administering an analgesic medication 1–2 hours before the resolution of the PNB may help reduce the occurrence of rebound pain. In ambulatory surgery, patients should be educated to take opioids at the earliest signs of block regression.

- **Combined PNBs:** The utilization of combined PNBs may decrease the occurrence of rebound pain. Following arthroscopic rotator cuff surgery, axillary and suprascapular ultrasound-guided PNBs reduced the incidence of rebound pain. Moreover, combined ultrasound-guided brachial plexus block and suprascapular nerve block have been shown to more effectively mitigate postoperative pain than a single-injection block within 36 hours after arthroscopic cuff surgery.

Suggested Reading

1. Admassie BM, Debas SA, Admass BA. Prevention and management of rebound pain after resolution of regional block: a systematic review. Ann Med Surg (Lond). 2024;86(8):4732–7.
2. Anastase DG18 how can we manage the rebound pain? Reg Anesth Pain Med. 2024;49:A397–9.
3. Barry GS, et al. Factors associated with rebound pain after peripheral nerve block for ambulatory surgery. Br J Anaesth. 2021;126(4):862–71.

Transient Neurologic Symptoms After Spinal Anaesthesia

71

Nishkarsh Gupta and Prateek Maurya

Case Scenario

A 24-year-old morbidly obese patient undergoes a short-acting spinal anaesthetic with 3 mls 5% Lidocaine for a day case hysteroscopy. After successful motor and sensory blockade onset, the patient was placed in the lithotomy position. The procedure took 45 minutes and was completed uneventfully. Postoperatively in the recovery room, on regression of the spinal anaesthesia, the patient complains of intense back pain radiating to the lower extremities. Opioids needed to be administered to control the pain. What could be happening?

1. What could be the diagnosis?

Transient Neurologic symptoms.

2. What is the differential diagnosis?
   - Drug error- Chlorhexidine contamination, tranexamic acid injection
   - Lower back pain following spinal anaesthesia
   - Postdural puncture headache,
   - meningeal symptoms,
   - neuropathic pain, and radicular symptoms.

Any patient who develops neurological symptoms following neuraxial anaesthesia, including TNS, should be referred to the anaesthesiology department for immediate evaluation and management. Severe cases or patients at risk of acute deterioration should be referred to the emergency department and/or for urgent neurosurgical consultation.

3. What are transient neurological symptoms (TNS)?

TNS is defined as
   - Symmetrical bilateral pain in the back or buttocks, or pain radiating to the lower extremities after recovery from spinal anaesthesia.
   - Symptoms typically appear within 24 hours of spinal anaesthesia and can last for 2–5 days, resolving completely without any lasting effects.
   - There should be an absence of abnormal neurological findings upon examination or imaging.

4. What is the incidence of TNS?

The incidence of TNS varies depending on the local anaesthetic used. A network meta-analysis (NMA) included 24 trials; the risk of developing TNS with lidocaine for spinal anaesthesia was increased compared to bupivacaine, prilocaine, or procaine; and similar compared to 2-chloroprocaine and mepiva-

N. Gupta (✉) · P. Maurya
Onco-Anesthesia and Palliative Medicine, All India Institute of Medical Sciences, New Delhi, India

S. Phillips et al. (eds.), *Regional Anaesthesia*, https://doi.org/10.1007/978-3-032-05165-3_71

caine. Approximately one in five participants who received spinal anaesthesia with lidocaine developed TNS.

Incidence of TNS varies in the literature, and is around 30% with 4% Mepivacaine, 3% when using hyperbaric bupivacaine, and 27% with 5% hyperbaric lidocaine.

5. What are the pathophysiological mechanisms for the development of TNS

There is no evidence that TNS is associated with any specific neurological disease, and the precise cause of TNS remains unknown. The proposed mechanisms are:

- Neurotoxicity of local anaesthetics: High concentrations of local anaesthetics like lidocaine and mepivacaine may have a neurotoxic effect, leading to TNS. In vitro studies have demonstrated that lidocaine can cause irreversible conduction block in isolated nerves. The transient neurotoxic effect of hyperbaric lidocaine 50 mg/ml is probably the main reason for TNS after spinal anaesthesia.
- Musculoskeletal factors: Profound muscle and ligament relaxation caused by high doses of local anaesthetics may result in straightening of the lordotic curve, and even transient spondylolisthesis, and may contribute to postoperative musculoskeletal pain and the development of TNS when the patient is lying on the operating table.
- Positioning during surgery: The lithotomy position may contribute to TNS by stretching the cauda equina and sciatic nerves, thus decreasing the vascular supply and increasing vulnerability to injury.
- Individual physical characteristics: Anatomical configuration of the spinal column affects the spread of subarachnoid anaesthetic solutions that move under the influence of gravity. Both lumbar lordosis and thoracic kyphosis differ between individuals, particularly concerning the lowest point of the thoracic spinal canal.
- Solution baricity: The greater the baricity of the solution, the greater the chance of gravity-determined spread restriction. This, together with tiny gauge pencil-point needles with one side hole near the tip, could pool the concentrated local anaesthetic solution.
- pH and preservatives: low pH and the presence of the antioxidant bisulfite were implicated in the early reports of TNS with the use of 2-chloroprocaine, which was then abandoned.

6. What are the risk factors?

The incidence of TNS is lower when bupivacaine, levobupivacaine, prilocaine, procaine, and ropivacaine are used compared to lidocaine. The use of 2-chloroprocaine and mepivacaine has a similar risk to lidocaine in terms of TNS development after spinal anaesthesia.

7. What is the treatment for TNS?

- Painful symptoms attributed to TNS disappear spontaneously and typically cease by the fifth postoperative day.
- NSAIDs: Ketorolac may prevent and/or mask symptoms of TNS.
- Analgesics: People with TNS may have higher pain scores and use more analgesics postoperatively; opioids and multimodal analgesia may be needed.
- Severe cases or patients at risk of acute deterioration should be referred for urgent neurosurgical consultation.

8. What is the prognosis and outcome of TNS?

The prognosis for TNS is generally good, with symptoms typically resolving entirely within 2–5 days without any lasting effects. Although TNS can cause higher pain scores and functional impairment, it does not necessarily have a negative influence on patients' decisions to receive spinal anaesthesia subsequently.

9. How can you prevent TNS?

- Use alternative local anaesthetics to lidocaine: The risk of developing TNS after spinal anaesthesia is lower when using bupivacaine, levobupivacaine, prilocaine, procaine, or ropivacaine.
- 2-chloroprocaine might be a viable alternative to lidocaine for day surgery of short duration and obstetric procedures since this local anaesthetic has a rapid onset of action, is quickly metabolised, and has low toxicity.
- Intraoperative positioning, such as the lithotomy position, should be performed for the shortest possible duration and with caution.
- Adoption of multimodal analgesia, routine use of nonsteroidal anti-inflammatory drugs (NSAIDs), and dexamethasone may prevent and/or mask symptoms of TNS.
- Patients should be informed of TNS as a possible adverse effect of local anaesthetics for spinal anaesthesia.

Suggested Reading

1. Forget P, Borovac JA, Thackeray EM, Pace NL. Transient neurological symptoms (TNS) following spinal anaesthesia with lidocaine versus other local anaesthetics in adult surgical patients: a network meta-analysis. Cochrane Database Syst Rev. 2019;12(12):CD003006.
2. De Weert K, Traksel M, Gielen M, Slappendel R, Weber E, Dirksen R. The incidence of transient neurological symptoms after spinal anaesthesia with lidocaine compared to prilocaine. Anaesthesia. 2000;55:1020–4.
3. Hiller A, Karjalainen K, Balk M, Rosenberg PH. Transient neurological symptoms after spinal anaesthesia with hyperbaric 5% lidocaine or general anaesthesia. Br J Anaesth. 1999;82(4):575–9.
4. Sankar A, Behboudi M, Abdallah FW, Macfarlane A, Brull R. Transient neurologic symptoms following spinal anesthesia with isobaric mepivacaine: a decade of experience at Toronto Western Hospital. Anesthesiol Res Pract. 2018;2018:1901426.

Index